AN INTRODUCTION TO
HEALTH
PSYCHOLOGY

AN INTRODUCTION TO
HEALTH
PSYCHOLOGY

SECOND EDITION

ROBERT J. GATCHEL
University of Texas
Health Sciences Center

ANDREW BAUM
Uniformed Services University
of the Health Sciences

DAVID S. KRANTZ
Uniformed Services University
of the Health Sciences

Foreword by **JEROME E. SINGER**

Random House, New York

This book is dedicated to Robert Garrett Gatchel, Jessie Slater Sachs, Michael K. Douma, and Della E. Krantz.

Second Edition
987654321
Copyright © 1989 by Newbery Award Records, Inc.

Library of Congress Cataloging in Publication Data

Gatchel, Robert J., 1947–
  An introduction to health psychology.

  Bibliography: p.

  Includes index.

  1. Medicine and psychology. I. Baum, Andrew.
II. Krantz, David S. III. Title.
R726.5.G38 1988   616.08   88-18231
ISBN 0-394-37931-7

Cover and Text Design: Sandra Josephson
Manufactured in the United States of America

CONTENTS

IIIIIIIIIIIIIIIIIIIIIIIIIIIIIIIIIIIIIIIIIIIIIIIIIIIIIIIIIIIIIIIIIIIIIIIIIIIIIIIIIIIIIIIIIIIIIIIIIIIIIIIIIIIIIIIIIIIIIIIIIIIIIIIIIIIIII

FOREWORD

There was a time when textbooks were considered original scholarly works. Their mission, then as now, was to present a field in an orderly fashion to the student. Their stock in trade was organization and the systematic arrangement of theories, research results, and intelligent discussion. Textbooks still do this and they are undoubtedly better at many aspects of presentation than they were in the past. Graphics, photographs, diagrams, even sidebars and boxes to make footnotes exciting, are all now highly developed forms of exposition.

In other ways that have evolved, it is more debatable whether there have been improvements. No textbook can be truly comprehensive and still be portable, so inevitably the authors must be selective in what they include. This selectivity extends to every aspect of the text: what topics to cover, what studies to use as examples, what theories to discuss, what emphasis to give to each selection, what level of readership to write for, are just a few of the many choices that must be made.

In the good old once upon a time, authors used these choices to shape textbooks to their own points of view. The selection and arrangement of materials was made with an eye toward advancing the field, and not just educating the student. Thirty years ago, major texts in almost every area of psychology were well known scholarly achievements. They were acknowledged for their points of view, were advocates for various theoretical positions, and were recognized as benchmarks in reviewing fields of research. Many had chapters that reviewed topics in ways that today would appear in a *Psychological Bulletin* article. In general, such texts were idiosyncratic, pleasing like minded readers, and often alienating those readers who disagreed with their basic premises and orientation.

For better or worse, texts are now different. Their intended audience is more clearly the student and less the instructor. Their selection of materials is now guided not by the authors' perspective, but rather by the publishers' market research as to what coverage is desired by a broad spectrum of adopting instructors. If one successful text has a section on a particular topic, soon all texts in the field report on that topic, lest they be at a competitive disadvantage in the marketplace. Similar market forces have made texts less critical. They are more apt just to report research as a series of studies rather than to discuss strengths and weaknesses of individual studies as a prelude to synthesizing them into a coherent conclusion.

This evolving set of changes in textbooks has both advantages and disadvantages. No one can fault student-oriented texts. After all, it is the students, not the instructors, who must learn from the books, and special viewpoints often are lost on those students who are getting their initial exposure to a particular area.

Less than a decade ago, the field of health psychology provided an opportunity for textbook authors to combine the best of the old and the new. At that time health psychology was just beginning to emerge as a separate subdiscipline in psychology. To be sure, there have long been psychologists who were interested in health and medical issues related to psychology and who did research and published on these topics, but they were not regarded as engaged in a particular specialty, such as clinical psychology, social psychology, or physiological psychology. In the late 1970s this began to change and a distinctive health psychology began to develop. It went under a variety of names, such as medical psychology or behavioral medicine. Signs of its independent growth began to appear. Specialized journals, focused professional societies, and a health psychology division of the American Psychological Association all date from this time as markers of the inception of the field.

The same *zeitgeist* that produced an independent health psychology also produced a number of new courses, both graduate and undergraduate, in this field. As is often the case as a new area becomes popular, many of the teachers of the first courses are at somewhat of a loss as to how to organize the course and how to select and present the materials. Instructors find that textbooks are extremely useful at this juncture in providing the framework for a new instructional venture in an incipient field. The first version of this text, *An Introduction to Health Psychology,* by Robert Gatchel and Andrew Baum, was the initial major textbook in health psychology.

In writing that initial text, Gatchel and Baum had a prodigious challenge and a marvelous opportunity. On the one hand they were challenged by the mass of material on factors relating health and medical issues to psychological processes. It had be sorted, arranged, codified, and put into didactic form. On the other hand, they had the opportunity to help structure a new field. To the extent that textbooks now copy the format of previous successful books, texts that follow theirs would adopt their organization, and, in pragmatic fashion, the field would be defined by what was in the textbook.

The Gatchel and Baum text made the most of its opportunity and met its challenge. The book has made a significant contribution by the way it has defined topics and by the inclusion of various perspectives in its discussions of areas of health psychology. The second edition, in which David Krantz joins the author team, continues to take advantage of these opportunities and builds on the record of accomplishment initially laid down.

For example, American psychology is in a period where the relationship of basic research to practice and application are strained, to say the least. The emergence of insurance companies and other third party payers has changed the face of clinical psychology. Without altering the nature of the services that they provide, many clinical psychologists now define themselves as health psychologists. This redefinition is made necessary by insurance plans that will reimburse clients for "medical services" but not for "mental health services." The redefinition of health psychology to embrace standard clinical psychological practice is understandable, but creates considerable terminological confusion in the field. One could imagine a text with the title *Health Psychology* that is entirely clinical in content; alternatively, one could imagine a parallel text, with the same title, that deals only in basic mechanisms and research. This text has integrated the appropriate aspects of each phase of the psychological spectrum as required by the problem being addressed. As a result chapters such as Chapter 3, dealing with stress, present the basic concepts and theories of stress, review the research literature critically, but also include ways of coping with and managing stress. In cold print this seems simple enough; a quick scan of the volumes of published stress material also shows how rare is such a balanced comprehensive review.

Perhaps the most important contribution of this text is the way in which it presents both the biomedical and the psychosocial components of the problems presented. Too often these differing approaches are pictured as opposing, mutually exclusive, ways of viewing a phenomenon. Thus, biofeedback is presented as an alternative to other more invasive treatments, such as pharmacotherapy. In reality, of course, the use of biofeedback is equally effective as a complement to other treatments, effective not because it eliminates other therapies but because it serves as an adjunct to them, such as lowering the dosage level of a drug and minimizing side effects.

By conceptualizing health psychology as part of a larger biosocial fabric, Gatchel, Baum, and Krantz have highlighted the concept that psychological mechanisms are not an alternative to medical ones. It is true that some psychosocial factors can be described in purely behavioral fashion—such as a personality based lifestyle that is a risk factor for one or another disease—but ultimately the behavioral factor must work through the same biological mechanisms as a purely biomedical factor. For example, if people must cope with the death of a spouse while not having a good social support network, they may be at risk of illness or death. The ways in which these risks are expressed are most likely through a compromised or suppressed immune function. The path from the critical event, the spouse's death, to illness involves both social and biological steps. A full picture of what is happening needs both biological and psychosocial explanations. No really meaningful understanding of the process can be gained by casting it one or the other explanation on a mutually exclusive basis.

For the purposes of a health psychology textbook the implications of this perspective are that health psychology must include as part of its discussions of psychosocial factors in health and disease background materials on endocrinology, immunology, and pharmacology, to name just a few of the requisite biomedical materials. The first edition of this text set the standard for a comprehensive treatment of topics by including this material. This edition continues to give an integrated view of the role of psychological factors in health.

Anyone who has written a review article, whether for a professional journal or for a term paper, comes to realize that the mastery of the materials is the easy part: organizing the material for a lucid, coherent, and sensible presentation is the difficult part. This is where *An Introduction to Health Psychology* is brilliant. The first edition was the pacesetter in its field. This edition once again defines health psychology in terms of the topics to be covered, the mixture of basic and applied materials to be incorporated, and the perspective that social and biological views of a phenomenon are but differing aspects of one thing and are to be unified in the presentation. Starting with an overview of mind and body, continuing through behavioral factors in cardiovascular diseases, stress, smoking, eating, and a variety of other illness-specific topics, the text also discusses behavioral mechanisms and factors, such as

control and learned helplessness. Applied topics, prevention, assessment, and biofeedback, for example, are presented in turn.

All in all, this text sets the standard for the field; it is exemplary in coverage,
organization, and perspective. It is a wonderful throwback to the vanished texts of
yesteryear in making a scholarly contribution as well as educating its readers.

Jerome E. Singer

PREFACE

||||||||||||||||||||||||||||||||||||||||||||||||||||||||||||||||||||||||||||||||||||||||||||||||||||||||||||||||||||||||||||||||||||||||||

Behavioral medicine is the broad interdisciplinary field of scientific investigation, education, and practice that concerns itself with health, illness, and related physiological dysfunctions. *Health psychology,* on the other hand, is a more discipline-specific term used to refer to psychology's primary role as a science and profession in the rapidly developing field of behavioral medicine. Psychologists have always been concerned with issues of illness and health. However, until recently they generally limited themselves to mental health settings and issues such as psychotherapy, mental retardation, and schizophrenia. This focus has changed rapidly during the past fifteen years, with an increased involvement in all areas of health and illness, not just mental health. This text provides a comprehensive review of the many medically related topics and areas that are being dramatically influenced by the new health psychology specialty.

We have taught courses in behavioral medicine and health psychology over a period of years to a varied audience—psychology students, medical and dental students, nurses, and other health care providers and trainees. Our experience has provided us with the opportunity to explore the best method for presenting the field as a meaningful whole to a diversified audience. We have attempted to provide a balanced mixture of material on basic theory, assessment, treatment, and specific practical, applied issues. The reader will be exposed to important psychological theories, concepts, and assessment/treatment methods of psychology as they apply to the area of health and illness. In presenting this material, we were cognizant of the fact that we would be addressing readers who differ in terms of backgrounds and expertise in psychology as well as in terms of basic psychobiological principles and service delivery experience. As a consequence, we have been careful to clearly express important concepts and terms in a manner that does not require a strong background in these areas and to provide basic material where needed. We have tried to present material in clear, understandable language without introducing complicated jargon or, conversely, oversimplifying basic concepts and issues.

The new edition features updated discussions of the material that was reviewed in the first edition and expanded or new coverage of three central issues in health psychology. Chapter 5 represents a summary of research and practical issues of behavioral factors in cardiovascular disease, which has historically been one of the most important areas in the development of the field. Chapter 6 is new, covering the emerging area of psychoneuroimmunology, behavioral factors in the etiology and treatment of cancer, and of AIDS, a vitally important area for behavioral study. Finally, Chapter 13 is a summary of research and practice of prevention, important to the aspects of health psychology concerned with health promotion and the minimization of disease.

We have organized the text in such a way that readers will first be introduced to the important concepts and issues in the field of health psychology. After an introduction and historical overview of the field in Chapter 1, we provide a summary of physiological bases of behavior and health in Chapter 2. We thought it would be beneficial to provide a "short course" in basic human physiology early in the text, since throughout the book we refer to various physiological factors and mechanisms when discussing concepts and phenomena. We then discuss basic concepts and behaviors that span the entire field of health psychology: stress (Chapter 3), control, and learned helplessness (Chapter 4).

Starting in Chapter 5, which deals with cardiovascular disorders, we turn to more specific areas within the field of health psychology. Chapter 6 considers psychological aspects of immunoregulation, cancer, and AIDS. The prevalence and significance of psychophysiological disorders are dealt with in Chapter 7, followed by a discussion of the impact of hospitalization and patient behavior on health and illness in Chapter 8. A review of psychological assessment techniques that can be employed in medical settings is presented in Chapter 9. This review is provided not only for clinicians in the reading audience, but also to introduce nonclinicians to procedures they are likely to encounter in their research and training activities. Chapter 10 reviews the various cognitive-behavioral treatment procedures that have been effectively employed with problem behaviors often seen in medical settings. Pain and its treatment are discussed in Chapter 11. In Chapter 12 we discuss three common appetitive problem behaviors that have significant health consequences—obesity, problem drinking/alcoholism, and smoking. We have selected these topics in order to provide vivid examples of how comprehensive psychological approaches can be applied to help us better understand the biological and psychosocial factors involved in these problem behaviors and thus treat the behaviors more effectively. The text concludes with discussion of health psychology contributions to the promotion of health and prevention of disease.

No text of this type is possible without the aid of many dedicated people. We are especially grateful to a number of colleagues who read drafts of the original text and provided helpful criticism and suggestions: David S. Holmes, Russell A. Jones, Mary Ellen Olbrisch, Paul B. Paulus, James W. Pennebaker, and Shelley Taylor. Extensive revisions were made as a result of their expert comments. Critical readings of sections of the new edition by Neil E. Grunberg and Carol S. Weisse were also extremely helpful. We would like to thank and acknowledge the great amount of help and support we received from the staff at Random House, particularly from Rochelle Diogenes and Tom Holton. Their persistence and expertise were greatly appreciated. We would also like to thank Mary Cranford, Shera E. Raisen, Rebecca A. Raymond, and Kitti Virts for their valuable assistance in the preparation of the book.

R.J.G.
A.B.
D.S.K.

AN INTRODUCTION TO
HEALTH PSYCHOLOGY

1 OVERVIEW

||||||||||||||||||||||||||||||||||||||||||||||||||||||||||||||||||||||||||||||||||||||||||||||||||||||||||||||||||||||||||||||||||||||

Traditionally, psychology and medicine have had little to do with each other. The "health" in psychology was mental health rather than a holistic mental and physical well-being. With the growing realization that psychological variables are important in health and illness, however, a new association between psychology and medicine has developed, as psychologists have begun to participate more actively in the diagnosis, treatment, and prevention of medical problems. Moreover, psychologists have brought their special research skills and technology to bear on major problem areas including the causes of illness, the nature of threats to health, and the care and management of patients and health care. Before more specifically defining and discussing this growing area, which is most commonly referred to as health psychology or behavioral medicine, we will briefly review how medicine and psychology have been linked historically.

THE MIND–BODY RELATIONSHIP: A HISTORICAL OVERVIEW

The relationship between the mind and the body has long been a controversial topic among philosophers, physiologists, and psychologists. Are experiences purely mental, purely physical, or an interaction of the physical and the mental? As Gentry and Matarazzo (1981) point out, the view that there are delicate interrelationships, such as the dry mouth and racing heart associated with fear or anger, or the headache triggered by emotional stress, can be found in ancient literary documents from Babylonia and Greece. The ancient Greek physician Hippocrates proposed one of the earliest temperamental theories of personality. He proposed that four bodily fluids or humors were associated with specific personality attributes or temperaments. An excess of yellow bile was linked to a choleric temperament. It was assumed that this yellow bile prompted an individual to become chronically angry and irritable, hence the word choleric (angry), which literally means bile. An excess

1

of black bile was considered to cause a person to be chronically sad or melancholic, hence the term melancholy, which literally means black bile. The sanguine or optimistic temperament was the result of excess blood in the system. Finally, the phlegmatic temperament, characterized by calm, listless personality attributes, was seen as being due to an excess of the bodily humor phlegm.

Of course this humoral theory of personality was long ago abandoned, along with a number of other prescientific notions. On a historical level, however, it points out how physical or biological factors have been seen through the ages as significantly interacting with and affecting the personality or psychological characteristics of an individual.

The traditional historical view of the interrelationship between mind and body lost favor in the seventeenth century. With the advent of physical medicine during the Renaissance, the belief that the mind influences the body came to be regarded as unscientific. The understanding of the mind and soul was relegated to the areas of religion and philosophy, while the understanding of the body was considered to be in the separate realm of physical medicine. This perpetuated the dualistic viewpoint that mind and body function separately and independently. Before this time, civilization's physicians, serving the multiple roles of philosopher-teacher, priest, and healer, had approached the understanding of mind-body interactions in a holistic way.

The individual usually credited with the development of the dualistic viewpoint and the resultant move away from the holistic approach was the French philosopher René Descartes. Descartes argued that the mind or soul was a separate entity parallel to and incapable of affecting physical matter or somatic processes in any direct way. This Cartesian dualism of mind and body became the preeminent philosophical basis of medicine. Although Descartes did indicate that the two entities could interact (he proposed that the pineal gland located in the midbrain was the vital connection between the mind and body), his basic tenet of dualism moved the newly independent field of medicine away from a holistic approach that emphasized psyche-soma interactions and toward the mechanistic pathophysiology approach that has dominated the field until relatively recently.

The discovery in the nineteenth century that microorganisms caused certain diseases produced further acceptance of the dualistic viewpoint. During this new scientific era of medicine, mechanical laws or physiological principles became the only permissible explanations of disease. Such an orientation, though, left a great many disorders unclassifiable. As McMahon and Hastrup (1980) note:

> There gradually emerged . . . an ambiguously defined diagnostic category designed to accommodate what we know today as "psychosomatic" disorders. This category was called "nervous". . . . The apparent influence of "emotions of the mind" in such conditions made their etiology an enigma. It was agreed that if a physician had evidence that a patient was "only nervous," he should "stop further inquiry. He is then without the pale of rational medicine. . . . According to the received view, that which was caused by a psychological variable could itself be nothing but psychological. Thus the "nervous" condition became dissociated from physiological processes, and a

somatic complaint "of nervous origin" was understood as having no physical basis. (p. 206)

Strict dualism mellowed somewhat during the mid-nineteenth century, primarily because of the work of Claude Bernard. Bernard was one of the first prominent physicians to emphasize the contributions of psychological factors to physical ailments. Subsequently, Sigmund Freud was very influential in stressing the interaction of psychological and physical factors in various disorders. Though emphasis was still placed on the body, microorganisms, and biological determinants of illness, gradually we were becoming aware of other sources of influence.

THE DEVELOPMENT OF PSYCHOSOMATIC MEDICINE

The twentieth century has seen a great deal of growth toward an integrated, holistic approach to health and illness. The major arena of this integration has traditionally been the area of psychophysiological medicine, which, as we will see, is based on the belief that social and psychological factors are important in the etiology (origin and development) and maintenance of many illnesses and in the treatment of these illnesses. The growth of this area of inquiry was partially a result of an increasing number of instances of illness that did not fit the solely biomedical view of health and disease and partially the result of gathering evidence that, in response to the environment, the psyche and the body often act as one.

In the early 1900s, efforts were being made by psychologists to integrate a psychological approach to health and illness into the field of clinical medicine. As Gentry and Matarazzo (1981) indicate:

> *The symposium on "The Relations of Psychology and Medical Education," sponsored by the American Psychological Association, at its 1911 annual meeting is a prime example of such an attempt. . . . The psychologists participating in this symposium, Shepard Ivory Franz and John Broadus Watson, and their physician-colleagues, Adolph Meyer, E. E. Southard, and Martin Prince, agreed (a) that medical students enter training with too little knowledge of psychology; (b) that such knowledge is essential to proper medical training; (c) that in fact courses in psychology should precede courses in psychiatry and neurology; and (d) that more hours should be devoted to psychology in the medical curriculum. (p. 6)*

Two decades later, however, this new role for psychology was still under discussion and little practical progress had been made (see Bott, 1928). The role of psychological factors was being recognized, but little was being done about them. It would take many years for the connections among psychological factors, illness, and the psychological processes underlying disease states to be studied more carefully and explained.

Initial discoveries of the importance of psychological factors in health-relevant matters were made largely by psychiatrists and psychodynamically oriented psychologists. For example, one of the first major controversies was whether personality factors were related to specific diseases (see Dunbar, 1943). Ruesch (1948) reported that a pattern of infantile behaviors characterized many patients, and others found associations between personality and the incidence of psychophysiological illness (see Deutsch, 1953). Oral and anal conflict, unconscious motives, maternal conflict, and the like seemed to find expression in health and susceptibility to illness.

Psychological input was not substantial during the early development of psychosomatic medicine. This was due in part to the inability of psychiatry and psychology to integrate practices and knowledge on a general level. However, it was also due to the way in which psychology developed. Psychology was founded as a narrow field concerned primarily with the subjective analysis of the structure of sensation and mental events. As this concern gave way to the study of purposive behavior, mental abilities, and functional aspects of behavior, the way was temporarily cleared for input into other areas. But the behaviorist revolution, with its interest in learning theory and its tendency to reduce behavior to its constituent, observable elements, sidetracked this growth. And so, for the greater part of the first half of this century, psychology remained insular.

Since World War II, psychology has grown in new directions. Renewed emphasis on the physiological bases of behavior, successful application in areas ranging from architecture to law, and the transcendence of the "schools" of psychology have all helped to bring about a richer and more open discipline. The expectation that psychology can contribute to many other fields is now firmly entrenched, and psychological input into matters of health and illness has increased greatly.

Not all of the initial work in health psychology was done by psychiatrists. Wolff (1950), for instance, made particularly important contributions to the study of health and illness with his extensive studies of the role of stress and adaptation in the development of disease states. He viewed illness as being caused by a number of factors, one of which was failure to adapt to the changes and stresses that are a normal part of life. Failure to adapt led to emotional and biological responses that could facilitate the onset of disease. Further, the particular ways in which people responded psychologically were linked to specific organs in the body and specific kinds of ailments.

Wolff's work remains of interest today, as does that of several other pioneering researchers (see Alexander, 1950; Graham, 1972) who were important in linking psychological and physiological realms of inquiry and in demonstrating how emotional factors influenced functioning by organ systems. Psychophysiological research provided basic evidence of the relationships between emotion and physiological responses (see Ax, 1953), and physiological research suggested that emotional and cognitive factors are extremely important in eliciting specific patterns of bodily response to threat (see Mason, 1975).

During the last decade, psychological contributions to medically relevant topics have become an important part of medical science, with the growing interest in treating patients as "whole" human beings and the realization that psychological factors are important in the course of almost any disease. In a comprehensive overview of the field of psychophysiological medicine during the 1970s, Lipowski (1977) noted a great resurgence of interest in this field. Indeed, most professionals today take the position that mind and body are not separate entities. A change in emotional state will be accompanied by a change in physiological response, and a change in physiological functioning will frequently be accompanied by alterations in emotional affect. In clinical treatment today, a holistic approach is advocated, with the view that to understand comprehensively health and disease, it is important to study people as "individual mind-body complexes ceaselessly interacting with the social and physical environment in which they are embodied" (see Lipowski, 1977, p. 234).

Gentry and Matarazzo (1981) have labeled this renewed orientation a reemergence rather than the emergence of a psychological approach to medical diagnosis and treatment. With the development of more effective psychological treatment and research technologies tailored specifically for medically relevant issues, there has been a dramatic reemergence of psychology in the study of health.

THE CHANGING NATURE OF HEALTH AND ILLNESS

The importance of mind-body interactions and of research on the relationships between behavior and health is further suggested by the changing nature of health care and threats to good health. Since 1900, life expectancy for both men and women in the United States has increased by 50 percent, a change made possible in part by breakthroughs in treating and preventing infectious illnesses such as polio, influenza, rubella, and smallpox (Matarazzo, 1985). With the elimination of these diseases through vaccination, "new" diseases became more prominent and now account for most deaths in this country. Cancer deaths, for example, have tripled since 1900, and heart disease, cancer, and acquired immune deficiency syndrome (AIDS) have become major killers. These diseases have no "magic bullet" cure or vaccine but are, in some respects, diseases caused by lifestyle and behavior. Diet, smoking, exercise, stress, and substance use are all behavioral factors that are associated with development of today's most feared illnesses. Califano (1979) noted that, at the turn of the century, 580 deaths out of every 100,000 U.S. citizens were due to influenza, pneumonia, diphtheria, tuberculosis, and gastrointestinal infections. Today these diseases account for only 30 deaths per 100,000 citizens. This rapid decline in deaths from infectious agents, he argues, has been accompanied by increased numbers of deaths from diseases caused or facilitated by preventable, behavioral factors such as smoking (see Figure 1.1).

Within the past decade, observable changes in the lifestyles of Americans reflect directly on these behavioral factors associated with heart disease, cancer, and other modern illnesses. Data from the 1981 Surgeon General's report (Harris, 1981) suggest that many people have taken steps to exercise, change their diets, quit smoking, and so on. Though some of these trends are not positive, as in recent increases in smoking among teenage girls, most reflect a growing awareness of lifestyle as a determinant of health (see Figure 1.2).

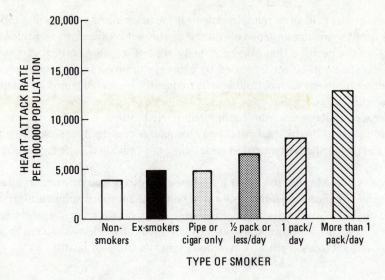

Figure 1.1   Age-adjusted rates of first heart attack for white males aged 30–59, United States, categorized by smoking status.
Adapted from J. A. Califano, Jr. *Healthy People: The Surgeon General's Report on Health Promotion and Disease Prevention.* Washington, D.C.: U.S. Government Printing Office, 1979.

METHODOLOGICAL DEVELOPMENTS

How does one go about studying the relationships between psyche and bodily tissue damage or resistance? The following example will demonstrate the complexity of the problem.

Assume that you are interested in the relationships between personality and illness. You first devise a personality scale that distinguishes people along a personality dimension, dividing people into "X" and "Not-X" categories. You develop the hypothesis that all people with the "X" trait are more likely to develop high blood pressure than are those without this trait. You therefore assemble a pool of 2,000 potential subjects, carefully matched on a number of variables such as education and income, and administer your personality scale to each subject. You recruit 500 people in each category, then you take each subject's blood pressure and inquire as to his or her history of high blood pressure (or lack thereof). When you tabulate your data, the findings are remarkable—not only do 70 percent of the "Xs" have a history of high blood pressure while only 10 percent of the "Not-Xs" have such a history, but the mean blood pressure of "Xs" is 20 mm of mercury higher than that of the "Not-Xs." Such results initially prompt you to believe that you have discovered the cause of high blood pressure.

The only problem with these results is that they have *not* demonstrated that your personality trait causes high blood pressure. Your evidence is correlational in nature—it shows that the personality trait "X" is related to high blood pressure, but it does not show that the factors are causally linked. It is possible, for example, that a third factor is also coincidentally related to blood pressure. This is a common

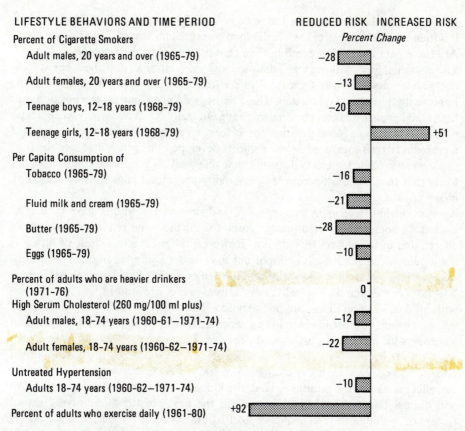

LIFESTYLE BEHAVIORS AND TIME PERIOD

Percent of Cigarette Smokers

Adult males, 20 years and over (1965–79)   −28

Adult females, 20 years and over (1965–79)   −13

Teenage boys, 12–18 years (1968–79)   −20

Teenage girls, 12–18 years (1968–79)   +51

Per Capita Consumption of

Tobacco (1965–79)   −16

Fluid milk and cream (1965–79)   −21

Butter (1965–79)   −28

Eggs (1965–79)   −10

Percent of adults who are heavier drinkers (1971–76)   0

High Serum Cholesterol (260 mg/100 ml plus)

Adult males, 18–74 years (1960–61–1971–74)   −12

Adult females, 18–74 years (1960–62–1971–74)   −22

Untreated Hypertension

Adults 18–74 years (1960–62–1971–74)   −10

Percent of adults who exercise daily (1961–80)   +92

REDUCED RISK   INCREASED RISK
Percent Change

Figure 1.2   **Recent changes in lifestyle behaviors that affect health.**
Adapted from P. R. Harris. *Health United States 1980.* U.S. Department of Health and Human Services Pub. No. (PHS)81-1232. Washington, D.C.: U.S. Government Printing Office, 1981.

problem in psychology, but it takes on a special significance in studies of health and illness. For example, based on your data, can one refute the possibility that high blood pressure causes personality trait "X" to develop? The answer, of course, is no. Being an "X" may cause people to develop high blood pressure, but it is equally possible that finding out that they have high blood pressure causes people to develop trait "X."

There are a number of ways to improve upon the above basic research design. The study we have outlined is a **retrospective study,** in which people are asked to recall past events or in which present conditions are used to explain these events. This is relatively easy to do. **Prospective studies,** in which an attempt is made to predict future events, are more costly and time consuming. A prospective version of your study might entail, for example, administering your personality inventory to your 2,000 subjects, recruiting 500 "Xs" and 500 "Not-Xs," and then following up all 1,000 regularly over five years to determine which ones do develop high blood pressure. Once a year, blood pressure is recorded from all subjects, and they are asked about diagnosis of high blood pressure. Suppose that only 10 of the subjects have high blood pressure when the scale is initially administered. After five years, it is found that 150 subjects have high blood pressure and that of these 120 are "Xs." Are these data any more revealing than those obtained in the retrospective study? The answer is yes. Although the data are still correlational, and therefore still do not provide a solid basis for causal inferences, they allow you to eliminate one important alternative explanation. These findings do not argue for the position that high blood pressure causes personality change to trait "X." You have predicted who would develop high blood pressure (or at least 80 percent of them) on the basis of a personality trait measured *before* subjects developed this problem. Since the trait assessment preceded subjects' learning that they had high blood pressure, it is not likely that the relationship between personality and blood pressure was caused by blood pressure.

As we shall see, many retrospective and prospective studies have been conducted. In some cases, retrospective studies yield the same results as prospective efforts, and in some cases they do not. However, the prospective study of illness is not a guaranteed panacea. It is important to consider a number of other problems. Choice of indicators is one potential problem—if one is interested in a specific illness, how does one define it? Typically, only extreme cases are studied, as many people with mild cases of an illness are undiagnosed. Thus, someone with very high blood pressure would be more likely to have a recorded history of high blood pressure than someone with moderately high blood pressure. Another problem is the sheer complexity of the human body and the number of factors that can influence health. Blood pressure is regulated by many biological systems. The sympathetic nervous system can affect it, as can the pituitary gland, the kidneys, and several other systems. (We will discuss these physiological systems in the next chapter.) Identifying causal factors or spelling out their sequence is often impossible given our present state of knowledge. These complexities are a formidable obstacle to studying the causes and development of illness.

Another problem facing the psychologist in studying health and illness is choice of variables and the operationalization of these variables. Operationalization refers to the translation of concepts into methodology. In learning psychology, for example, the conceptual variable motivation or hunger may be operationalized as food deprivation for twenty-four hours. The operational definition is believed to reflect the conceptual variable, but one cannot be sure that this reflection is accurate. If we are interested in studying causes of lower back pain or of headache, we normally must rely upon subjects' reports of discomfort. However, there is no assurance that these reports are comparable or that they reflect the same sensation in all patients. Using physiological measurements strikes most of us as being more objective, and the assumption is often made that such recordings are more reflective of a given condition than are self-reports. However, physiological activity can usually be interpreted in many ways. Thus data that we believe are indicative of a particular condition may instead be related to another. We should never assume that physiological response data are necessarily any more reliable than self-report data.

Selection of appropriate subject groups is another important problem that needs to be considered. Biases in selection can undermine our best research efforts. In a recent study of stress at Three Mile Island, for example, this problem was particularly evident (Baum et al., 1981). If we are interested in the health consequences of the stress caused by the Three Mile Island nuclear accident, who should be studied? The "experimental" group—people exposed to this stress—could be drawn randomly from people living near the crippled nuclear plant. However, with whom should they be compared? What is the appropriate comparison group? If we decide that it should be people living one hundred miles away, we have not accounted for the fact that living near any power plant could be stressful. As a result, if it is found that the Three Mile Island group is more stressed than the comparison group, we will not be able to tell whether this stress is caused by living near Three Mile Island or by living near *any* power plant. In order to account for this, we could add a second control group—people living near a coal-fired power plant. Now, if the Three Mile Island group is more stressed than either control group, we can say that this stress is not caused by living near any power plant. However, another possibility still cannot be ruled out—that living near any *nuclear* plant is stressful. In order to eliminate this possibility, yet another control group drawn from people living near an undamaged nuclear plant must be added. If the data still show that Three Mile Island residents are more stressed than the control groups, we can then conclude that these differences are unique to the Three Mile Island incident.

There is yet another problem, more relevant to convincing people of the veracity of your findings than to generating the findings. Many disease states, such as cancer, heart disease, and hypertension, have a long recruitment period—they develop slowly and are often not detectable for many years. Thus it is very difficult to identify when this development began (if such a point exists), and as a result, it is hard to convince people that a particularly salient (and therefore recognizable) event was the cause. Returning to our Three Mile Island example, even if we find in ten years that in comparison to people living elsewhere four times as many Three Mile Islanders have hypertension, controlling for age and the like, how do we convince people that the presence of Three Mile Island was *the* cause?

In spite of the extensive and challenging problems in the field of health psychology, research has produced interesting and important findings. Interdisciplinary methodologies have evolved to deal with many of the problems. The future is an interdisciplinary one, in which psychology can make important contributions. The opportunity to offer input into an exciting and basic enterprise where the outcomes—life and death—are often more dramatic than psychologists are used to makes grappling with these thorny issues worth our time and effort. Like the efforts to apply psychology to environmental problems and other issues that consistently defied attempts to exert experimental control and rigor (Singer and Glass, 1973), the drive to apply psychology to health will ultimately be successful.

EMERGENCE OF BEHAVIORAL MEDICINE

Behavioral medicine represents the integration of the behavioral sciences with the practice and science of medicine. In an enlightening historical overview of the emergence of health psychology, Matarazzo (1980) points out how Schofield (1969) emphasized that although the research and services of psychologists traditionally were primarily in three health areas—psychotherapy, schizophrenia, and mental retardation—there was a growing opportunity and need for psychological research in a number of other health areas. Specifically, he mentioned that the 1964 report of the President's Commission on Cancer, Heart Disease, and Stroke indicated that these health areas were targets for well-funded research, treatment, and prevention programs. This potential research opportunity of psychology in the field of health stimulated the interest of the American Psychological Association and ultimately resulted in the development in 1978 of the Division of Health Psychology (Division 38 of the APA), which publishes its own journal, *Health Psychology.* Also within the decade, the Academy of Behavioral Medicine Research and the Society of Behavioral Medicine have been formed and the *Journal of Behavioral Medicine* established. Currently a great number of special courses, and even subspecialty areas of study, in behavioral medicine and health psychology are being developed in psychology, psychiatry, and other programs throughout the country.

Although behavioral medicine is now recognized as an important area, there is still some debate among professionals in the field concerning just what behavioral medicine is. A widely accepted definition was originally developed at the Yale Conference on Behavioral Medicine and later articulated by Schwartz and Weiss (1977). Their definition viewed the area as an amalgam of elements from behavioral science disciplines, such as psychology, medical sociology, and health education, that have relevant knowledge which can assist in health care, treatment, and illness prevention. They thus emphasized the interdisciplinary nature of behavioral medicine.

Subsequently, Pomerleau and Brady (1979) proposed a less broad definition of the field. They expanded upon the initial use of the term behavioral medicine by Birk (1973). Birk used the term behavioral medicine in the context of defining biofeedback as an approach to the treatment of medical disorders based on learning theory. Pomerleau and Brady argue that the main "core" of behavioral medicine should be viewed as the *experimental analysis of behavior,* based on learning theory, since it was this area that served as the key source and inspiration of much of the current research in the field. They go on to define the area as: (1) consisting of methods derived from the experimental analysis of behavior—specifically behavior therapy and behavior modification—that are clinically used in the evaluation, treatment, or prevention of physical disease or physiological dysfunction (e.g., essential hypertension, addictive behavior, obesity, etc.), and (2) emphasizing the conduct of research that will contribute to a better understanding, and the functional analysis, of behavior associated with medical disorders or health care problems.

Even more recently, Matarazzo (1980) has pointed out that the field of behavioral medicine should actually be broken down into specific areas. He suggests that the term **behavioral medicine** should be used for the broad interdisciplinary field of scientific investigation, education, and practice which concerns itself with health, illness, and related physiological dysfunctions. This is similar to the Schwartz and

Weiss (1977) definition. **Behavioral health**, he proposes, is a term to describe the new interdisciplinary subspecialty within behavioral medicine that is specifically concerned with the maintenance of health and the prevention of illness and medical dysfunctions in currently healthy individuals. For example, educational effects directed at the maintenance of good health through proper diet and exercise fall into this subspecialty. Finally, **health psychology** is a more discipline-specific term encompassing psychology's primary role as a science and profession in both of these domains. This is more akin to the Pomerleau and Brady definition, although they were more specific in their emphasis in the area of the experimental analysis of behavior within the field of psychology. Matarazzo's definition is much broader in scope:

> Health psychology *is the aggregate of the specific educational, scientific, and professional contributions of the discipline of psychology to the promotion and maintenance of health, the prevention and treatment of illness, and the identification of etiologic and diagnostic correlates of health, illness, and related dysfunction.* (Matarazzo, 1980, p. 815)

The authors of this text subscribe to Matarazzo's categorization, and therefore have adhered to it in their discussions of health psychology throughout the book. In the chapters that follow, we will present important areas of health psychology that have contributed, or that have the promise to contribute, significantly to our understanding of health and illness.

SUMMARY

This first chapter provides a brief historical overview of how medicine and psychology have been linked. Until recently, the concept of a dualism between mind and body dominated the field of medicine. Currently there is a movement toward an integrated, holistic approach to health and illness and a renewed effort toward employing psychological approaches to medical diagnosis and treatment. Psychology has a great deal to offer the study of health and illness, especially in methodology.

What exactly constitutes this burgeoning new area of behavioral medicine was also discussed. In light of Matarazzo's contention that the growing field of behavioral medicine should actually be broken down into specific areas, those areas were defined: the term *behavioral medicine* should be used for the broad interdisciplinary field of scientific investigation, education, and practice that concerns itself with health, illness, and related physiological dysfunctions; *behavioral health* describes the new interdisciplinary subspecialty within behavioral medicine that is specifically concerned with the maintenance of health and the prevention of illness in currently healthy individuals; and *health psychology* is a more discipline-specific term encompassing psychology's primary role as a science and profession in both of these former domains. Throughout this text, advances in the area of health psychology will be highlighted.

RECOMMENDED READINGS

Matarazzo, J. D. Behavioral health and behavioral medicine: Frontiers for a new health psychology. *American Psychologist,* 1980, *35,* 807–817.

Matarazzo, J. D. Behavioral health's challenge to academic, scientific, and professional psychology. *American Psychologist,* 1982, *37,* 1–14.

Matarazzo, J. D., Weiss, S. M., Herd, J. A. Miller, N. E., and Weiss, S. M. (Eds.), *Behavioral health.* New York: Wiley, 1984.

Schwartz, G. E., and Weiss, S. What is behavioral medicine? *Psychosomatic Medicine,* 1977, *36,* 377–381.

2 PHYSIOLOGICAL BASES OF BEHAVIOR AND HEALTH

||||||||||||||||||||||||||||||||||||||||||||||||||||||||||||||||||||||||||||||||||||||||||||||||||||||||||||||||||||||

In this chapter, we will review some physiological aspects of behavior and health that relate to the material in the rest of this book. We will briefly cover the nervous system, the endocrine system, the cardiovascular system, the respiratory system, the digestive system, the immune system, and genetic influences on behavior and health.

One of the first things we learn in health psychology is that mind and body are thoroughly intertwined. The physiological aspects of behavior and the ways in which physiological response can be altered by emotional response attest to this linkage. Without an understanding of both realms, our knowledge of each one suffers. For this reason, we cannot emphasize enough the importance of learning about the ways in which the body works. This chapter will provide the reader with a brief beginning.

SYSTEMS OF THE BODY

Stress and other aspects of behavior and health are mediated primarily by the nervous system and the endocrine system. These systems provide most of the regulatory and control functions in the body. They are both channeled through the hypothalamus, a section of the brain that regulates the internal functions of the body, including temperature, blood flow, and body weight. Extending down from the hypothalamus, the nervous system consists of billions of neurons (nerve cells) that communicate with one another and carry messages to and from all parts of the body. Interfacing with the nervous system at a number of places, the endocrine system uses chemical messengers to stimulate, slow, or otherwise govern response by organ systems.

THE NERVOUS SYSTEM

Most views of the nervous system refer to two levels of organization. The first is the central nervous system and the second is the peripheral nervous system. These classifications are further subdivided. For example, the peripheral system is often described as having somatic and autonomic components.

13

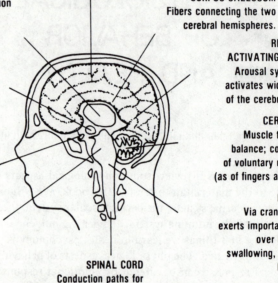

CEREBRUM
(Surface: cerebral cortex)
Sense perception; voluntary
movements; learning, remembering,
thinking; emotion; consciousness.

THALAMUS
Sensory relay station
on the way to the
cerebral cortex.

CORPUS CALLOSUM
Fibers connecting the two
cerebral hemispheres.

**RETICULAR
ACTIVATING SYSTEM**
Arousal system that
activates wide regions
of the cerebral cortex.

HYPOTHALAMUS
Control of visceral
and somatic functions,
such as temperature,
metabolism, and
endocrine balance.

CEREBELLUM
Muscle tone; body
balance; coordination
of voluntary movement
(as of fingers and thumb)

PITUITARY GLAND
An endocrine gland.

PONS
Fibers connecting
the two hemispheres
of the cerebellum.

MEDULLA
Via cranial nerves
exerts important control
over breathing;
swallowing, digestion,
heartbeat.

SPINAL CORD
Conduction paths for
motor and sensory
impulses; local reflexes
(e.g., knee jerk).

Figure 2.1   Cross section of the brain—major structures of the brain and their functions.
Adapted from Ernest R. Hilgard, Richard C. Atkinson, and Rita L. Atkinson. *Introduction to Psychology,*
Sixth Edition. Copyright © 1975 by Harcourt Brace Jovanovich, Inc. Reprinted by permission of the
publisher.

The Central Nervous System

The central nervous system (CNS) is the command post of the body. Under most
circumstances, it regulates and integrates all other bodily functions. It consists of
only two parts—the brain and the spinal cord. But these two parts are enormously
complex.

The brain, the large mass of nervous tissue located beneath the skull, is organized in layers emanating out from the center. Toward the middle are the areas
responsible for bodily processes and survival. The brain stem, located at the point
where the spinal cord widens as it enters the skull, is regarded as the center for
regulating life-support systems. Included in or near this core are several structures.

Hypothalamus controls visceral (organ) functions, including temperature, metabolism, eating, and endocrine function.
Thalamus directs sensory information received by the brain.

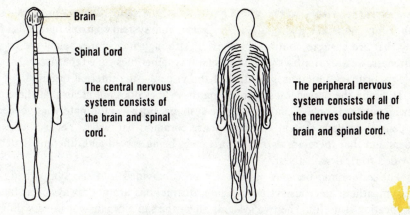

Brain

Spinal Cord

The central nervous system consists of the brain and spinal cord.

The peripheral nervous system consists of all of the nerves outside the brain and spinal cord.

Figure 2.2   Central and peripheral nervous systems.

Medulla regulates breathing, digestion, and other basic processes.
Reticular activating system arouses parts of the cortex and is involved in sleep.
Cerebellum governs muscle tone, balance, and coordination of bodily movements.

These brain areas function to assure survival of the organism.

Surrounding this central area of the brain is the limbic system, which includes the hippocampus, olfactory bulbs, septum, and amygdala. The limbic system is believed to play a role in emotions, but detailed information is not available. The outer area of the brain farthest from the core is the cerebral cortex. Here reside such intellectual abilities as learning, memory, and consciousness.

The spinal cord is also a mass of nervous tissue, but it occupies the vertebral canal that runs through the center of the body. It is protected by bony structures and is organized in segments. Each segment is associated with specific muscles, organ systems, or functions.

Within the spinal cord cell bodies are responsible for receiving and transmitting sensory and motor information. Sensory information is received from nerves emanating from the periphery and channeled to the brain. Information from the brain is similarly transmitted from the brain to the peripheral nerves that reach the cord. In this way, the spinal cord serves as the link between the brain and the rest of the body.

The Peripheral Nervous System

All of the other nerves in the body (outside the CNS) constitute the peripheral nervous system. Of the many ways of viewing this massive system's components, the most common involves distinguishing between the somatic and autonomic nervous systems. Although both are composed entirely of peripheral nerves, they serve different functions. The **somatic system** connects with voluntary muscles and consists of nerves between sensory and motor organs. Thus walking or lifting an arm is governed by the somatic nervous system. This system also provides the central nervous system with its only access to external information through sensory input.

The **autonomic system**, on the other hand, connects with involuntary muscles—such as the lungs, stomach, and kidneys. The autonomic system controls functions of the body that are basic to continued survival. Although it operates below the level of awareness, we are often aware of its effects. It is sometimes called the **visceral system** since its primary function is control of the viscera—the internal organs.

Dividing the peripheral system along these lines does not mean that there is no overlap between somatic and autonomic systems. Both are ultimately influenced by the central nervous system and may share common pathways. Yet it is useful to understand that there are two basic processes being served and different structures provided to deal with them.

The autonomic nervous system can be subdivided into the sympathetic and parasympathetic nervous systems. Again, distinctions are not always clear but the classification is useful. The two systems affect the same organs but in very different ways (see Table 2.1).

The **sympathetic nervous system** is a catabolic system responsible for arousing or mobilizing the body for action. It stimulates organs that must increase activity in order to ready an organism to act and inhibits organs that are not involved in such a mobilization. For example, it increases heart rate and blood pressure, increases conversion of stored energy to usable energy, constricts blood vessels, and reduces blood flow to the skin (to reduce bleeding in case of injury) and to the gut while it

TABLE 2.1   Comparison between the Sympathetic and the Parasympathetic Nervous Systems

	Sympathetic	Parasympathetic
General Function	Catabolism	Anabolism
Activity	Long-lasting	Short-acting
Specific Actions		
Pupil of eye	Dilates	Constricts
Salivary glands	Scanty, thick secretion	Profuse, watery secretion
Heart rate	Increase	Decrease
Contractility of heart (force of ventricular contraction)	Increase	—
Blood vessels	Generally constricts	Slight effect
Bronchial tubes of lungs	Dilates lumen	Constricts lumen
Sweat glands	Stimulates	—
Adrenal medulla	Secretes epinephrine and norepinephrine	—
Genitals	Ejaculation	Erection
Motility and tone of gastrointestinal tract	Inhibits	Stimulates
Sphincters	Stimulates	Inhibits (relax)

Based on A. C. Guyton. *Textbook of Medical Physiology,* Philadelphia: Saunders, 1981, p. 715.

dilates vessels to the muscles and generally increases blood flow to areas that will be needed to act. As we will see in the next chapter, this readying of the body, described by Cannon (1927) as the fight-or-flight response, is basic to stress. For the present it is sufficient to think of the sympathetic system as being responsible for arousing an organism and preparing various organs to meet an emergency quickly and with maximum strength.

While the sympathetic nervous system is concerned with arousal, the **parasympathetic nervous system** is concerned with calming or reducing arousal of various organisms. In a sense the two are opposites—the parasympathetic system counteracts arousal (the sympathetic system) when it is no longer needed. (See Figure 2.3.) It is an **anabolic system** in that it restores the body's reserves of stored energy. After the sympathetic system has increased heart rate, the parasympathetic system slows it down. Since both systems affect the same organs, it is sometimes difficult to know which system is responsible for an effect.

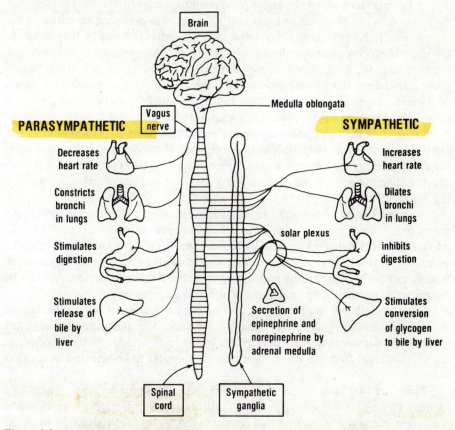

Figure 2.3 The sympathetic and parasympathetic nervous systems, though affecting the same organs, have different effects.

Adapted from Ernest R. Hilgard, Richard C. Atkinson, and Rita L. Atkinson. *Introduction to Psychology,* Sixth Edition. Copyright © 1975 by Harcourt Brace Jovanovich, Inc. Reprinted by permission of the publisher.

Not all the differences between the two systems are based on function. The activity of the sympathetic nervous system is generally an all-or-nothing response. That is, the entire body is affected together—all organs are affected at once. Sympathetic arousal is also relatively long-lasting. Endocrine functions associated with sympathetic activity, as we will discuss in the next chapter, serve to extend the arousal generated. Parasympathetic activity is short-lived and much more specific, and individual organs can be affected in a more or less isolated manner.

Related Endocrine Activity

As noted earlier, the sympathetic nervous system, because of its association with arousal, was readily implicated in the stress response. This activity is accomplished mainly through one of its primary ganglia, the adrenal medulla. Stimulation of the sympathetic nervous system causes the adrenal medullae to secrete large quantities of two neurotransmitter hormones, epinephrine and norepinephrine (also known as adrenaline and noradrenaline). These two substances are called catecholamines. Epinephrine is secreted only by the adrenal medulla while norepinephrine is primarily released by sympathetic neurons and also serves as a neurotransmitter in the sympathetic nervous system. Once released by the adrenal medulla, they enter the bloodstream and are carried throughout the body. Norepinephrine in the bloodstream causes the same effects as does sympathetic stimulation; as a result, it supports and extends the arousal generated by the nervous system because the effects of norepinephrine in circulating blood last much longer than do those generated directly by norepinephrine released at synapses in the sympathetic nervous system. Norepinephrine increases heart rate and other coronary activity to a limited extent, constricts most blood vessels, inhibits gastrointestinal activity, and increases a number of other bodily functions. Although epinephrine is similar in its effects, it is more effective than norepinephrine in stimulating the heart and less effective in constricting blood vessels.

A second system often implicated in stress is the hypothalamic-pituitary-adrenal cortex axis. The activities of these adrenal systems are depicted in Figure 2.4. The adrenal glands (located above each kidney) are made up of two parts: the medulla, which we have already considered, and the adrenal cortex. As we have noted, medullary activity is caused by and similar to sympathetic stimulation. Activity by the cortex is stimulated by secretions of the pituitary gland.

When stimulated, the pituitary gland secretes a number of hormones. One of these is adrenocorticotrophic hormone (ACTH), which stimulates the adrenal cortex and controls the secretion of corticosteroids by the cortex. Although these hormones are very different from the catecholamines, they appear to be involved in stress as well.

There are two basic forms of corticosteroids: the glucocorticoids, which help regulate levels of glucose in the blood, and the mineralocorticoids, which affect utilization of mineral substances and regulate electrolytes in the blood. Most of the glucocorticoid secretion in humans is cortisol. Cortisol has a number of effects on carbohydrate metabolism. It also inhibits inflammation of damaged tissue. More important for our purposes, cortisol appears to accompany stress. Most situations that are considered stressful, including trauma, heat, cold, and even sympathetic

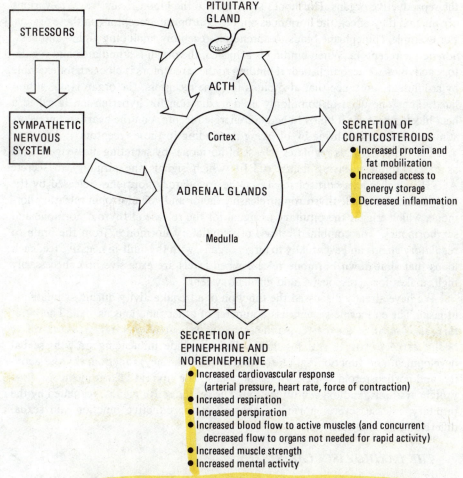

Figure 2.4   Diagram of stress-related activities of the adrenal glands.

stimulation, elicit large increases in cortisol secretion. The exact role played by cortisol in the stress response is not as clear as is that played by the catecholamines. It is likely that cortisol speeds the body's access to its energy stores of fats and carbohydrates, thereby supporting arousal. It is also not clear whether the increased secretion of cortisol is caused by parallel activation of the pituitary and the sympathetic nervous system or is stimulated first. However, it is clear that both systems are related to the stress response.

THE ENDOCRINE SYSTEM

The adrenal glands are part of the endocrine system and generally serve as a complementary system to the nervous system in regulating bodily function. The endocrine network is made up of several glands that secrete hormones directly into the circulating bloodstream, and includes the adrenals, the pituitary, thyroid, and the reproductive organs. Hormones secreted into the bloodstream travel to various organs that they affect; the hormones bind to appropriate receptors on these organs. For example, epinephrine binds to adrenergic receptors, including alpha- and beta-adrenergic receptors. When binding is achieved, the organ is stimulated and regulatory activities are accomplished. If binding to these receptors is blocked, for example by a different substance that also binds to these receptors, the organ is not stimulated. Thus one class of commonly used medication for hypertension is called a beta-blocker because it binds to beta-adrenergic receptors on the heart and prevents stimulation by epinephrine by blocking its binding to these receptors.

The hypothalamus regulates release of hormones by secreting messengers such as corticotropin releasing factor (CRF), which signals the pituitary to secrete ACTH, which elicits cortisol release. Other regulatory hormones released by the hypothalamus include thyrotropin releasing factor and gonadotropin releasing hormone, which trigger the pituitary to signal for the release of thyroid hormone and sex hormones. The combined release of stimulatory hormones, from the brain to regulatory glands and eventually to target organs, with the built-in negative feedback loops that shut down hormone release when levels are excessive or unnecessarily high, makes for a responsive and efficient system.

We have already discussed the function of adrenal activity during sympathetic arousal. The endocrine system has a number of other functions as well. The pituitary, also known as the master gland because of its central importance in controlling bodily activity, has several functions. These include influencing growth, sexual development and functioning, reproduction, renal (kidney) function, thyroid activity, and corticosteroid release by the adrenals. The thyroid affects metabolic rate, protein systhesis, and oxygen utilization. The reproductive glands, regulated by the pituitary, release several hormones that affect reproductive function and sexual differentiation and activity.

THE CARDIOVASCULAR SYSTEM

The cardiovascular system consists of the heart, the arteries that carry oxygenated blood to the various parts of the body, the capillaries, and the veins that return blood to the heart. (See Figure 2.5.) The heart, generally thought of as the most important muscle in the body, is responsible for circulation of blood throughout the body.

The heart is composed of four parts, or chambers, that work in sequence to bring blood into the heart and then pump it out again. Blood, after passing through the body, enters the right atrium and then the right ventricle. This blood has little oxygen left and so is sent into the pulmonary artery and through the lungs, where it disposes of wastes and is replenished with oxygen. It then returns to the left atrium of the heart through the pulmonary vein. The heart pumps the oxygenated blood from the left ventricle into the arterial system, through which it carries nutrients to all of the body.

The motion of blood through the heart is governed by the opening and closing of valves that connect the various chambers and by the regular sequence of contraction and relaxation of the heart muscle. The phases of contraction and relaxation are referred to as the **cardiac cycle**, and consist of systole and diastole. During

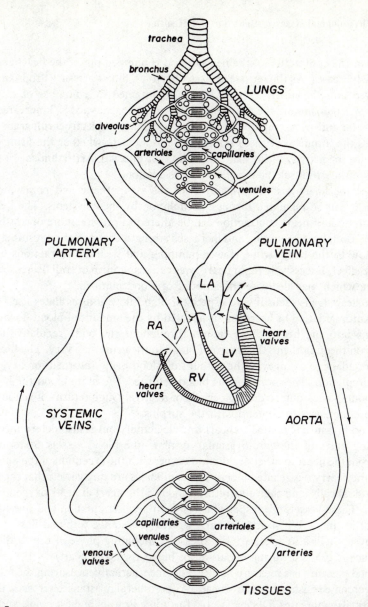

Figure 2.5 The cardiovascular system. The heart, blood vessels, and lungs provide for exchange of gases between the atmosphere and the tissues. The right and left side of the heart are two pumps arranged in series on the same circuit. The oxygenated blood (arterial blood) returning from the lungs by the pulmonary veins enters the left atrium (LA) and the left ventricle (LV). Contraction of the latter expels the blood into the aorta, which ramifies into numerous arteries for distribution of the blood to the tissues. The end branches of the arteries (arterioles) give rise to the exchange vessels (capillaries) where oxygen and foodstuffs pass to the tissues and carbon dioxide and waste products are taken up by the blood (venous blood). The capillaries reunite to form the venules and veins, which return the venous blood to the right atrium (RA) and right ventricle (RV). The contraction of the right ventricle propels the blood into the pulmonary artery and its branches. In the pulmonary capillaries the carbon dioxide diffuses to the small air sacs (alveoli), and oxygen is taken up from the latter by the blood. The presence of valves in the heart and the limb veins ensures forward movement of the blood.

From J. T. Shepherd and P. M. Vanhoutte. *The Human Cardiovascular System: Facts and Concepts.* New York: Raven Press, 1979, p. 3.

21

systole, or the contraction of the heart, blood is pumped out of the heart and blood pressure increases. As the muscle relaxes (**diastole**), blood pressure drops and blood is allowed into the heart. This rhythm is maintained in a number of ways. The primary mechanisms are the atrioventricular and sinoatrial nodes, innervated by the sympathetic and parasympathetic nervous systems. An **electrocardiogram** (EKG) measures the impulses of these nodes and can indicate whether the firing pattern (and hence the activity of the heart) is normal or unusual. **Arrhythmias** are unusual patterns of heart-muscle contraction and relaxation.

Since the heart is innervated by both the sympathetic and parasympathetic systems, it can be regulated through stimulation by these systems. The heart rate or the strength of heart contraction can be altered to provide more or less blood to the body. Both faster pumping and increased strength of contraction result in greater blood flow to the body, while slower pumping and weaker contractions have the opposite effect. Excessively rapid heart rates can result in an overall decrease in heart strength, which may decrease the amount of blood pumped.

The heart is also sensitive to aspects of blood flow and regulates itself accordingly. Autoregulation of heart rate is affected by the amount of blood flowing from the veins into the heart. Since tissues throughout the body regulate the blood circulation through them, the return of blood in the veins may vary. The heart must therefore adapt to changes in the amount of blood being returned for oxygenation and recirculation. The more venous blood returned, the more blood the heart will have to pump back out, so during periods of relatively high returns of venous blood, heart rate increases to contend with the surplus.

Blood pressure is related to heart muscle activity but is also determined by the remaining parts of the cardiovascular system—the blood vessels. **Arteries** carry blood from the heart to other organs and tissue; with the exception of the pulmonary artery, they carry oxygenated blood. The **capillaries** are tiny vessels that carry blood to individual cells, and the **veins** return blood to the heart after its oxygen has been used up. These vessels are responsible for peripheral circulation and may dilate or constrict at times. When arteries narrow, their resistance to blood flow increases. Other events will also affect arterial pressure, including phase of the cardiac cycle (resistance is greatest during expulsion of blood from the heart).

Blood pressure is a measure of this resistance, actually measuring the force built up to overcome resistance in the arteries. As peripheral resistance increases, the force necessary also increases. During systole this force is at its highest point, and during diastole it falls to its lowest. Thus systolic blood pressure is higher than diastolic blood pressure.

There are a number of ways to increase or decrease arterial pressure, but we will not deal with them. It is sufficient here to understand that blood pressure is related to the rate at which the heart is pumping, the resistance in the arteries, and various other bodily processes. It is regulated by several systems and reflects generally upon cardiovascular function.

The heart, being living muscle tissue, must receive nourishment. The coronary arteries carry oxygen-rich blood to the heart and cardiac veins and return the used blood to the circulatory system. Most coronary arteries are on the surface of the muscle. When these arteries narrow or become blocked, heart attacks or other dangerous conditions result. As we will see in Chapter 5, coronary artery disease is a leading cause of death in the United States.

THE RESPIRATORY SYSTEM

Closely linked to the cardiovascular system, the **respiratory system** provides the blood with oxygen and rids it of carbon dioxide before it is pumped through the body. As we have already noted, blood returns to the heart full of carbon dioxide waste, and it must exchange this waste for oxygen before it can be recirculated. This process occurs in the lungs, the most important organ of the respiratory system.

The respiratory system includes the nose, mouth, pharynx, trachea, lungs, diaphragm, and a number of abdominal muscles. When we breathe, air is brought in through the nose and mouth, then passed to the lungs through the pharynx and trachea. Once the air reaches the lungs, it exchanges its oxygen for carbon dioxide with the capillaries in the lungs.

Respiration is controlled by both voluntary and involuntary muscles. Unlike the heart, the lungs can be stopped voluntarily—we do this when we hold our breath. We cannot do it very long, however, because there is a respiratory center in the medulla of the brain that monitors the carbon dioxide levels in the blood and initiates respiration involuntarily when necessary.

THE DIGESTIVE SYSTEM

The digestive system, or **gastrointestinal (GI) tract**, is responsible for processing the food that we eat. Extending from the mouth, salivary glands, and esophagus, through the stomach, large and small intestines, and the anus, the digestive system is a long, complex, and poorly understood system. As food passes through this GI tract, it is broken down into various nutrients by chemicals and juices (e.g., saliva) that are secreted by organs along the way. These nutrients are absorbed into the bloodstream and carried to other areas of the body.

Our understanding of the GI tract suffers from its relative inaccessibility to measurement. Much of what we do know comes from studies in which gastric fistulas—artificial openings at the surface into the stomach through which the stomach can be seen—have been placed in a patient. These studies have suggested that the GI tract is sensitive to emotions—during periods of anger or fear, for example, gastric changes were observed. The nature of these changes has never been clear; many appear to involve simultaneous sympathetic and parasympathetic activation.

THE IMMUNE SYSTEM

Unlike many of the systems already discussed, the complex array of immune organs and cells are not primarily concerned with transporting nutrients or signaling the body to work in special ways. Instead, the immune system is responsible for providing defense against pathogens and "foreign" agents—particles and substances that do not "belong" in the body. Bacteria, viruses, abnormal cells, transplanted tissue, and allergens are all subject to attack by the immune system. The exterior defenses of the body, including the skin, and local initial defenses against entry of pathogens in the body (see Figure 2.6) protect us against most organisms. For example, microorganisms are trapped by cilia and mucus in the nose and trachea, and the "mucociliary escalator" removes foreign particles from the lungs. Some pathogens may penetrate these systems, however, and require more complex defenses.

The task of the immune system is enormous, and to meet this challenge, it has evolved into a very complex system. Among other things, it must learn to discriminate between what belongs in the body—what is "self"—and what is foreign—"not self." The targets of much of immune system activity are **antigens**, defined as any substances or organisms that are "not self," that are foreign or that have been altered so as to no longer "belong." Thus pollen that we breathe, viruses that infiltrate our bodies, bacteria, cancer cells, and infected cells (e.g., cells that normally would be considered "self" in which a virus is living) are antigens, and set off immune reactions. The process by which the distinctions between antigens and particles that belong in the body are made is complex. We will deal briefly with this process.

The complexity of the immune system is quickly seen in the number of different organs and cells **(leukocytes)** that are involved in combating antigens. (See Figure

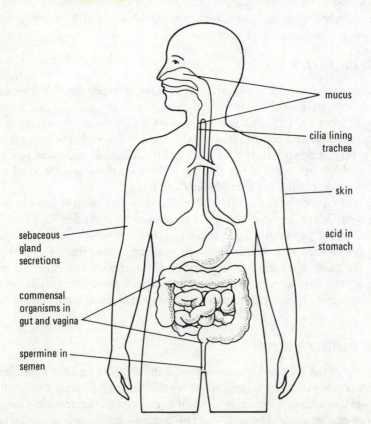

Figure 2.6 Exterior defenses. Most of the infectious agents that an individual encounters do not penetrate the body's surfaces, but are prevented from entering by a variety of biochemical and physical barriers.
From I. Roitt, J. Brostoff, and D. Male. *Immunology.* St. Louis: C. V. Mosby, 1985.

2.7.) Several parts of the body are involved in the production and regulation of leukocytes, or white blood cells, that are the primary mechanisms of immune system function. These cells are produced in the **bone marrow,** soft tissue found in the center of many bones. Some migrate to the **thymus,** located in the center of the chest. Slowly shrinking in size as an individual grows older, the thymus helps to develop some lymphocytes and produces several substances involved in immune system function. These cells, called T-lymphocytes, are agents of **cell-mediated immunity;** cells that mature in other immune system organs, known as B-lymphocytes, are agents of **humoral** immunity.

Lymphocytes are what many people call white blood cells. As noted, there are two types, B-cells and T-cells. The former produce **antibodies;** upon contact with an antigen, B-lymphocytes produce a number of plasma cells, each of which produces antibodies and secretes them into the bloodstream. The antibodies produced by plasma cells derived from the same B-cell are identical and are tailored to combat a particular antigen.

Antibodies are made up of one of five types of **immunoglobulin** (Ig), each of which has a different function or mode of action. The most common is IgG, and its primary function is to cover antigens with a substance that facilitates destruction by other immune cells. IgM is effective primarily against bacteria. IgA is located primarily in fluids such as saliva, and destroys antigens as they enter the body. IgE attaches itself to other immune cells and directs them to act when encountering an appropriate antigen while IgD exerts an effect on cell activity.

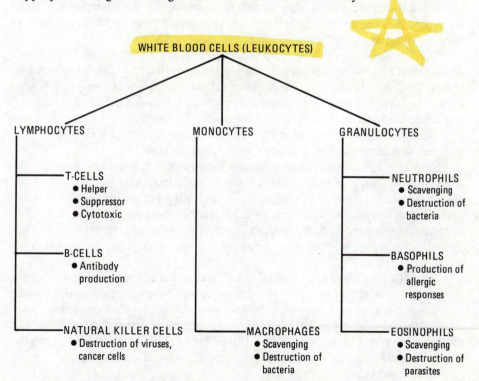

Figure 2.7   **Cells of the immune system.**

The ability to produce specific antibodies to combat a particular antigen is dependent on prior presentation of the antigen to B-cells. The B-cell must first "meet" an antigen; it is introduced by macrophages, which bring markers of encounters with antigens to the B-cells. In this way, B-cells become sensitized to particular antigens and are capable of secreting antibodies designed to combat them. Antibodies cannot penetrate living cells, so they are not as effective in combating viruses that have found cellular hosts and are living with a cell membrane. They do, however, provide an effective defense against antigens in the bloodstream. Some surround antigens and destroy them, others coat them with a substance that makes the antigen attractive to scavenger cells, which then destroy them, while still other antibodies are primarily responsible for neutralizing the toxins produced by pathogens. Some antibodies can also prevent viruses from entering host cells, making them more vulnerable to assault by other antibodies.

T-lymphocytes act as controllers in the immune system. (See Figure 2.8.) Some, called **helper cells**, function to activate B-cells and other components of the immune system, while others, called **suppressor cells**, reduce activity by these cells. This is a very simple description of these functions; the processes by which the T-lymphocytes carry out their regulatory functions are extremely complex and not altogether clear. However, we know that some T-lymphocytes are more concerned with killing antigens than with regulating immune processes. Called **cytotoxic cells**, these lymphocytes bind with antigens and destroy them. Other T-lymphocytes are involved in delayed hypersensitivity reactions. If we divide these T-lymphocytes according to their functions, we can see that there are regulatory T-lymphocytes (the helper and suppressor cells) and effector cells (including those that kill antigen and reject foreign tissues and grafts).

The T-lymphocytes secrete **lymphokines**, which are different from the antibodies secreted by plasma cells. Among the lymphokines that have been identified are interleukin-2 and interferon, which direct cellular immune reactions. Interferon appears to initiate or regulate antiviral activity by cells, inhibit replication of viruses, and affect the function of a variety of immune cells. Interleukin-2 also affects an array of immune functions, and there is some evidence that these lymphokines are involved in communication with other systems in the body.

Natural killer cells are large granular lymphocytes that exhibit spontaneous killing activity against a wide variety of targets. Unlike most lymphocytes, they do not require sensitization to an antigen before they kill it but are nonspecific in their mission to destroy tumor cells, normal cells that have become host to a virus, and metastasizing cancer cells in the bloodstream. Natural killer cells function much like cytotoxic T-lymphocytes but do so naturally, without prior acquaintance with the target.

Natural killers make up a relatively small proportion of total lymphocyte populations, but their ability to target and destroy tumor cells or normal bodily tissue that has become infected appears to be very important. Many components of immune defense are unable to detect and/or eliminate viruses after they have taken up residence in a host cell, and the immunosurveillance function against tumor growth shown by natural killers may represent a primary natural defense against tumor growth and metastasis.

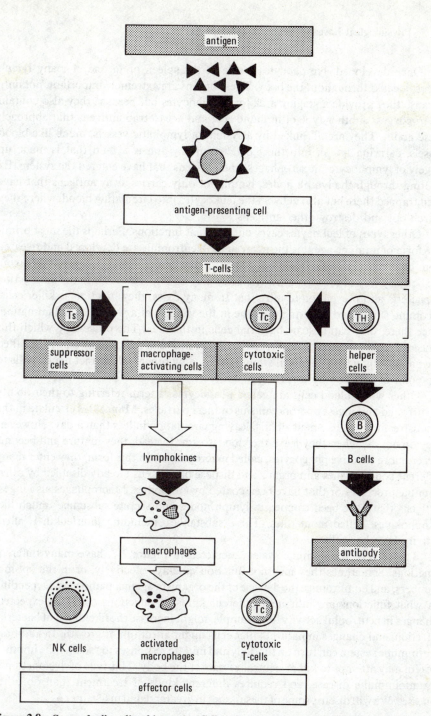

Figure 2.8 Scope of cell-mediated immunity. Cell-mediated immune responses follow antigen presentation and activation of T-cells. Activation is regulated by suppressor and helper cells. Certain T-cells (macrophage activating cells) elaborate lymphokines, which activate macrophages to enhance their phagocyte and bactericidal functions. Cytotoxic T-cells are activated by antigen and receive help from helper T-cells. Helper cells also cooperate with B-cells in the production of antibody.
From I. Roitt, J. Brostoff, and D. Male. *Immunology.* St. Louis: C. V. Mosby, 1985.

Once developed, lymphocytes reside in the spleen or in one of many **lymph nodes,** located throughout the body. These organs are extremely important, not only because they provide a staging area for lymphocytes but because they also contain **macrophages,** another type of immune cell, and act to trap antigens that approach these nodes. They are all linked by a system of lymphatic vessels, much like blood vessels, carrying **lymph** into the bloodstream. Lymph is a fluid that is made up largely of lymphocytes, macrophages, and antigens that have entered the system. By filtering through the lymph nodes, lymph not only carries away antigens that have been trapped there but also delivers the leukocytes into circulating blood, where they search out and destroy other antigens.

Other types of leukocytes carry out different functions. Perhaps the most primitive form of immune agent is the **neutrophil.** Neutrophils are developed and released from bone marrow and circulate for about a day before losing potency and leaving the body by way of several pathways. They play an important role in the destruction of bacteria and prevention of infection. In many cases, they function as killer cells, becoming sticky and adhering to tissue in the vicinity of a wound or inflammation. Once there, they can destroy bacterial cells in the area. The process by which this process unfolds appears to be directed by other immune cells and by a process called **chemotaxis,** by which chemical stimuli released by other cells attract neutrophils to the point of invasion by a pathogen.

Other white blood cells are called **phagocytes,** a term referring to their ability to surround and ingest microorganisms or inert particles. **Monocytes** circulate in the bloodstream much like neutrophils, leaving circulation in less than a day. However, they do not die when they leave the bloodstream. Instead, they mature and become larger, more effective phagocytes, called macrophages. In this form, they enter many different bodily tissues and organs and dispose of antigens already disabled by other immune processes or that have been coated by antibodies. Macrophages also ingest antigens that have been trapped in lymph nodes and secrete substances much like lymphokines, called **monokines.** These substances, including interleukin-1, affect activity by other cells.

The cells of the immune system, depicted in Figure 2.7, have many different functions. Sometimes they may not function quickly, effectively, or in the optimal numbers, and compromise the defense of the organism against pathogens. Depending on what functions are inhibited, different kinds of infections could be expected. Changes in neutrophil activity, for example, might increase the likelihood of bacterial infection, and changes in natural killer cells might affect tumor growth. In addition, the immune system can turn on the body and initiate responses to "self"—the immune system may attempt to kill or neutralize part of the body. This type of dysfunction is an autoimmune disease, and requires different kinds of treatment than do other illnesses. We will discuss some of these issues in greater detail in Chapter 6.

GENETIC INFLUENCES ON HEALTH AND BEHAVIOR

Genetics have an effect on behavior and health. Darwin proposed that the great diversity among species was a result of variations adaptive to the environment being transmitted onto successive offspring. Favorable or adaptive variations in a plant or animal in a given environment would increase the probability that the plant or animal would survive to transmit those variations to offspring. Extinction of a species was the result of the failure of adaptive evolution; "survival of the fittest" was the result of successful adaptive evolution. Successive generations would thus be infused with qualities from past generations that fitted well into a particular environment. This principle was called **natural selection**.

Darwin suggested that each part of an organism produced in its cells substances called gemmules that contained a type of blueprint for that cell and the organism. These gemmules, he believed, were collected in the semen and were transmitted through sexual reproduction. While neither Darwin nor anyone else during that time fully understood the rudimentary mechanisms of heredity and genetics, Darwin's theory of evolution rested on the centerpiece of heredity and genetic transmission.

Among one of the many scholars and intellectuals who admired and studied Darwin's work, Galton was one of the first to study influences of genetics on behavior and intelligence. Indeed, Galton is often considered the father of eugenics (a term he coined), which is the study of human genetics with the goal of "improving" human characteristics. In 1869 he published a text entitled *Hereditary Genius* in which he presented some evidence suggesting that intelligence and talent were inherited characteristics. The general argument of this book, plus several of his earlier articles, was that certain talents and abilities tended to run in families. He studied a number of brilliant families and noted that they produced a larger than usual number of gifted individuals. Further, he noted that the closer the family relationship, the more likely the trait was to be expressed. Thus eminence in a given field was directly related to family membership, and a child's chances of being eminent increased as closer relatives had achieved this status. (Later in this chapter we will return to this issue of intelligence and heredity.)

Neither Darwin nor Galton understood the basic mechanisms of heredity and gene transmission. Mendel, however, carried out a detailed, lifetime study in an attempt to explain how inherited characteristics might be acquired. Using ordinary garden peas as his subject population, he worked for years in his monastery gardens, crossing certain shapes of peas with other shapes to produce **hybrids** (literally meaning a crossmating between two subspecies). Very generally, he found that given traits were passed on from one generation to the next in a rather systematic fashion that could be predicted mathematically. Mendel actually uncovered the basic workings of hereditary transmission; although neither he nor anyone else knew of the actual existence of genes, he was nonetheless aware of their effects. He concluded that inherited characteristics are determined by combinations of hereditary units received from each parent's reproductive cells, cells that we know as **gametes**. In addition, Mendel recognized that some gene factors are more potent than others for a given trait. For example, in the case of his plants, the color of pods and the form of pods were traits. Since each parent contributes a given gene for a particular trait, each trait is determined by pairs of genes. The gene from each parent may be either **dominant** or **recessive**. Parents having both dominant genes for a given trait would breed true, or produce offspring with the obvious expression of that trait. If one parent had the recessive gene, the parents would produce mixed offspring. In recessive inheritance, also noted by Mendel, neither parent may express the trait but both may have recessive genes for it; therefore, it could be expressed in an offspring. Thus Mendel observed that what you see is not always what you get. Even though an organism may not appear to have a particular trait (the trait is not expressed), the organism may possess recessive genes for that trait. The characteristics observed in the organism are called **phenotypes**; what the organism contains both expressed and nonexpressed is called **genotype**. A short plant has shortness as a phenotype (you can actually see the shortness), but this plant may contain recessive genes for tallness (the genotype). Mendel determined the phenotype through mere observation, but genotype was determined by looking at the inbreeding history of the organism.

Mendel's work showed that a single genetic trait seen in the offspring is a result of paired genes acquired from the parents, one coming from the germ cell of the female, the other coming from the germ cell of the male. An acquired trait is the result of two discrete bits of genetic information coming from each parent. The variation within and between species, a phenomenon that fascinated Darwin, was now partly explainable by Mendel's laws—it was a result of the passing on of genetic material from both parents.

BEHAVIORAL GENETICS

As we noted earlier, Mendel, Darwin, and other early researchers in the field of genetics were chiefly interested in how physical or anatomical features were transmitted from parents to offspring. In more recent years another focus has emerged—observation of *behaviors* that could be transmitted from parent to offspring. This field is called **behavioral genetics**. Behavior, in this usage, refers to numerous phenomena such as intelligence, aggression, emotionality, mental illness, and criminality. The three major methods of genetic investigation of humans are family studies, twin studies, and studies of adopted children.

Family Studies

Family studies assess each member of a family in order to determine whether the prevalence of a certain characteristic exceeds that found in the general population. Of critical importance in such studies is the requirement that the considered characteristic be precisely defined. If this requirement is not met, then meaningful comparisons with a norm cannot be made.

Family studies are generally the weakest kind of evidence to support the presence of genetic predisposition to a certain personality characteristic. Since family members have not only the same genes but also the same environment, it is impossible to determine whether the relationships found are due to genetic or environmental factors.

Twin Studies

Twin studies can provide a somewhat stronger test of the possible presence of genetic factors because they compare persons raised in a highly similar environment who are either genetically identical (**monozygotic twins**) or similar but not identical (**dizygotic twins**). Twin studies are the most popular method of evaluating human inheritance. Monozygotic twins develop from the same fertilized egg ovum and thus share the same set of inherited genes. As a result, they are often called **identical twins**. Because they are genetically identical, any observed differences between the twins can be attributed to environmental factors. Dizygotic twins develop from two separate fertilized eggs and, therefore, are not any more genetically alike than other brothers and sisters (that is, they share 50 percent of their genes). Any observed differences found between these **fraternal twins** can be ascribed to a combination of genetic and environmental factors. Any differences found between monozygotic and dizygotic twins raised in the same environment would be evidence for possible genetic involvement.

Twin studies, although strongly suggestive of the presence or absence of genetic factors, must be interpreted with some caution. We can argue that monozygotic twins not only are alike genetically, but also share a more nearly identical environment than dizygotic twins. They are of the same sex and commonly tend to be dressed alike, treated alike, and usually confused with each other by other people. One way of overcoming this potential argument is to examine monozygotic twins who were separated from each other very early in life and reared apart. But because of the time and expense involved in conducting such studies, only a small number of cases have been studied, primarily in the area of psychopathology. For example, in the investigation of schizophrenia, such studies have suggested a genetic predisposition for this disorder. However, the small number of cases involved in these studies prevents any definitive conclusion (Rosenthal, 1970).

Another point concerning twin studies is worthy of comment. Identical twins, in comparison with fraternal twins or normal siblings, have a greater risk of retardation and pregnancy and birth complications (Hanson and Gottesman, 1976). Such an observation raises some questions about identical twin studies and the possibility of genetic involvement because it is possible that trauma to the central nervous system (birth complications, for example), and not genetic factors, predisposes twins to develop certain forms of psychopathology and personality characteristics.

Adopted Child Studies
Finally, another type of study—the adopted child study—attempts to eliminate the possible developmental effect of being raised in a similar environment. Such studies examine children who were adopted away from their original biological family at birth and raised by another family. These persons have the genetic endowment of one family and the environmental learning experiences of another family. A number of meaningful comparisons can be made employing this method. For example, we can determine whether the adopted child resembled his or her biological parents with regard to the psychological characteristic in question. Other comparisons are also helpful in determining the impact of genetic endowment in a different environment.

Convergence
The strongest support for the inheritance of a particular personality characteristic or trait comes from the convergence of evidence from family studies, twin studies, and studies of adopted children. If it is found that there is familial similarity in a trait, if monozygotic twins are significantly more similar than dizygotic twins on that

trait, and if adopted children resemble their natural parents more than their adoptive parents, then some involvement of heredity for that trait is beyond dispute. In the field of personality, the only trait for which all three methods of investigation has been amassed is intelligence. The data strongly suggest that there is a significant inherited component in intelligence (Buss and Plomin, 1975).

ABNORMAL BEHAVIOR AND GENETICS: SCHIZOPHRENIA AS AN EXAMPLE

There is evidence to suggest the importance of genetic factors in various forms of abnormal behavior such as schizophrenia (see Mears and Gatchel, 1979). This evidence comes from the three major types of studies we have discussed: family studies, twin studies, and studies of adopted children. At the outset, we should point out that a major problem in such research is confusion concerning just what schizophrenia is and how it can be reliably diagnosed and measured. This psychotic disorder consists of a complex array of symptoms that may differ from person to person and that may change within a particular individual over time. The reader is referred to a thorough review of this problem provided by Mears and Gatchel (1979).

Family Studies
A number of family studies have demonstrated that the more closely a person is related to a schizophrenic, the higher the probability that that person will develop schizophrenia. Various family studies examining schizophrenia have been summarized by Rosenthal (1970). Although findings varied considerably among these studies with reported risk factors ranging from 0.2 to 12.0 percent, twelve of the fourteen studies revealed a risk factor for related individuals of above 1 percent, which is roughly the expected occurrence of this disorder in the general population. Of course, it can be argued that the effects of a schizophrenic's parent's bizarre and distressing behavior on a youngster during the developmental years may be traumatic enough to produce disordered behavior in the child.

Twin Studies
Kallman (1946) conducted one of the earliest large-scale studies that demonstrated a greater concordance rate of schizophrenia in identical twins than in fraternal twins. More recently, Ban (1973) and Rosenthal (1970) summarized the findings of various twin studies. These summaries indicated that the concordance rate for identical twins was approximately five times as great as the concordance rate for fraternal twins. However, as can be seen in Table 2.2, which summarizes the results presented by Rosenthal (1970), there is a great deal of disparity in the concordance rates reported in the various studies.

In spite of this disparity, it is readily apparent that the concordance rate is usually much greater for identical than for fraternal twins. Data such as these strongly suggest a genetic involvement in this disorder. However, in no instance has any study found a 100 percent concordance rate. Even though the measurement error involved in assessing schizophrenia will normally prevent the concordance rate from reaching 100 percent, these data imply that, although there may be a genetic component in schizophrenia, it is not the entire story.

TABLE 2.2   Concordance Rates in the Major Twin Studies of Schizophrenia

Study	MONOZYGOTIC (IDENTICAL) TWINS		DIZYGOTIC (FRATERNAL) TWINS	
	Number of Pairs	% Con-cordant	Number of Pairs	% Con-cordant
Luxemburger, 1928a, 1934 (Germany)	17–27	33–76.5	48	2.1
Rosanoff et al., 1934–35 (U.S. and Canada)	41	61.0	101	10.0
Essen-Möller, 1941 (Sweden)	7–11	14–71	24	8.3–17
Kallmann, 1946 (New York)	174	69–86.2	517	10–14.5
Slater, 1953 (England)	37	65–74.7	115	11.3–14.4
Inouye, 1961 (Japan)	55	36–60	17	6–12
Tienari, 1963, 1968 (Finland)	16	0–6	21	4.8
Gottesman and Shields, 1966 (England)	24	41.7	33	9.1
Kringlen, 1967 (Norway)	55	25–38	172	10
Fischer, 1968 (Denmark)	16	19–56	34	6–15

From D. Rosenthal. *Genetic Theory and Abnormal Behavior* New York: McGraw-Hill, 1970. Copyright © 1970, McGraw-Hill Book Company. Used with the permission of McGraw-Hill Book Company. See original source for full references.

Adopted Child Studies

If it could be determined that children who are born to schizophrenic mothers but are not exposed to the potentially traumatic experiences of being raised in a schizophrenic family still develop schizophrenia at the same rate as children who are born to schizophrenic mothers but are not adopted, then this would be convincingly strong support for the presence of a genetic predisposition.

Heston (1966) conducted a study in which fifty-eight adoptees born to hospitalized schizophrenic mothers were examined. Adopted individuals who did not have schizophrenic mothers (the control group) were simultaneously examined. These individuals were matched for age, sex, duration of time in child-care institutions, and type of placement. Independent diagnoses of these persons, made by several psychiatrists and based on a wide variety of information, demonstrated that schizophrenia was found only in those children who had schizophrenic mothers. In addition, Heston reported that approximately half of the children of schizophrenic mothers demonstrated major forms of psychopathology such as neuroses, psychopathy, and mental retardation.

Much larger scale adoptee studies were conducted by Kety, et al. (1971). These studies again indicated that children of schizophrenic parents who were adopted by other families had significantly greater schizophrenic characteristics than a matched control group of adopted children whose biological parents had no history of psychiatric hospitalization for schizophrenia.

Conclusions

Taking into account all the results found in family studies, twin studies, and adoptee studies, one is led to conclude that genetic factors play an important role in the etiology of schizophrenia. As Lindzey et al. (1971) conclude on the basis of a review of the literature on the role of genetic factors: "The presence of a genetic predisposition to schizophrenic-like disorders may now be regarded as firmly established" (p. 63). However, the fact that the concordance rates are far from 100 percent suggests the involvement of other factors in the disorder. In other words, genetic factors are necessary, but not sufficient. Currently, a widely held position proposes a diathesis-stress formulation of schizophrenia. It is assumed that some people genetically inherit a diathesis (or predisposition) toward the development of schizophrenia, but schizophrenia will actually develop only in those predisposed individuals who are exposed to particular stressful experiences for which they have not developed adequate coping behaviors. Meehl (1962) and Zubin and Spring (1977) have proposed such a diathesis-stress model of schizophrenia that is receiving widespread support.

SUMMARY

In this chapter, we have discussed the physiological systems involved with behavior and health. It is important to know both psychological and somatic aspects of the body and behavior in order to better understand the topics of health psychology.

Most aspects of body function are mediated by the nervous system and the endocrine system. The *brain* (part of the *central nervous system*) is the command post for the body. The *peripheral nervous system* extends out to the muscles and organs of the body from the spinal cord. At various points along the way, connections with the *endocrine system* coordinate the chemical support it gives to nervous system function. One of the most important links is between the endocrine system and the *sympathetic nervous system,* a subdivision of the peripheral nervous system that controls arousal and stimulation of bodily functions. The *parasympathetic nervous system* works to counter the effects of the sympathetic system. Endocrine activity supports the sympathetic nervous system through the use of long-lasting hormones that extend the arousal generated by the nervous system. Norepinephrine and epinephrine, hormones also called *catecholamines,* are produced in the *adrenal medulla.* The *adrenal cortex,* controlled by the *pituitary gland,* secretes a number of hormones that regulate glucose levels in the blood and spur other metabolic functions.

The *cardiovascular system* is responsible for circulation of blood through the body. The *arteries* carry oxygenated blood away from the *heart* to the *capillaries,* where it is used by the cells and where carbon dioxide is returned. The capillaries then carry the blood to the *veins,* which lead back to the heart. The heart is composed of four chambers that work in sequence to bring the blood into the heart and pump it out again. The motion of the blood through the heart is governed by the valves that connect the four chambers. The sympathetic and parasympathetic nervous system regulate the heart, and the heart is sensitive to blood-flow changes itself. Blood pressure is related to the activity of the heart and the contraction of the blood vessels.

The *respiratory system* provides the blood with oxygen and rids it of carbon dioxide. Respiration is controlled voluntarily and involuntarily—there is an area in the medulla that overrides voluntary control when necessary.

The *digestive system,* or *gastrointestinal (GI) tract,* is responsible for processing the food we eat. It includes the mouth, esophagus, stomach, large and small intestines, and anus. As food passes through the GI tract, various nutrients are absorbed into the bloodstream and carried to other areas of the body. The GI tract seems sensitive to emotion, and it appears to involve sympathetic and parasympathetic system activities simultaneously.

The *immune system* is responsible for protection of the body from germs, bacteria, and other pathogens that attempt to invade the body. Several lines of defense exist, beginning with cells and tissue designed to trap viruses or other "not-self" particles as they enter the body. Other components of the immune system neutralize, ingest, or kill these antigens once they have entered the body. The function of the immune system appears to be regulated by *T-cells* and the *lymphokines* that they secrete, but this direction is dependent on function by other *lymphokines, macrophages,* and *granulocytes.*

Genetics has an impact on behavior and health. Galton is considered the father of *eugenics,* the study of human genetics with the intent to improve the human species. However, there is no evidence that eminence is transmitted in a simple way. *Behavioral genetics* is the study of behavior transfer from parent to offspring. *Family studies, twin studies,* and *adopted child studies* are the three most common methods of behavioral genetic study. Some interesting research in behavior and genetics shows that schizophrenia may have a genetic component.

RECOMMENDED READINGS

Hassett, J. *A primer of psychophysiology.* San Francisco: Freeman, 1978.

Isaacson, R., Douglas R., Lubar, J., and Schmaltz, L. *A primer of physiological psychology.* New York: Harper & Row, 1971.

National Institute of Allergy and Infectious Disease. *Understanding the immune system.* Washington, D.C.: National Cancer Institute.

Obrist, P. *Cardiovascular physiology.* New York: Plenum, 1981.

Plomin, R., DeFries, J., and McClearn, G. *Behavioral genetics.* San Francisco: Freeman, 1980.

Roitt, I., Brostoff, J., and Male, D. *Immunology.* St. Louis: C. V. Mosby, 1985.

Thompson, R. *Foundations of physiological psychology.* New York: Harper & Row, 1967.

3 STRESS

||||||||||||||||||||||||||||||||||||||||||||||||||||||||||||||||||||||||||||||||||||||||||||||||||||||||||||||||||||||||||||||||||||||

Stress is an important concept in the study of psychology and health for a number of reasons. The term itself has become enormously popular as a lay explanation for any number of aches, pains, and maladies. We often speak of stress as if it were pressure, or some negative force that could explain unusual behaviors and sensations. Stress has been considered by researchers as a psychological or physiological precursor of illness, as an explanation for spontaneous outbreaks of inexplicable illnesses, or as a catch-all for emotional reactions, such as anxiety, discomfort, or depression. From a cursory reading of psychological and medical texts, we can derive a fairly broad definition of stress. Yet stress actually refers to a process that is not only specific but also central to the relationship between people and their surroundings.

As we shall see, the effects of stress include biochemical, physiological, behavioral, and psychological changes, many of which are directly related to health. After reviewing major theories of stress and discussing evidence supporting each, we will use a combination of these theories to provide a framework for discussing some of the specific causes and effects of stress.

THE MODERN CONCEPT OF STRESS

Stress is the process by which environmental events threaten or challenge an organism's well-being and by which that organism responds to this threat. The environmental events are called stressors. Under certain conditions, these events give rise to a stress reaction, characterized by such symptoms as fear, anxiety, and anger. Although they are easily recognized, these reactions may simply be side effects of the process—perceiving a threat, coping with it, and adapting to it. This adaptation sequence characterizes our daily lives—constant adaptation to sudden change in, or the gradual evolution of, our surroundings. Sometimes changes are minor and we adapt to them without even being aware of them. At other times, however, these changes are more severe and conscious effort is required to adapt to them. You may find that events such as moving away from home for the first time or studying for final examinations are associated with negative sensations and unusual behavior. On a different level, events such as loss of a loved one, natural disaster, loss of a job, or family problems are often translated into changes in mental and physical health. Stress may be viewed as one process by which stressors cause health-related change. When stressors occur, a complex physiological and psychological response is evoked, and it is this response that in many cases is used to explain negative outcomes.

Although there is still a great deal that we do not know about stress, research has revealed some important facts and relationships that help to explain its source (stressors), its characteristics, and its effects.

WHAT IS STRESS?

Lay definitions of stress are primarily concerned with two factors: the notion of pressure or tension and the implication that this pressure is aversive. Physical science conceptions of stress as a force acting on an object are reflected in this everyday use of the term. However, this is a fairly general definition, and most of us cannot define stress in much greater detail. Stress is pressure; stress is the tension created by pressure; stress is unpleasant.

One consequence of such general notions of stress is the fact that when people talk about stress they are often referring to only one part of it. If they focus on the pressure to which someone is exposed, they are looking outward at the environmental events and forces that affect people. If they focus on the effects of that pressure, the tension or mental state of the recipient of pressure, they are looking inward at biological and psychological events. In fact, stress is both.

Another factor contributing to the superficiality of general understanding of stress is that it cannot really be described as a thing the way most of us would like to describe it. As we have noted, it is a process, unfolding in a sequence of events and feelings and involving a number of factors that by themselves can be quite complex. It involves environmental and psychological events, interpretations of them, and behavioral and physiological responses. Stress is, as Lazarus and Launier (1978) suggest, a transaction between people and the environment.

As we have already suggested, stress is a complex process by which an organism responds to certain environmental or psychological events, called stressors, that pose challenge or danger to the organism. Stressors may be external to the organism, representing possible harm or loss, or they may be symbols of threat or other psychological representations of danger. Usually noxious, they may include anything from a disease germ to a tornado or earthquake. The kinds of dangers that they pose vary and their relative magnitudes are different, but they all evoke some kind of response from the organism. Response may be physiological, behavioral, cognitive, emotional, or a combination of all of these. Typically, physiological and emotional responses are tied to **arousal**—heightened brain activity and increased physiological responding. Stress elevates the body's state of activity, and this arousal is linked with cognitive variables to our experience of emotions; various interpretations of arousal may lead to different outcomes (see Schachter and Singer, 1962).

Appraisals of stressors are our evaluations of their effects and how best to deal with them. Cognitive and behavioral variables may also be linked to coping by which we attempt to remove the stressor or insulate ourselves from its effects. If coping is successful, the organism returns to normal physiological and psychological arousal as the threat is eliminated or minimized. When this occurs, the organism has adapted—either cognitively (by making itself unaware of the stressor or by reassessing the degree of threat) or behaviorally (by removing or reducing the threat).

Stress begins with our anticipation of or encounter with a stressor and unfolds as we become aware of its danger, mobilize to cope with it, and either succeed or fail in adapting to it. (This sequence is depicted in Figure 3.1.) The stressor's danger is evaluated, coping strategies are selected, the body mobilizes itself to combat the stressor, and coping is put into action. If adaptation is successful, the effects of the stressor diminish. If it is unsuccessful, stress persists, arousal is not reduced, and pathological end-states such as mental or physical illness become more likely.

There are a number of aspects of this depiction of stress that are not universally accepted. While most agree that a stressor and awareness of it are necessary to evoke a stress response, theories on the mechanisms by which awareness is made vary greatly. Some feel that appraisals and interpretation are necessary, while others assert that such structures are unnecessarily mentalistic. The evidence seems to

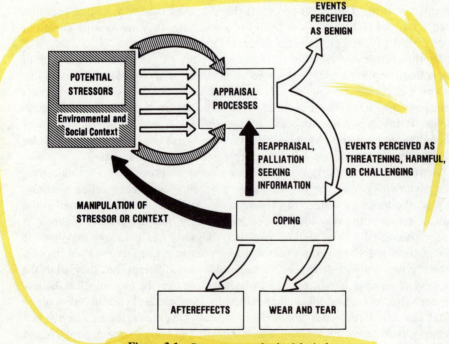

Figure 3.1 Stress as a psychophysiological process.

suggest that, although appraisal processes are often carried out automatically without direct awareness, some sort of appraisal must occur. There are many instances in which interpretation is necessary to explain response. We may not know right away if something is dangerous, especially if we have never seen it before. We learn properties of events that cause us harm, and we distinguish between those that we feel are threatening and those that we feel are not. It is very difficult to explain the variety of stress responses by different people to the same stressors without looking to some evaluation mechanisms.

EARLY CONCEPTIONS OF STRESS

Although interest in stress has become fashionable among the public only recently, stress has been of concern to the medical profession for centuries. Hippocrates separated suffering caused by disease (pathos) from the toil involved in resisting and fighting it (ponos). In doing so, he suggested a stresslike aspect of illness—the energy and wear caused by attempts to combat disease. Since then, many similar notions have appeared (Selye, 1956). It was not until the beginning of the twentieth century, however, that the notion of stress became formalized through the work of Walter Cannon.

Cannon was among the first to use the term stress and clearly suggested both physiological and psychological components of it. In studying emotions, he referred to "great emotional stress" to describe a powerful psychophysiological process that appeared to influence emotion (Cannon, 1914, 1928, 1929). He viewed stress as a potential cause of medical problems and felt strongly that emotional stress could cause disturbances of a physiological nature. As mentioned in Chapter 2, he provided a simple description of the readying function of the sympathetic nervous system—a threatened organism readies itself for "fight or flight" by producing a heightened arousal state. This is accomplished partly by secretion of epinephrine and other chemicals produced by the body, which increase the speed and intensity of response. When you are suddenly confronted with danger—you realize that you are driving your car off the road at high speed—you experience sensations (such as rapid heart rate and respiration) as your body readies itself to respond. In this case, such arousal may increase the speed with which you can respond—get the car back on the road. In some instances, where resistance is feasible, arousal will increase ability to resist, while in others it will enhance ability to flee.

By 1935 Cannon had clearly defined stress in terms of emotional and physiological response to dangers. In his portrayal of the effects of voodoo or of breaking a taboo, he allowed for psychological contributors to this syndrome. He argued that this perspective is important because it offers "insight into the strength and endurance of an organism, and, thus, its ability to resist the operation of disturbing forces" (1935). Critical stress levels were defined as threats or dangers that affect an organism sufficiently so as to disrupt homeostasis (organic stability or equilibrium) and throw the organism off balance. Thus stress can cause disruption of emotional and physiological stability as well as aid in survival.

Cannon's work is, in some ways, a forerunner of Selye's work on biologic stress (see Selye, 1976). However, his insistence on psychological aspects of the stress response makes it more compatible with more recent descriptions of stress (see Frankenhaeuser, 1971; Mason, 1975).

SELYE'S BIOLOGIC STRESS MODEL

Hans Selye's research on stress, spanning a forty-year period, was a watershed for stress research. He did much to popularize the notion of stress and to bring it to the attention of scientists in many disciplines. In doing so, he compiled an extensive empirical literature, much of which has come from his laboratory (see Selye, 1976).

Selye's work began accidentally—in studying sex hormones, he found that injections into rats of extracts of ovary tissue caused an unexplainable triad of responses: enlargement of the adrenal glands (which secrete catecholamines and corticosteroids) shrinkage of the thymus gland, and bleeding ulcers. Following up on this discovery, Selye found that extracts of other organs caused the same triad of responses, and that substances not derived from bodily tissue also caused these responses. Eventually he found the same nonspecific responses to be characteristic of such disparate events as injection of insulin, application of heat or cold, exposure to X-rays, exercise, and so on. Each time an alien agent was applied, changes in the adrenal and thymus glands and in the acid-sensitive stomach lining were observed. The response was nonspecific because it appeared to be caused by *any* noxious or aversive event.

Nonspecific Response

Selye's notion of nonspecific response has come under more fire than any other aspect of his theory. Because nearly everything he did to the organisms was associated with the same pattern, Selye believed that stress was a specific syndrome (it followed certain specific patterns and affected specific organs) but that it was *nonspecifically induced* (Selye, 1956). He felt that the specific syndrome of stress was caused by many or all agents. Thus the opening curtain of a stress response would be the same regardless of what specific event had signaled it.

Selye (1956) illustrated this notion by comparing stress response to a burglary:

> Suppose that all possible accesses to a bank building are connected with a police station by an elaborate burglar-alarm system. When a burglar enters the bank, no matter what his personal characteristics are—whether he is small or tall, lean or stout—and no matter which door or window he opens to enter, he will set off the same alarm. The primary change is therefore nonspecifically induced from anywhere by anyone. The pattern of the resulting secondary change, on the other hand, is highly specific. It is always in a certain police station that the burglar alarm will ring and policemen will then rush to the bank along a specified route according to a predetermined plan to prevent robbery. (p. 58)

Using this notion of nonspecific response, Selye defined the stress syndrome as all of the nonspecifically induced changes induced by a noxious agent. Stress itself was considered a specific state that was the "common denominator of all adaptive reactions in the body." The occurrence of a stressor (e.g., injection of a pathogen) aroused a response set involving, among other things, the original triad.

Criticisms of Selye's theories (see Mason, 1975) focus on the fact that this notion of nonspecificity seems to rule out psychological mechanisms in determining response to a stressor. As we shall see, many of these criticisms are appropriate. Yet it is possible to allow for appraisal in this process if we assume that the nonspecific nature of stress is limited to our initial responses to a stressor. Selye has described a syndrome involving alarm, resistance, and exhaustion. If the alarm response alone is seen as nonspecific, then interpretation may still affect subsequent response.

At this point, we have two pieces of Selye's puzzle: a triadic response that appears to be nonspecifically induced and a notion of stress as a syndrome of response to noxious agents. In order to describe the processes involved in these events, Selye devised the **general adaptation syndrome (GAS)**.

The General Adaptation Syndrome

The GAS consists of three stages of response (see Figure 3.2). First, as the organism becomes aware of a stressor or the presence of noxious stimulation, the **alarm reaction** is experienced. Here the organism prepares to resist the stressor. Adrenal activity and cardiovascular and respiratory functions increase and the body is made ready to respond. When reserves are ready and circulating levels of corticosteroids have increased, the organism enters a **stage of resistance**, applying various coping mechanisms and typically achieving suitable adaptation. During this stage, there is a relatively constant resistance to the stressor, but there is a decrease in resistance to other stimuli.

When these reactions are repeated many times or when they are prolonged because of a recurring problem, the organism may be placed at risk for irreversible physiological damage. Selye believes that this is the result of a third stage of the GAS, **exhaustion**. Adaptive reserves are depleted by long-term or repeated conflict with stressors, and resistance is then no longer possible. The result of exhaustion is likely to be the onset of **diseases of adaptation,** illnesses such as kidney disease, arthritis, and cardiovascular disease. For example, cardiovascular damage and arthritis may be made likely by prolonged elevated levels of catecholamines (see Ross and Glomset, 1976), and high concentrations of inflammatory corticosteroids may figure in the onset of arthritis. There is also some evidence that prolonged stress can affect immunity.

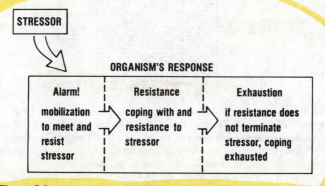

Figure 3.2   **Diagram of Selye's three-stage general adaptation syndrome.**

The picture that Selye draws for us of a rise and fall in response to threat is a useful one (see Figure 3.3). Relying primarily on pathogens (e.g., disease-producing microorganisms) as stressors, he was able to show that the sequence of alarm and resistance is characterized by a focusing of adaptive abilities on the noxious agent. But Selye also believed that these adaptive abilities are limited. Under most conditions we can cope with a stressor—we resist and overcome it, and our physiological state returns to normal. Repeated, prolonged, or sufficiently strong stressors may deplete our ability to resist further. When adaptive reserves are gone, we enter a state of exhaustion and run the risk of stress-related illness. Resistance results in wear and tear on the body that can use up its ability to resist.

Thus the GAS describes the stages of bodily response to various stressors. The alarm reaction is clearly nonspecific, as Selye's parallel bank robbery situation illustrates. The initial response, as in the police response, may also be nonspecifically induced. It is possible that later response may vary with the nature of the stressor and the individual in question. However, to Selye, the GAS is set off by stressors that all share a common property of noxiousness and that all result in the same basic response. As a result, there is no need for a decision-making component—the organism mobilizes upon recognition of threat by a noxious agent.

The importance of the GAS is in its depiction of how stress can lead to resistance and physiological damage. Research has indicated that stressors cause many of the kinds of changes Selye outlined. For example, Levi (1965) has linked aggression-

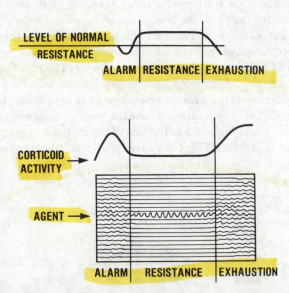

Figure 3.3 Selye's general adaptation syndrome reflects changes in resistance and adrenal cortical response. In the top figure, general level of resistance is depicted as it increases during alarm, levels off, and falls during exhaustion. In the middle figure, changes in cortical activity are depicted during these stages. The lower figure portrays the narrowing of response to a stressor as an appropriate system is chosen and subsequent widening of response as exhaustion in that system occurs.

Adapted from H. Selye. *The Stress of Life.* New York: McGraw-Hill, 1956. Copyright © 1956, McGraw-Hill Book Company. Used with the permission of McGraw-Hill Book Company.

provoking stimuli to increased adrenal activity, and Theorell (1974) has shown that major changes in people's lives are related to increased catecholamine levels. Situations of overload, involvement, or lack of control are likely to result in increased physiological response as well (see Frankenhaeuser, 1976). The specific mechanisms by which the body may mobilize and resist, however, are still under investigation.

PSYCHOBIOLOGIC STRESS

Concern with stress theory widened following the popularization of Selye's work. The psychoendocrinology of Cannon and the biologic stress system of Selye found interested researchers in psychology, psychiatry, physiology, and other areas of biology and medicine.

A major development in stress research in the 50 years since Selye's works were first published has been an integration of psychological mechanisms into what essentially remains a biological model. Pointing out that many people assume that emotional factors are a part of Selye's stress model, John Mason (1975) questioned the scope of the GAS and its linkages with psychosocial stimuli. Selye had psychological stress representing a subset of a unitary, nonspecific response to anything noxious. Mason disagreed, arguing that stress is neither nonspecific nor unitary and that psychological awareness of noxious events may be necessary for stress to occur.

As we have noted, Selye's nonspecific response was based on the fact that the triad of responses he first observed—enlargement of the adrenal glands, shrinking of the thymus, and ulceration of the stomach—occurred in the presence of any event; nonspecific aversive events caused this response. Since then, researchers have found evidence of specific responding or patterning of adrenal corticosteroids for different stressors. For example, Mason (1975) reported different patterns of epinephrine, norepinephrine, and corticosteroid secretion associated with stressors varying in uncertainty or anger and fear elicitation. We will not deal with this issue in great detail. It is enough to recognize that Mason was concerned with the role of aversive events in evoking secretion of hormones and transmitters by the adrenal glands. More important, he clarified the role of psychosocial stimuli in stress.

Psychological distress, according to Mason, precedes adrenal-pituitary response and may be necessary for a physiological reaction to occur. There may be circumstances in which the nonspecific stress response occurs without psychological input, but the best evidence suggests that awareness of a noxious condition and attempts to deal with it are crucial. This awareness need not be conscious in the common use of the term because of the body's ability to attack foreign substances unbeknown to the individual. Mason's own work has shown that physical stressors, such as application of heat, do not elicit adrenal activity when psychological factors involved in perception and sensation of the stressor are eliminated (see Mason, 1975). Another study compared two groups of dying patients, one composed of people who remained in a coma until they died and the other made up of patients who remained conscious until they passed away. Autopsies indicated that the conscious group showed symptoms of stress, such as enlarged adrenal glands, while those who were not conscious showed no such symptoms (Symington et al., 1955).

Marianne Frankenhaeuser and her colleagues have conducted many studies that reveal a strong psychological component of stress. Returning to Cannon's work, Frankenhaeuser focused on epinephrine and norepinephrine, attempting to extend the readying function Cannon spoke of to everyday coping with nonemergencies. For example, she has demonstrated that these bodily substances can affect emotional and cognitive functioning and that they are secreted in response to purely psychological events (Frankenhaeuser, 1972). In one study, increases in levels of epinephrine and norepinephrine were associated with decreasing amounts of control over electric shock (Frankenhaeuser and Rissler, 1970), and in another, both understimulation (not having enough to do) and overstimulation (having too much to do) were associated with rises in epinephrine and norepinephrine levels (Frankenhaeuser et al., 1971).

An interesting study by Patkai (1971) showed that increased output of the "stress hormones" epinephrine and norepinephrine is associated not only with noxious or aversive events but also with pleasant but uncontrollable events. Subjects each participated in four sessions. During one session they played a game of chance—a modified bingo game that was generally regarded as being pleasant. In another session they viewed gruesome surgery films, and in a third, unpleasant and tedious tasks were performed. Subjects also spent one session in "neutral inactivity" to provide a control for their other experiences. Epinephrine secretion among subjects was highest in the pleasant but uncontrollable setting (playing the game), next highest in the less pleasant conditions (tedious task session, film session), and lowest in the inactivity session. Both pleasant and unpleasant events evoked biochemical symptoms of stress (see Figure 3.4).

Frankenhaeuser's work is important because it demonstrates the pervasive role of psychological factors in eliciting a primary physiological symptom of stress. This physiological response is in turn associated with psychological responses—emotionality and cognitive ability. It also suggests a kind of nonspecificity not unlike Selye's. The same bodily response—secretion of epinephrine and norepinephrine—seems to occur in the face of a wide range of psychological events. Included in the list of stressors that elicit this response are urban commuting, job dissatisfaction, loss of control, conflict, taking examinations, noise, anticipation of an aversive event, and boredom (see Collins and Frankenhaeuser, 1978; Frankenhaeuser, 1972, 1977, 1978; Johansson, 1977; Lundberg and Frankenhaeuser, 1976; Singer, Lundberg, and Frankenhaeuser, 1978).

Up to now, social and psychological variables have been progressively added to biological aspects of stress to create a more complete view. The biological bases of stress are important because they are responsible for much of what we feel or do under stress. However, the psychological side, in terms of both causes and effects, is of great importance as well. If psychological factors can actually alter bodily functioning in ways that may facilitate illness, for example, an important link between psychology and health has been revealed.

PSYCHOLOGICAL STRESS

Against the backdrop of physiological response to threat, Lazarus and others have added a psychological dimension to the stress concept. The notion of psychological

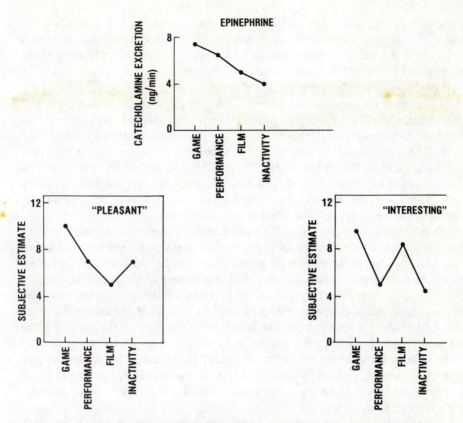

Figure 3.4   Mean epinephrine levels and ratings of pleasantness for the bingo game (pleasant condition), task and film (less pleasant conditions), and inactivity sessions. Higher levels of epinephrine were associated with pleasant and unpleasant events.

From P. Patkai. Catecholamine excretion in pleasant and unpleasant situations. *Acta Psychologica*, 1971, *35* 352–363.

appraisal—that the stress process can be initiated or influenced by psychological events—is not inconsistent with the models already described, but historically the research traditions have developed independently of each other. Only now are researchers working to put physiological and psychological research together. Lazarus's theories are almost as exclusively psychological as Selye's are physiological, yet their compatibility seems clear.

By pointing out that stressors can be psychological, Lazarus (1966) made the study of stress more complex and challenging. Like other aspects of behavior, psychological stressors cannot be measured directly. Instead, they must be inferred from responses or defined in terms of the situations in which they arise. Stress can be measured in many ways, including asking people how they feel, observing performance on tasks, or measuring levels of epinephrine and norepinephrine. Since stress causes negative mood states, performance deficits on some tasks, and increased secretion of catecholamines by the adrenal glands, stress may be measured by observing these effects. Similarly, stressors may be grouped or labeled in terms of where they occur, what they entail, or their characteristics. As a result, we can discuss occupational stress, urban stress, and the like. The problem is that the impact of the death of a parent, losing a job, or being exposed to crowding is greater than the sum of its effects. What does it mean to experience such stress?

Lazarus (1975) emphasizes the role of perception and cognitive appraisal in the stress response. He suggests, for example, that unless we perceive a situation as threatening, we will not experience stress. Thus the animals in Selye's experiments may have had to perceive danger before an alarm reaction and subsequent phases of the GAS could occur. In support of this hypothesis, we can return to the study by Symington et al. (1955) that found that patients who were dying from injury or disease showed no stress response, as measured by adrenal activity, as long as they were unconscious. It is possible that blocking a person's ability to appraise a situation as stressful can prevent the onset of the stress response.

Over the course of more than 20 years, Lazarus has evolved a model of stress that recognizes the significance of psychological stress (see Figure 3.1). Lazarus argues that in order for an event to be a stressor, it must be appraised as threatening. We evaluate the pressures we encounter, and only those appraised to be threatening evoke the stress response. If you fail an examination, a number of factors will enter into your appraisal of the event. You may consider how much the failure will affect your final grade, whether you feel the failure was your fault or the fault of a bad test, how failure will affect your self-image, or the extent to which you care about grades or tests. If the failure will not count toward your grade, if it does not threaten your self-esteem, or if you do not care how you did on the exam, you probably will not experience stress. If, on the other hand, the failure is perceived as threatening, stress is more likely.

A series of studies conducted by Lazarus and his associates during the 1960s provided support for this perspective. In one, Lazarus et al. (1965) had subjects view a gruesome and stressful film depicting such woodshop accidents as a worker cutting off a finger and a worker being killed by a wooden plank driven through his body. Subjects were told either that the events had been staged and no one was really being hurt or that the events were real but the film would help improve safety in such settings. A third group of subjects was given no explanation.

Both sets of instructions were effective in reducing arousal during the film, presumably because they allowed appraisal of the film in a less threatening manner. It can be argued, for example, that subjects who were told that the film had been staged would not find the film as gruesome as those who believed that the carnage was real. These results are similar to those of an earlier study (Speisman et al., 1964) in which subjects were shown a film depicting primitive initiation rites that included rather unpleasant genital surgery. Subjects saw the film accompanied by one of the three soundtracks. One group heard narration emphasizing pain, mutilation, and possible disease consequences (trauma condition); another group heard a script in which the pain and consequences were denied and the participants in the rites were depicted as willing and happy (denial condition); and the third group heard a detached description of the rites from an anthropological perspective (intellectualization condition).

The results showed that stress responses were reduced for subjects in the denial and intellectualization conditions, relative to subjects in the trauma group.

Once again, instructions in the second and third conditions allowed subjects to appraise the situation as less threatening, while the instructions given to trauma subjects emphasized those aspects of the film that were more likely to be seen as stressful.

These studies, and a number of other studies conducted by Lazarus and his colleagues (see Lazarus and Alfert, 1964; Nomikos et al., 1968; Koriat et al., 1972), provide convincing evidence that stress is not well understood in situational terms alone. The films that different groups of subjects saw were the same, and the settings in which they saw them were comparable. By altering the interpretations people made while viewing the films, Lazarus and his colleagues were able to observe different stress reactions.

Some of these studies suggested another source of variance in stress reactions—personality dispositions or tendencies to appraise events in particular ways. In the study of responses to the film depicting genital surgery, Speisman et al. found that subjects predisposed to use denial as a means of coping with aversive events showed more stress in response to the detached intellectualization soundtrack than to the denial soundtrack. The opposite was true of those who tended to cope by intellectualizing a threat. Differences in appraisal were still found to be responsible for variations in the magnitude of the stress response, but a different source of these differences was implicated—situational and personality-based variation in the ways in which a stressor was appraised.

The role of appraisal processes in the stress process has been widely demonstrated and generally accepted. Recent work has focused on long-term coping and on the kinds of appraisals that can be made. Lazarus and Launier (1978) identify a number of possible appraisals, including evaluation of an event as *irrelevant* (the event in question will not affect me), *benign* appraisals (the event is positive), and harmful or threatening interpretations which may lead to stress. Stressful appraisal may involve evaluation of harm or potential loss; threat of danger, harm, or loss; and challenge.

Lazarus's conceptualization has proven to be an important contribution to the development of a thorough understanding of stress. When exposed to a potentially stressful situation, we appraise the setting and make judgments about how threatening it is to us. After a situation is judged to be threatening and stressful, secondary appraisals are made. No longer concerned with assessment of danger, we turn our attention to the dangers or benefits of different modes of coping with perceived threats. The perception of danger motivates a search for coping responses that will reduce this threat.

Consider an example of this sequence in a familiar and relatively low-threat event. You feel as if your peers at college exclude you from their activities. When impromptu parties come up, you are the last to find out. People go to the movies without inviting you to come along or go to dinner without waiting for you. You feel isolated from your fellow students. If you are the kind of person who derives self-esteem or gratification from being part of the "gang," you are more likely to appraise this as threatening and aversive than if you prefer the role of "loner." Let us say you are of the former persuasion. You are upset by the situation and wish to respond. During a second appraisal of the situation you may consider several approaches. You can do nothing or even withdraw further—the benefits of which are that you do not have to expend energy or risk the rejection that might result from a blatant attempt to join the group. The costs of this coping option are continued isolation and loss of self-esteem. On the other hand, you may make a strong effort to join the group, risking embarrassment and rejection for the possible benefit of being accepted into the group. A third alternative might be to slowly increase your participation in the group. The risks and benefits are similar to those of the second alternative except that the risk of embarrassment is reduced and the period of time before you can feel that you "belong" is greater. You may try to find out why you are being treated as you are so that you understand it better. Finally, you may reinterpret the situation, deciding that you do not want to join the group. By reinterpreting rejection by the group in a positive light, you may reduce loss of self-esteem, but you are still not a member of the group.

Thus your response to the situation will depend on two kinds of appraisals. First, you must interpret the situation and consider its potential threats, harm, or challenge. Second, you must consider your response choices. Obviously, evaluation of your choices is based on your interpretation of the situation and the nature of the threat you see. By weighing the costs and benefits of these choices, you select a coping strategy.

Coping behavior is, therefore, an important part of the stress response. Lazarus proposed that stress responses can take manipulative or accommodative forms. They may be *direct action* responses, where the individual tries directly to manipulate or alter his or her relationship to the stressful situation. Thus people may change the setting, flee, or otherwise remove the physical presence of the stressor. Alternatively, people may *seek information* about the situation so that they can understand it and predict related events. They may also do nothing—*inhibition of action* may be the best course of action in some situations. Finally, *intrapsychic or palliative coping* may be necessary. Here the individual accommodates the stressful situation by reappraising the situation or by altering his or her "internal environment." Taking drugs, using alcohol, learning to relax, creating or using psychological defense mechanisms, and engaging in meditation are examples of this kind of coping (Lazarus and Folkman, 1984).

Early stress research emphasized the biological and nonspecific responses associated with a variety of stimuli (see Selye, 1956); subsequent theory and research has come to focus on appraisal and contextual cues in the elicitation of stress responses (see Lazarus, 1966; Mason, 1975). The evolution of psychological mechanisms as a part of the stress process helps to explain variations in responses to stress. While some divergent responding is based on biological predispositions (see Levi, 1978), many other instances are explainable in terms of differences between stressors, contexts in which they occur, perceived abilities to cope with them, and the like (Coyne and Lazarus, 1980; Kanner, Coyne, Schaefer, and Lazarus, 1981). Clearly, styles of coping with stress as well as psychosocial supports and assets will affect response to stressors and ultimate consequences of exposure to them (see Baum, Singer, and Baum, 1981).

In the next sections of this chapter, we will consider factors that affect stress. Differences in stressors, appraisal, and response will be discussed in their relationships to one another. It should be remembered that, although presented as discrete factors, they cannot be isolated in practice. Aspects of one necessarily affect the others.

STRESSORS

Although some events are threatening to almost no one, most carry a range of potential problems. Some or all of these problems may be appraised as stressful under some conditions. The properties of the stressor can affect the appraisal made of it but cannot ordinarily determine reactions directly.

Lazarus and Cohen (1977) have described three general categories of stressors drawn along a number of dimensions, including how long the stressor persists, the magnitude of response required by the stressor, and the number of people affected. Cataclysmic events are stressors that have sudden and powerful impact and are more or less universal in eliciting a response. These events usually require a great deal of effort for effective coping. War, natural disaster, and nuclear accident are unpredictable and powerful threats that generally affect all of those touched by them. The drought in the American southeast and the more common tornadoes, hurricanes, and other natural disasters (Baker and Chapman, 1962; Baum et al., 1980; Pennebaker and Newtson, 1981; Sims and Bauman, 1974) can all be considered in this category of stressors. Imprisonment, torture, and concentration camp experiences are also forms of cataclysmic events and appear to engender substantial effects (see, Schmolling, 1984). One study suggested that concentration camp survivors who had developed cancer showed poorer coping than cancer patients who had not been in camps and that concentration camp survivors may be more vulnerable to stress associated with the disease (Baider and Sarell, 1984).

The powerful onset of a cataclysmic event may initially evoke a freezing or dazed response by victims. Coping is difficult and may bring no immediate relief. When a severe storm hits an area or when an earthquake occurs in a region, it can be extremely frightening and dangerous, it can cause severe disruption of people's lives, and it can cause damage or loss whose impact will not fade for years. But because the actual event is brief, the severely threatening aspects of such a stressor dissipate rapidly. Some cataclysmic events cause little physical damage and do not fade quickly. At Love Canal in upstate New York, for example, the discovery of toxic wastes and dangers to area residents was a slow process with little physical destruction. Of course, a storm or a quake will leave destruction in its wake, but people can confront harm and loss they have already sustained with the knowledge that "the worst is over." As they go about recovering from the disaster, they know that things will get better and better each day. When recovery is allowed to proceed without return of the stressor, rebuilding progresses and full recovery is generally achieved. In the cases of Three Mile Island and Love Canal, where rebuilding is not what is needed (nothing was actually destroyed) and the damage already done is less important than the damage that may yet come, recovery may be more difficult.

The fact that cataclysmic stressors usually affect large numbers of people at one time is also important in rate of recovery. Individuals have no specific immunity—many homes are damaged, many people are injured, and so on. Because people helping each other seems like a logical way of speeding recovery and rebuilding, disasters often lead to an increase in social cohesion in affected communities (see Quarantelli and Dynes, 1972). People draw together after a disaster, providing each other with comfort as well as support and assistance in recovery. Centers for homeless victims may be set up, and people housed in them may form attachments with one another. People may help one another search through debris for personal belongings, may help the police maintain order, or may render assistance in many ways. Sometimes whole communities will band together to meet threats or repair damage already incurred. Of course, not all major disasters dissipate quickly, and residents cannot band together to fight a stressor indefinitely. When a disaster persists in an apparently unresolvable manner, it can lead to problems of a different kind.

Similar to cataclysmic events, personal stressors are strong and may be unexpected. **Personal stressors** include those events that are powerful enough to challenge adaptive abilities in the same way as do cataclysmic events, but that affect fewer people at any one time. This distinction is important; affiliative and socially comparative behaviors have been identified as styles of coping with a focused, specific threat (see McGrath, 1970; Schachter, 1959), and social support has been shown to moderate the effect of stress (see Cobb, 1976). In other words, having people around to provide support, help, comparison for emotional and behavioral responses, and other assistance can reduce the negative impact of a stressor. With cataclysmic events, people are able to share distress with others undergoing the same difficulties; the second class of stressors, however, affects fewer people at a time, resulting in fewer people with whom to share. These events include response to illness, death (see Greene, 1966; Hackett and Weisman, 1964; Parkes, 1972), or losing one's job (Kasl and Cobb, 1970). The death of a parent, for example, is generally an intensely painful loss, and it is not always anticipated. The event itself is acute—the death and immediate period of grief are relatively short—even though, like a disaster, it may leave scars or problems that continue for years. Usually the occurrence of the stressor and its immediate aftermath are the low points of the experience. Things gradually improve, and people may begin to cope with the loss of a loved one by believing that things will continue to improve steadily. Again, the point of severest impact occurs early, and coping can progress once the worst is over.

Of course, things do not always get better with time. But in general, the magnitude, duration, and point of severest impact of cataclysmic events and personal stressors are similar. The biggest difference between the two types of events is the extent of impact, or the number of people affected. One affects large numbers of people, while the other affects relatively few. Coping with the death of a parent may be more difficult if one is alone than if one has a large family with whom to share the grief. Losing a job is usually an individual loss, although groups may be affected in some cases. When many people are laid off at once, they can share and help one another. Under normal circumstances, however, the unemployed individual has few people with whom to compare and commiserate.

Background stressors are persistent, repetitive, and almost routine stressors that are part of our everyday lives. Lazarus and Cohen (1977) have labeled this third group of stressors daily hassles—stable, repetitive, low-intensity problems encountered daily as part of one's routine.

Daily hassles are different from other stressors in many ways. First, they are by themselves considerably less powerful than the stressors noted previously. Cumulatively, over time, they may pose threats equally serious, but individually the stressors do not generally pose severe threats. Second, they are chronic. Their impact persists over relatively long periods of time, and the effects of exposure are gradual. Thus living in a very noisy neighborhood may not pose severe threats all at once—one exposure to noise is easily coped with and not particularly threatening. However, noise is not usually a one-time event. Rather, it is repeated often and may persist indefinitely. In this context, the notion that things are getting better may not be common—the point at which the worst is over may never occur as things slowly become worse and worse. People can cope with individual episodes of noise even if it is uncontrollable (see Glass and Singer, 1972), but the cumulative effects of chronic exposures to noise over time appear to be more severe (Cohen, 1980). Another approach to background stressors is provided by Burks and Martin (1985) in a study of ongoing, everyday problems and hassles that are often neglected in studies of life changes. These kinds of stressors were seen as more chronic than most life events, and cumulative effects were expected. The types of everyday problems measured by Burks and Martin were different from those measured in studies of daily hassles (see, Kanner et al., 1981). Daily hassles are typically defined as relatively minor events that may be chronic or acute, but in this study attention was focused more on chronic problems of more substantive consequence. A sample of 281 college students completed a life events survey, an everyday problems scale that included items such as "too much schoolwork," "parents having marital difficulties," "dissatisfaction with housing," "carrying on a long-distance relationship," and "not having enough money," and a symptom checklist. Results suggested that symptom reporting was more strongly related to everyday problems than to life events, though both were associated with symptom reporting.

Other chronic stressors include job dissatisfaction (Frankenhaeuser and Gardell, 1976; Kahn and French, 1970), neighborhood problems (Harburg et al., 1973), and commuting (Singer, Lundberg, and Frankenhaeuser, 1978). Theorell et al. (1985) have reported greater systolic blood pressure elevations among those in high demand–low control occupations (such as waiters, drivers, and cooks) than among those in more controllable or less demanding settings. Crowding, especially encountered repetitively in one's neighborhood, on commuter trains, or in apartment buildings, may form part of an individual's background. In dormitory settings, for example, it is unlikely that a single episode of unwanted contact in which you encounter someone you do not like will present severe adaptive demands. Rather, the sum total of instances of unwanted contact may be responsible for the stress experienced if these encounters are repeated often or cannot be avoided (Baum and Valins, 1977). Chronically high levels of social interaction on the job may also cause problems; over a two-year period, higher levels of social contact were associated with increased serum triglycerides and uric acid levels (Howard, Cunningham, and Rechnitzer, 1986).

Finally, the benefits of sharing with others in order to cope may not be as important here. Even if large numbers of people are affected, the duration and magnitude of individual exposure may be so brief as never to raise the need for affiliation. Crowded subway rides are episodic bouts with stress. However, the stress is not severe and can usually be coped with (although it may become increasingly difficult to do so over time). Such an aversive experience probably will not be of sufficient intensity to cause people to band together to provide each other with support and comfort.

Consider the worker who must get up at 5 A.M. each morning, commute an hour each way to work on a crowded train, and work in a noisy and congested area of a big city. Each individual crowded train ride or encounter with noise may not present much of a problem. Combined, these two daily occurrences may pose more of a problem, but they can be adapted to as well. Add other problems encountered regularly, and the cumulative adaptive difficulty becomes more demanding. Although adaptation may still be possible, the background level of stress becomes higher. As exposure becomes more chronic and these problems are encountered regularly, costs may continue to mount. At some point these daily hassles may exceed one's adaptive abilities, resulting in too much wear and tear on the body and placing one at risk for major psychological and physiological response to acute stressors. The worker with a high background stress level may overreact to unrelated stressors or may become so responsive that he or she shows exaggerated responses to them. Thus he or she may overreact to a child's disobedience, a friend's carelessness, or some insignificant hassle with a neighbor.

In sum, background stressors are chronic, affect large numbers of people *on an individual basis,* and alone do not require a great deal of coping. In fact, some stressors are not always noticeable, as in the case of air pollution (see Evans and Jacobs, 1981). Yet the cumulation of stress over a long period of time may result in deceptively severe consequences. Regular and prolonged exposure to low-level stress may require more adaptive responses in the long run than exposure to other stressors. Background stressors generally push an individual's adaptive abilities toward their limit; by requiring that people allocate attention and effort to them, they may gradually reduce an individual's ability to cope with subsequent stressors.

Chronic stressors are not necessarily of small magnitude like hassles of many everyday events. Some may be substantive and may result in long-term disruption and problems. For example, residents of the area around Three Mile Island are faced with the chronic threats inherent in believing that they were exposed to radiation. The consequences of such exposure are long term; they take years to become detectable, and people who think they were exposed may worry about the possibility that they or their children will develop cancer or show genetic abnormalities. This can produce a chronic uncertainty that may give rise to persistent stress. Research has shown that some of these people have exhibited chronic elevations in blood pressure, cortisol, catecholamines, and symptom reporting over a period of several years (Baum, Gatchel, and Schaeffer, 1983; Davidson and Baum, 1986).

Part of the problem at Three Mile Island appears to be the involvement of toxic substances of which radiation is often considered a prime example. Other studies suggest that the presence of toxins appears to intensify or prolong stress responding (Fleming, 1985). Another instance of this is provided by a study of mothers who took diethylstilbestrol (DES) while pregnant (Gutterman, Erhardt, Markowitz, and Link, 1985). During a twenty-five year period (1948–1971), DES, a synthetic estrogen, was used to improve prenatal child health and reduce spontaneous abortion, but use was stopped after studies indicated a risk for female children of cervical/vaginal cancer (Gutterman et al, 1985; Herbst, Ulfelder, Poskanzer, 1971). However, by the time DES use was halted, millions of women had taken it and many of them had children who were apparently at risk for a host of health threats. The results of questionnaire assessment of the psychological well-being of a sample of these mothers suggested few symptoms of chronic stress and, for the most part, good adjustment. However, when other chronic stressors were present, psychological health was affected by a history of DES use. Thus, for example, women who had used DES had poorer mental health when they were exposed to other threats or problems as well (Gutterman et al., 1985).

It should be clear that some stressors are very intrusive, physical, and universally threatening (such as natural disaster), while others are more culturally determined, less universal, and more psychological. Crowding and spatial invasion, for example, are culture-bound in that responses to varying densities and proximities are specific to cultural norms and meanings (see Aiello and Thompson, 1980; Hall, 1966). These kinds of stressors are based on psychological processes involved in appraisal and are far less universal than such things as earthquakes or floods.

APPRAISAL

Factors that affect the way we interpret stressors include environmental, social, and psychological variables. Individuals who possess great wealth, coping skills, or resources (e.g., friends, material) may not be as prone to appraise a given event as threatening. As a result, they tend to be less affected by the stressor. The upper-middle-class resident of a large city, for example, may be less likely to experience difficulty from urban stressors than a poorer resident, as he or she may be better able to avoid aversive urban conditions. Attitudes toward the sources of stress will also mediate responses. If we believe that a stressor will cause us no permanent harm, our response will probably be less extreme than if the danger carries the threat of lasting harm. If our attitudes are strongly in favor of something that may also cause us harm, we may reappraise threats and make them less alarming. Thus the dedicated urbanite might interpret crowding as exciting and "alive," jokingly proclaiming "We've got nature under control—we use asphalt." The array of environmental and psychological variables associated with each encounter with stress determines response.

Harm/loss assessments typically involve analysis of *damage that has already been done* (Lazarus and Launier, 1978). The properties of a sudden event such as a tornado may predispose people toward this type of appraisal, since damage is done very quickly and people will be more concerned with existing damage than with the possibility of more. Of course, harm and threat appraisals can be coexistent if more tornadoes and damage are predicted. Bereavement is also likely to reflect a harm/loss evaluation, although when someone has been chronically ill bereavement may also occur in anticipation of loss. Further, loss may imply threat, the second type of appraisal that can be made. In addition to the loss of the loved one, we may also perceive demands that will occur after death.

Threat appraisals are concerned with future dangers. If warning is given of the approach of a tornado, the tornado may initially be appraised as a threat. The stress of moving away to college, of learning to live with a roommate, and of similar events is largely anticipatory. Likewise, waiting to take an exam may be more stressful than taking it or even than failing it. The ability to foresee problems and to anticipate difficulties allows us to solve or prevent their occurrence. It also allows perception of threat and anticipatory stress.

Challenge appraisals focus not on the harm or potential harm of the event but on the possibility of overcoming the stressor (Lazarus and Launier, 1978). Some stressors may affect us beyond our ability to cope, but we all have a range of events within which we are confident of our ability to cope successfully. Stressors that are evaluated as challenges fall within this range. The event may be seen as potentially harmful, but we feel that we can prevent harm from occurring. The magnitude of the stressor, our estimates of our coping resources, our styles of coping with problems—all of these determine whether an event is seen as challenging or threatening.

MEDIATING VARIABLES

SOCIAL SUPPORT

One mediator of stress is social support, the feeling that a person is cared about and valued by other people and that he or she belongs to a social network (see Cobb, 1976). The notion that people need to be embedded in groups of people who provide love and a sense of belonging is not new. Many philosophers have spoken of the social needs of people, and psychologists have postulated needs for social caring and nurturance (see Fromm, 1955; Maslow, 1954; Murray, 1938). Many have long believed that interpersonal relationships can somehow protect us from many ills. However, the effects of having or not having social and emotional support have not always been clearly shown.

The fact that social support can be measured in a number of ways makes research difficult to interpret or integrate. The number of people an individual sees on a regular basis can be directly observed, or people can estimate this number (see Berkman and Syme, 1979; Killworth and Bernard, 1976; Ludwig and Collette, 1970). For a broader definition of social support, estimates of the number of people one considers to be friends, the types of nonfriend contacts, such as clergy or family, and the importance of each (see Caplan, Cobb, and French, 1975) can be collated. A number of other measures include evaluations of broad social networks at home and at work, the perceived importance of social ties in general, and the degree to which these relationships satisfy various needs (Pilisuk and Parks, 1980). Problems arise because almost all measures of social support are based on what people say and are therefore susceptible to self-report bias (e.g., someone with few friends may be reluctant to admit it). In addition, the more objective measures of support, such as counting numbers of friends, provide no information about the quality of relationships. When measuring social support, one must specify the kinds of social ties one wants to assess in order to obtain reliable estimates of the quantity and quality of supports provided.

Further complicating study of social support is the fact that we derive many kinds of support from people. Wills (1985), for example, presents an analysis of types of social support based on the function served by each kind. **Esteem support** refers to the effects of other people in increasing feelings of self-esteem: we may feel better about ourselves if a group of friends and acquaintances thinks well of us. We may also get necessary information from social interaction, which Wills calls **informational support. Social companionship** is defined as support derived from social activities, and **instrumental support** refers to the physical aid one can get from friends. If your car breaks down, your friends may bolster your self-esteem by assuring you it was not your fault (esteem support), provide information about how to get it repaired (informational support), take you with them to a party (companionship), or give you a ride to the garage to get your car towed (instrumental support). All or some of these functional aspects of social support may be important in any given situation.

A number of other categorizations or types of social support have been discussed, and most of these analyses suggest that their relative effectiveness in reducing stress is determined by the degree to which they meet the needs of a specific situation (see Cohen and McKay, 1984; Cohen and Wills, 1985). To some extent, the functions of social support depend on how it helps us: Does having social support help us cope with stressors, or does it help by making us less likely to experience stress at all? Is social support beneficial only when we are experiencing a stressor, or is it beneficial all of the time? Could it be that stress is not reduced by having social support but that stress is increased when we do not have it?

These issues have led to the formulation of two basic mechanisms by which social support affects stress. One posits that social support is beneficial regardless of whether we are stressed and that not having social support is stressing by itself. This hypothesis is called the **direct** or **main effect hypothesis** and stands in opposition to the alternate, **stress-buffering hypothesis,** which views social support as beneficial because it buffers or helps us cope with stress (Cohen and McKay, 1984; Cohen and Syme, 1985). Evidence actually supports both views; sometimes social support appears to be helpful to people regardless of stress and having little support generates stress on its own, while in other cases positive effects of having social support show up only when we are under stress. Differences in findings may be attributable to the outcome variables used (e.g., psychological, physiological), to the nature of the situation studied, to the characteristics of the people involved, and other variables (Fleming et al., 1982; Wills, 1985). Both the direct and stress-buffering models of social support describe the relationship between one's social reality and stress (Cohen and Syme, 1985).

Research on social support and recovery from illness has shown such beneficial effects as reduction of the degree to which stress can lead to the onset of illness (see Chen and Cobb, 1960). Chambers and Reiser (1953) suggest that emotional events or crises are sometimes responsible for the onset of episodes of cardiac failure and showed that supportive behavior by attending physicians can have a facilitating effect on recovery from heart attack. Studies on surgical patients (see Chapter 8) also show the positive effects of supportive information on patient recovery, and a study by Whitcher and Fisher (1979) has demonstrated the therapeutic benefits of socially supportive interventions. Supportive touch by nurses improved recovery among surgery patients, primarily for women.

The effects of social support are not confined to the recovery of the ill. Studies of grief and bereavement after the death of a loved one have indicated that psychological adjustment is affected by social support (see Parkes, 1972). One study (Burch, 1972) demonstrated that married men (who presumably derive social support from their nuclear families) whose mothers had died were better able to deal with this trauma than were single or divorced men. The probability of suicide was also found to be higher for the single or divorced men. Extending this, Burch found that close ties with nonnuclear family also reduced the probability of suicide.

Other studies that have considered social support as it affects pregnancy and birth, hospitalization, job loss, and response to the threat of death or injury also provided evidence of the beneficial effects of social support. One study provided tentative evidence that birth complications were less likely among women reporting high social support than among those having low social support (Nuckols et al., 1972). Supportive behavior by parents and staff has been associated with adjustment to hospitalization among children (see Jessner, Blom, and Waldfogel, 1952), and alcoholism and depression have been related to relatively low social support (Brown, Bhrolchain, and Harris, 1975; Jackson, 1954). Similarly, studies have shown that social support helps people cope with the stress of losing one's job (Cobb et al., 1969; Gore, 1973). Clearly social support can have potent effects on responses to stress, but what are the mechanisms by which stress is mediated by social support?

Among the explanations that have been offered, Cobb (1976) notes the possibility that social support helps people to be flexible and alter roles and identities as stressors demand. Others have considered the role of affiliation in reduction of distress (see Schachter, 1959), and it is reasonable to assume that opportunities for social comparison and affiliation are related to social support. Membership in a social network may assure beneficial role and comparison levels, and may affect the degree to which we view an event as stressful or may help us choose the "best" way of coping with a stressor.

EXERCISE

A number of ways of reducing stress have been devised, and we shall consider several of these in greater detail in Chapter 10. For now, it is important to note that there are some conditions or activities that appear to be associated with less stress in everyday life. Among these is exercise, which appears to be an effective means of keeping stress levels down (Cox, Evans, and Jamieson, 1979; Keller, 1980; Sinyor et al., 1983). In one study, regular exercisers and those who did not exercise frequently were exposed to a laboratory stressor; those who exercised showed stronger, more rapidly recovering hormonal responses to the stressor (Sinyor et al., 1983). In a recent example, Brown and Lawton (1986) conducted a study of 220 adolescent women in order to determine relationships among stressful life circumstances, measures of physical and psychological well-being, and exercise. The primary assumption regarding exercise was that regular physical exertion would result in less susceptibility to the negative effects of stress. Findings showed first that life events were related to reported illness and that illness reports were related to depression. Exercise was negatively associated with depression and positively associated with age. More important, those women reporting high stress exhibited more stress-related illness if they did not exercise regularly.

Other research on exercise has also been reported, much of it dealing directly with cardiovascular risk factors. Subjective reports of mood are more positive among exercisers, and reduction of anxiety or depression can be achieved by initiating physical training programs (see Berger, 1984; Folkins, 1981; Markoff, Ryan, and Young, 1982).

DISPOSITIONAL VARIABLES

Research has suggested that there may be sex differences in the way in which our bodies respond during stress. A meta-analysis of studies of acute stress responding, for example, suggests that men may respond more strenuously to stressors than do women, particularly if one considers systolic blood pressure response (Stoney, Davis, and Mathews, 1987). Stress hormones, such as catecholamines, have also been studied and evidence suggests that men exhibit greater epinephrine response during stress but show norepinephrine and cortisol responses comparable to women (Frankenhaeuser, 1983). More recently, Stoney, Mathews, McDonald, and Johnson (in press) found that women show smaller increases in low density lipoprotein cholesterol and blood pressure during three different stressful tasks. Low density lipoprotein cholesterol increases during stress, and high levels of this cholesterol fraction have been associated with atherosclerosis and coronary heart disease, suggesting one possible reason for differential vulnerability to cardiovascular disease among men and women (Kannel, Castelli, and Gordon, 1979; Stoney et al, 1987).

The existence of "high stress" or "high risk" personalities, or of other personal variables that affect appraisal of stressors, has been considered in many studies. Grinker and Spiegel (1945) noted that only a relatively small number of air combat crews serving during World War II ever developed serious stress-related disorders. Some of the airmen studied had previously established neuroses that made them more susceptible to the stress of battle. In more recent years this vulnerability notion has been used to provide an explanation for selective onset of schizophrenia (see Zubin, 1976), illness (Kobasa, 1979), and other stress-related disturbances (see Cobb, 1976; Kasl and Cobb, 1970).

Coping styles or behavior patterns have also been identified, and these styles appear to affect the ways in which events are appraised as well as which types of coping are involved. Work on a number of these dimensions—repression-sensitization, arousal seeking, screening, and denial—has indicated that people differing in these areas may not interpret situations in the same way (see Byrne, 1964; Janis, 1958; Mehrabian, 1977; Zuckerman, 1971). A study by Baum et al. (1981), for example, suggests that individuals who handle overload by screening and prioritizing demands are less susceptible to the effects of crowding than are people who do not cope in this way.

There are other stress-relevant coping styles. As we will see in Chapter 5, individuals who manifest a Type A behavior pattern respond to stress as if it were control-threatening and interpret most threats to control as stressful. Their appraisal of events is particularly sensitive to anything that might reduce their control over a situation. The time urgency, competitiveness, and hostility that accompany this response, together with the enhanced likelihood of experiencing stress and physiological concomitants of that stress, may cause Type As to be at a higher risk for coronary heart disease. We shall discuss this pattern in more detail in Chapter 5.

CONTROL

Perceived control is a powerful mediator of stress, providing individuals with a sense that they can cope effectively to predict events and so determine what will happen. Glass and Singer (1972) considered the effects of perceived controllability and predictability in their studies of stress due to noise. The perception that the noise could be accurately anticipated, or even turned off if desired, facilitated adaptation with minimal aftereffects. Subsequently, Sherrod (1974) found the same relationship for stress due to crowding; and Rodin, Solomon, and Metcalf (1978) found that providing control reduced crowding stress. The degree to which control operates by influencing appraisal of the stressor, however, is more speculation than fact.

A study by Staub, Tursky, and Schwartz (1971) bears some relevance to this point. Subjects who were given perceived control over shock reported less discomfort than did subjects who did not have perceived control of the intensity or administration of the shock, even though all subjects actually received the same number and intensity of shocks. The perception of control seemed to affect perception of the stressor used in this study.

Somewhat more direct evidence of control influencing appraisal of stressors comes from the growing literature on cognitive control. By providing subjects with information about a stressor prior to subjects' exposure to it, researchers have been able to reduce the threat appraisal made when the stressor is experienced. Studies have found that accurate expectations reduce stress (Baum, Fisher, and Solomon, 1981; Langer and Saegert, 1977). Inaccurate or violated expectations result in some negative response, but they appear to be remedied quickly when people realize what has happened and form new expectations (Greenberg and Baum, 1979). We shall consider these topics in greater detail in the next chapter.

PHYSIOLOGICAL ASPECTS OF THE STRESS RESPONSE

Despite the sometimes overwhelming nature of stressors or the likelihood that they will be appraised as threatening, stress cannot be defined without reference to the response made by the organism. These physiological, cognitive, and behavioral reactions or effects are important aspects of the stressor-stress process.

Physiological and biochemical measurements of stress allow inferences about emotional states and provide markers of those bodily responses most affected by stress. As noted earlier, catecholamines and corticosteroids, secreted by the adrenal medulla and cortex respectively, are involved in stress responding (see Cannon, 1929; Frankenhaeuser, 1973; Glass et al., 1980; Mason, 1975), and the refinement of measurement techniques (see von Euler, 1956; Nagatsu, 1973) allows estimates of their levels to be drawn from urine and blood samples. Catecholamine secretion also reflects sympathetic arousal; the adrenal medulla is innervated by the sympathetic nervous system, and secretion of epinephrine and norepinephrine appears to be part of sympathetic arousal. Thus secretion of catecholamines is also associated with systemic reactions in the body (Ax, 1953). Increases in cardiovascular reactivity (i.e., faster heart rate, higher blood pressure), changes in muscle potential, and measures of skin conductance have also been used to show the effects of stress. At this level, the stress response seems to be fairly nonspecific—that is, physiological arousal and related somatic changes are similar for most stressors, although some research has suggested patterning of endocrine responses to different situations. Generally speaking, many stressors appear to cause the same kind of general physiological response.

These somatic consequences of stress are important for a number of reasons. First, increased catecholamine and corticosteroid secretion is associated with a wide range of other physiological responses, such as the aforementioned changes in heart rate, blood pressure, breathing, muscle potential, inflammation, and other functions. Prolonged or sudden elevation of circulating catecholamines may damage body tissue, as is suggested for the pathogenesis of atherosclerosis (see Schneiderman, 1983). Catecholamines also appear to affect cognitive and emotional functioning, and elevated levels of epinephrine or norepinephrine in the blood may affect mood and behavior.

In order to view this link more fully, we must review Cannon's work on the "emergency function" of catecholamines. Cannon (1929, 1931) suggested that epinephrine has a salutary effect on adaptation. By arousing the organism, epinephrine provides a biological advantage to the organism, enabling it to respond more rapidly to danger. When we are extremely frightened or enraged, we experience an arousal that may be uncomfortable but which readies us to act against the thing that frightens or angers us. Thus stress-related increases in catecholamines may facilitate adaptive behavior. In fact, studies have shown superior performance on some tasks among subjects injected with epinephrine (Frankenhaeuser, Jarpe, and Mattell, 1961) and also among people who produce larger amounts of catecholamines in the face of challenge (see Frankenhaeuser, 1971). However, arousal has also been associated with impaired performance on complex tasks (see Evans, 1978).

There may be cognitive benefits of stress, but it is also evident that the "fight or flight" model, derivable from Cannon's work, is inadequate for predicting response to danger in our complex society. Aside from the wear and tear on our bodies generated by repeated or prolonged stress, a number of less desirable outcomes are likely when stress does not abate readily. Most of the research that finds support for facilitating aspects of stress has considered acute situations in which adjustment leads to a decrease in stress. The consequences of unabated stress or repeated exposure to stress, as in the case of background stressors, have only recently come under study. Among these consequences are decrements in ability to cope with subsequent stress, aftereffects, and, in some cases, physiological dysfunction, tissue damage, or death.

Thus physiological responses to stress may be both specific and nonspecific and may be chronic or acute. Those responses that are short-lived—either because adaptation is achieved or because the stressor was brief—resemble Cannon's mobilization response. When frightened by a loud noise or exposed to a highly threatening but rapidly unfolding situation (e.g., we see a car heading right for us at high speed, and it speeds by just missing us), the organism is alerted to the danger and readies itself to respond. After the danger has passed, we become aware of a racing heart, sweatiness, and the like. Since the danger has been averted, these symptoms soon pass. However, when stress responses are repeated or prolonged, the alarm reaction is no longer functional. If adaptation is not achieved, prolonged arousal can lead to tissue damage and diseases of exhaustion (Selye, 1976).

Other biological changes occur as a direct or indirect consequence of stress. The extent to which they are part of the adaptive response itself or products of these responses is sometimes unclear. Immune system changes do not appear to be adaptive. Though suppression of immune system activity could reflect a conservation of energy, it may instead be a product of neural and hormonal changes that are part of the stress response. We shall discuss these issues in greater detail in Chapter 6.

EMOTIONAL AND PSYCHOLOGICAL ASPECTS OF THE STRESS RESPONSE

Emotions can be part of stress or can occur independently. They are usually thought of as powerful responses to positive or negative events. Emotional response is not unlike the stress response—heightened sympathetic arousal, sensations in the viscera, unhappiness, and excitement can all be characteristic of emotion. And, like stress, emotions typically motivate people to try to dispel, avoid, overcome, or prolong the source of emotional arousal. This seems like an awfully complicated way of defining such a common state. We are all familiar with emotions—we are sometimes sad, sometimes happy, and sometimes angry. Yet the true nature of emotions is still a matter of debate. As with many things, the common is more mysterious than the unusual.

So, how can emotions be defined? The classical view, espoused by many philosophers before the advent of modern psychology, was that emotions are experienced by the mind, and that associated bodily responses (e.g., the sensations accompanying arousal) follow this mental event. This view emphasizes the subjective—the feelings that people experience. It also focuses on the individual's reaction to something, rather than on the event that sets the whole thing off. Our understanding of emotions was initially slowed by failure to realize that they involve a cause-and-effect process, and by hesitancy to integrate the physiological with the psychological.

In 1890 James challenged the traditional view that bodily response followed emotion. Instead, he argued, conscious emotional response followed the body's reactions to an event. He considered the viscera to be central to the emotional response. The sight of a threatening or emotional stimulus caused a physiological reaction that was interpreted in terms of an emotion. If James is correct, we infer emotion from arousal or internal upset. When we see a dangerous situation before us, our bodies react and we are provided with sensations associated with distress. Fear is then experienced, partly as a consequence of these sensations.

James was not the only one to derive such a theory. Lange (1922) published a similar account of emotion. As a result, this basic position is known as the James-Lange theory of emotion. The experiences that we call emotions derive not from our psychological interpretations of external events but rather from our interpretations of visceral responses to the events.

This perspective has received both criticism and support. Research has indicated, for example, that when animals or patients have had the neural connections between visceral receptors and the sensation centers of the brain severed, they are still capable of emotional reactions such as fear (see Cannon, 1914, 1929). Yet a study by Schachter and Singer (1962) suggests that emotional response is heavily determined by the prior or simultaneous occurrence of physiological arousal.

Schachter and Singer gave subjects injections of epinephrine, which produced sensations associated with arousal. Those subjects receiving the injections of epinephrine were told either that it was epinephrine or that it was another substance that would not cause any side effects. The subjects then waited with another person (a confederate of the experimenter), who played a set role during the waiting period. In different conditions, the confederate behaved as if angry or euphoric.

The logic behind this experiment is elegantly simple. If physiological arousal is involved in emotions, the injection should elicit emotional response after it has caused physiological arousal. However, Schachter and Singer believed that interpretation of the arousal was also important. When subjects began to experience arousal but knew that they had received an injection of epinephrine, they could attribute the arousal to the shot and make no further inferences about it. In such a case, there would be no emotional response. However, when the injection was described in such a way as to eliminate it as a cause of the arousal, subjects had to search further for an explanation for the arousal. The most readily available source of information was the behavior of the other person in the room. Thus, when the injection was not described as causing arousal, subjects should interpret it as an emotional response and label it in accord with the confederate's behavior.

This is what Schachter and Singer (1962) found. When the shot was labeled as epinephrine, emotional interpretations were not made. When the shot was not described as causing arousal, subjects experienced emotions consistent with the confederate's behavior, reporting anger or happiness depending on how the confederate behaved.

The plasticity of emotion is not unlimited. The implications of these theories, however, include the fact that different emotions are not the result of different types of physical sensations but rather how they are labeled. Research has both supported and contradicted this position (see Dutton and Aron, 1974; Marshall and Zimbardo, 1979; Maslach, 1979; Schachter and Singer, 1979). It appears that in at least some cases arousal and labeling jointly determine emotion.

We have considered these theories because emotion is an important part of the stress process. The nonsomatic feelings that we have when stressed—anxiety, fear, anger, and so on—are emotional responses to threat or harm. The physiological systems through which emotion and stress appear to be channeled are similar, and both are heavily influenced by sympathetic arousal. More important, response to stress is likely to be affected by emotional responses associated with an event. If we respond angrily, our coping is likely to be more forceful or direct and active than if we respond with sadness and despair.

Anxiety disorders are emotional problems that are characterized, as the term suggests, primarily by the presence of anxiety. Anxiety is defined as a generalized state of fear or apprehension. The afflicted individual will begin to experience anxiety and distress in everyday situations that do not normally elicit such behavior from other persons. These disorders are distinguished by diffuse and often severe "free-floating" anxiety that may not be related to any one immediate situation or object threat. The individual may not be able to identify the source of fear or apprehension. Physiological symptoms, reflective of heightened autonomic nervous system arousal, include elevated heart rate and blood pressure level, sweating, intestinal distress, and muscular tension and weakness. Anxious individuals also report symptoms such as insomnia, worry, forgetfulness, difficulty in concentrating, irritability, and frequently mild depression. Besides their clinically high level of anxiety, these individuals often experience acute episodes of panic.

Depressive disorders are marked by disturbances of mood that can cause a great deal of debilitating distress for the afflicted person. Depression is characterized by a dejected mood, loss of desire to do things, general tiredness, and inability to concentrate. It can be a significant problem that seriously interferes with an individual's everyday functioning. With the intensification of a dejected mood, the individual often loses interest in the world and lacks the motivation and desire to get involved in tasks. The future looks bleak, and the person believes that nothing can be done to change this condition. Moreover, the depressed individual may experience crying spells; loss of appetite, weight, sleep, and sexual desire; and a desire to avoid people.

Nonpathological but generally negative psychological consequences of stress are not as severe or debilitating as these "clinical" consequences. However, decreases in problem-solving abilities, increases in general negativity, impatience, irritability, feelings of worthlessness, and emotionality may all accompany a stress response.

As we have already noted, stress can cause cognitive deficits as well as improved performance. Cognitive deficits may in turn be caused by behavioral strategies that are used for coping—we may "tune out" loud noise or narrow our field of attention (see Cohen, 1978; Deutsch, 1964). We may also be unable to concentrate or unwilling to put effort into a task (see Glass and Singer, 1972). At this level, response may become more specific to the stressor being experienced. Behavioral aspects of the stress response may reflect the specific causes of discomfort as the organism copes with the stressor.

Coping behavior seems to be related directly to characteristics of the source of stress. People may respond to crowding caused by a surplus of people by withdrawing and avoiding social contact, while they may respond to crowding caused by inadequate amounts of space by becoming aggressive (see Baum and Koman, 1976).

By the same token, they may respond actively to job loss if the loss was caused by a lack of effort rather than of ability, or under certain conditions they may become helpless. For example, response to being in a crippling accident appears to be specific to different levels of self-blame (see Bulman and Wortman, 1977). The type of strategy chosen for dealing with stress also seems to be related to the kind of problems confronted during exposure to a stressor.

Aftereffects, on the other hand, do not appear to be specific to certain stressors; they appear to reflect more general effects. Defined as consequences that are experienced after exposure to a stressor has terminated, these effects fit into Selye's (1976) notion of limited adaptive energy. As exposure to stress increases, the adaptive reserves are depleted, causing aftereffects and reductions of subsequent coping ability. Evidence for the existence of poststressor effects comes from a number of sources, including research on the effects of noise (see Glass and Singer, 1972; Rotton et al., 1978; Sherrod and Downs, 1974; Sherrod et al., 1977), crowding (Evans, 1979; Sherrod, 1974), and electric shock (Glass et al., 1973). However, explanations for these effects are not as clear.

Aftereffects that have been found to occur after exposure to a stressor include decreases in cognitive ability, reduced tolerance for frustration, aggressiveness, helplessness, decreased sensitivity to others, and withdrawal (Cohen, 1980). These postexposure consequences appear to be affected by perception of control during exposure to the stressor, with fewer aftereffects following experiences in which participants felt that they had control (Cohen, 1980). One explanation for this is that aftereffects are related to the amount of effort expended in coping with a stressor. Since perceived control appears to ease the difficulties posed by a stressor, it should reduce the effort needed to adapt and, therefore, reduce aftereffects. Thus costs of adaptation may be reflected by aftereffects, and we should expect to find them when people have successfully coped.

That aftereffects occur is fairly well established. Why they occur, however, is not as clearly understood. The notion of adaptive costs or depletion of adaptive reserves has not been firmly established (see Glass and Singer, 1972), and other explanations have received equivocal support. For example, some aftereffects may be maladaptive instances of persistent coping behavior. If someone is chronically exposed to a stressor and learns a coping response very well, he or she may automatically behave in this manner. This kind of habitual responding, regardless of whether the stressor is present, can lead to some of the aftereffects noted.

Psychological effects that linger or persist may also reflect consequences of adaptation. Calhoun (1967, 1970) has referred to refractory periods, in which an organism recovers from a bout with a stressor, as crucial to the effects of population density in animal populations. If recovery is interrupted by another encounter, increased stress-relevant problems are likely. Further, depletion of catecholamines in the brain as a result of severe or prolonged stress has been associated with death in studies using animals (see Weick, Ritter, and Ritter, 1980). Population density has also been associated with health in a number of settings. In one study, stress associated with population density appeared to contribute to death rates (Paulus, McCain, and Cox, 1978).

POSTTRAUMATIC STRESS

Posttraumatic stress disorder (PTSD) is a diagnostic category in the DSM-III (*Diagnostic and Statistical Manual of the American Psychiatric Association,* third edition) that includes several characteristics. First, an individual with PTSD has experienced a threat or event that is so severe and overwhelming as to be considered outside the range of normal human experience. These events are similar to Lazarus and Cohen's (1977) cataclysmic events and include war, torture, and disasters. Other events, such as rape, are comparable to Lazarus and Cohen's second category of powerful but more personal stressors and may also give rise to PTSD. Individuals diagnosed as having PTSD are highly responsive to stimuli that are reminiscent of the event that caused the problems, exhibit guilt about the event, show evidence of social withdrawal, and reexperience the event over and over in dreams, nightmares, and daydreams.

The fact that PTSD has become a diagnostic category only recently does not mean that it is new. It may well reflect a new name for an "old" ailment, as syndromes such as "shellshock," similar to PTSD, have been noted for centuries. Railroad accidents during the industrial revolution and after were associated with symptoms among victims that defied traditional medical explanation. Called railway spine because many thought that the symptoms were caused by microlesions of the spine sufferred in the accidents, this syndrome included inexplicable pain and weakness, psychological malaise, and general disability (see Trimble, 1981). Industrial accidents were also associated with these symptoms, and some argued that the problems victims experienced were psychological rather than physical.

One of the major proponents of the organic theory of these ailments was John Erichsen, who asserted that the symptoms observed in trauma victims were caused by molecular changes in the spinal cord due to concussion or twisting (Erichsen, 1882). Among the case studies presented was one in which a sixty-year-old man, traveling on a railroad, had one of his fingers crushed in the door of a car. The painful injury was treated, and the victim went home "faint and exhausted with the shock." There was contusion and laceration of the finger but the bones were not broken, and since the patient was in excellent health at the time, prognosis for recovery was good. However, within a month the victim lost a substantial amount of weight, "became weak and never seemed completely to rally from the shock that he had sustained." He developed shooting pain in his arm and began to twitch. Following this, he experienced fatigue, numbness, and spasms in parts of his body far removed from the original accident site. He quit his job, grew steadily worse, and, within eighteen months, he died. Erichsen (1882) concluded that the cause of death was damage to the nervous system spreading outward from the primary site of the injury.

Erichsen continued to write about injuries to the spinal cord and nervous system, but not everyone agreed with him, and, in 1883, Herbert Page, a London surgeon, rebutted his views about railway spine. Page argued that there was little evidence to support the organic bases of the diseases that Erichsen noted and that nervous shock was not a function of molecular disruptions of the spinal cord. In 1885 Page began to include psychological dimensions in his description of disorders following accidents, using fear and alarm to explain sequelae of these traumas. The horror of experiencing a railway accident was part or all of the syndrome (Trimble, 1981), and Page argued that "the medical literature abounds with cases where the gravest disturbances of function, and even death . . . have been produced by fright and by fright alone" (Trimble, 1981, p. 26). Over the next forty years the debate continued with new advocates of both positions entering into the argument. Twentieth-century warfare, however, was more influential in the debate than were the debaters' well-constructed positions, as war exposed people to new and unspeakable horrors.

However, the tendency to attribute unusual behavior and symptoms to organic causes persisted. During World War I, for example, cases of PTSD-like syndromes were referred to a shell shock because it was widely believed that the concussion of huge artillery shells used in that conflict caused central nervous system damage resulting in observed symptoms. Mott (1919) suggested that these symptoms were caused by physical damage to the brain caused by carbon monoxide or changes in air pressure. However, this did not explain cases of shock or distress among those not exposed to the exploding shells, and Southward (1919), in reviewing 589 cases from World War I, concluded that most were psychological in origin and not due to organic changes. Several researchers reported the same conclusions based on studies of World War II victims; they viewed the symptoms as part of a neuropsychoactive disorder (see Kardiner, 1941; Ross, 1941).

More recently recognition of the psychological effects of extreme stress and trauma has led to different views of the lingering or chronic consequences of these events. Vietnam veterans, for example, have been studied and treated for PTSD, and their seemingly high incidence of PTSD may have contributed to the evolution of PTSD as an independent diagnostic category. It is difficult to determine whether the Vietnam war generated more cases of post-traumatic stress than did previous ones because researchers and clinicians were more aware of it in the 1960s and 1970s than they had been before and were therefore more likely to find it. However, there are several aspects of the Vietnam conflict that could have made combat there more traumatic, difficult, or stressful.

In Vietnam, there were no battlelines as in previous wars, and progress was not measured as often in terms of territory gained as in body counts—how many of the enemy were killed. The nature of guerrilla warfare also mixes soldiers and civilians so that distinction between them is blurred. Civilians were frequently "combatants in disguise" and soldiers were forced to treat all or most as possible enemies. This led to atrocities, such as at My Lai, and to situations in which harmless-looking civilians were shot or arrested. The method by which individual tours of duty were determined may have resulted in emphasis on personal survival rather than group goals and could have undermined the cohesiveness of combat units. Finally, and perhaps most important, was the divisiveness in the United States and the lack of support given the war. Returning veterans were not usually treated like heroes, and in many cases they were victims of discrimination and objects of disdain. These events may have worked together to create an unusually severe stress response among some soldiers, resulting in disturbance and distress.

The issue of whether Vietnam was worse than other wars is not as important as are the causes and consequences of trauma during combat. Studies of Vietnam veterans many years after their experiences there have revealed persistent physiological response patterns much like those associated with stress. One study reported that PTSD patients exhibited substantially higher levels of epinephrine and norepinephrine in their urine than did other psychiatric inpatients, while another found evidence of lower levels of cortisol in PTSD patients than in patients with major depressive disorders and other inpatients (see Mason et al., 1986). Other studies have found that, among veterans with PTSD, sympathetic reactivity to events reminiscent of combat was greater than among control subjects (Blanchard et al., 1982; Brende, 1982; Malloy et al., 1983). Studies of disaster victims also reveal lasting stress symptoms associated with the posttraumatic stress syndrome including correlated reports of intrusive thoughts and dreams and levels of sympathetic arousal (Davidson and Baum, 1986). Psychological distress, including anxiety and depression, is also found in chronic stress situations, suggesting that PTSD may represent an extreme consequence of lasting stress caused by unusually severe stressors.

STRESS AND ILLNESS

Chapters 5, 6, and 7 are devoted to exploring the link between stress and illness, demonstrating the relationships among stress, behavior, and such illnesses as coronary heart disease and cancer and the links to psychophysiological disorders such as hypertension and hives. Research clearly indicates that behavioral factors and stress are involved in the development of many illnesses. Before turning to these points, basic issues in stress and illness will be considered.

MECHANISMS OF BEHAVIORAL INFLUENCE

Krantz et al. (1981) have classified behavioral links to illness into three basic mechanisms: direct psychophysiological effects, health-impairing habits, and reactions to illness.

The first is consistent with notions of stress, including all direct alterations of bodily processes and tissues by psychosocial events. Thus events such as stress can cause neural and endocrine change that alters the normal functioning of the organism (e.g., changing cardiovascular reactivity or immune system functioning). These physiological changes, in turn, cause illnesses ranging from coronary heart disease to gastrointestinal disorders and cancer. We have seen abundant evidence that stress can cause a number of physiological and biochemical changes. Now we shall see that some of these changes can be linked directly to illness.

The evidence for the second mechanism, the effects of habits or lifestyles, is also formidable. Cigarette smoking, diet, lack of exercise, coping styles, and other aspects of one's lifestyle have been linked to both physiological changes and the onset of illness.

The third mechanism is concerned primarily with behavioral factors that affect the treatment of illness. Reactions to illness, such as one's willingness to report symptoms or seek medical attention, obviously affect the course of an illness. If an individual fails to report noticeable changes in bodily function or delays reporting these changes, the likelihood of an illness progressing to a point where it is more difficult to treat will increase. In addition, response following diagnosis of disease is also important. Failure to follow treatment regimens or change lifestyles will usually retard recovery or cure.

In practice, the three mechanisms are difficult to separate completely and should not be thought of as exclusive or independent processes. Stress and the physiological effects that accompany it may be exacerbated or moderated by one's characteristic coping style or reaction to being ill. However, the distinctions among these mechanisms are important in explaining the ways in which behavioral factors can affect health and illness.

RESPONSE TO STRESS

Traditionally illness has been viewed as a biomedical phenomenon. Sickness is caused by germs or by some internal malfunction. Many health professionals have tended to assume that illness is simply a matter of biology and not affected or caused by what we do or how we respond to the demands of our environment. Yet there are a number of illnesses that do not fit the biomedical model—diseases caused, at least partly, by our behavior patterns and our psychological response to our surroundings. Hypertension and heart disease are not contagious; they do not seem to be caused by germs or pathogens. Rather, they develop over the course of a person's life and are apparently caused by a number of factors including diet, working habits, smoking, and response to stress. As Eliot and Buell (1981) have noted: "These disease states [coronary and hypertensive heart disease] appear to be the major epidemic afflictions of industrialized communities in the 20th century. Indeed, the prevalence of coronary heart disease and hypertension parallels the increasing complexity of social systems and social order whether we are speaking of animals or mankind" (p. 25).

The study of links between psychological factors and disease states is relatively new. However, research has already identified a number of relationships. In an attempt to include some psychosocial contributions to disease in the etiology of illness, researchers have devised the diathesis-stress model of illness (Levi, 1974). This model is a relatively simple statement of the ways in which psychosocial, environmental, genetic, and physiological elements should be considered in the description of disease. (See Figure 3.5.) All elements are *continually* interacting with one another. *Physiological predispositions* toward a certain illness (such as genetic weakness or biochemical imbalance), *psychosocial stimuli* (e.g., stress and how we respond to it), and previously experienced *environmental conditions* will jointly determine many disease states. Biological factors are still viewed as important, but other factors, including psychological variables, are also critical.

Research on the relationship between stress and illness has been conducted in several settings and at different levels. Early research on stress found that Londoners showed increased blood pressure during the initial phase of the mass bombing of London during World War II. The stress associated with incarceration in German concentration camps and prisoner-of-war camps was also studied. Survivors of concentration camp brutalities, for example, showed relatively permanent psychological adjustment problems and greater rates of physical illness than people of their

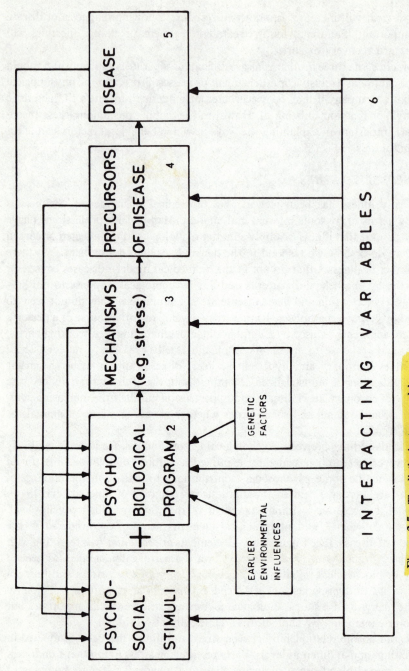

Figure 3.5   The diathesis-stress model. Based on A. R. Kagan and L. Levi. *Health and Environment—Psychosocial Stimuli.* Contribution to WHO document for the United Nations Conference on the Human Environment, Geneva, 1972. Reprinted with permission.

age who were not prisoners. Concentration camp survivors also showed a greater incidence of premature death in the years following their release (Bettelheim, 1960; Cohen, 1953). More recently, research has focused on the relationship between life change stress and illness.

LIFE CHANGE

A great deal of evidence of a stress-illness link has been provided by the study of life change or stressful life events. Research on life events is essentially concerned with correlating the frequency of change caused by different events and the onset of illness. The idea that such change could predispose illness is not new, but the study of life events is a fairly recent phenomenon, beginning in earnest with Holmes and Rahe's (1967) Schedule of Recent Experiences. This scale provided an extensive listing of events and changes that occur from time to time (see Table 3.1). (See Chapter 9 for further information on the SRE and other instruments.) Initially, respondents simply checked those events that had occurred in their lives in a given time period, and the number of events experienced was used as an index of life change for that period. Thus someone who had committed a misdemeanor, who had taken a vacation, and whose spouse had recently begun work was given a score of three, while someone who had gotten divorced and been fired from work received a score of two.

The problems with such a gross scoring method are obvious. Such a method indicates greater life change for the first person in the preceding example, while common sense suggests that change was greater for the second. Despite the fact that gross summation measures did show relationships to illness, numerous changes have been made. In some studies, weights—or relative degrees of life change caused by each event—were generated by panel ratings; other studies asked subjects to assign their own weights (see Holmes and Rahe, 1967; Rahe, 1975; Rahe et al., 1980).

Initial research using these scales was generally retrospective in nature. Subjects reviewed their experiences over a prior time period, and these recollections were translated into life change scores. These studies reported a consistent increase or clustering of life events causing change and requiring adjustment during the year preceding diagnosis of illnesses such as infectious disease, metabolic disturbance, and heart disease (see Garrity and Marx, 1979; Jacobs et al., 1970; Rahe, 1975). In a prospective study, Rahe, Mahan, and Arthur (1970) reported a linear relationship between life change and illness rates among enlisted men during six-month cruises aboard U.S. navy ships.

Other studies indicate that life change is associated with a wide range of behavioral and health outcomes, including accidents, academic performance, cardiovascular risk, drug use, and illness (see Bruns and Geist, 1984; Garrity and Ries, 1985; Rahe, 1987). There appears to be a great deal of evidence for the notion that life change and frequency of stressful life events are associated with the onset of illness.

To the extent that these measures reflect stress, stressful life event measures can predict illness. However, a number of major criticisms have led to attempts to devise alternative ways of assessing life events (see Dohrenwend and Dohrenwend, 1974; Rabkin and Struening, 1976; Sarason, de Monchaux, and Hunt, 1975).

TABLE 3.1   The Schedule of Recent Experiences

LIFE EVENT	VALUE
Death of spouse	100
Divorce	73
Marital separation	65
Jail term	63
Death of close family member	63
Personal injury or illness	53
Marriage	50
Fired at work	47
Marital reconciliation	45
Retirement	45
Change in health of family member	44
Pregnancy	40
Sex difficulties	39
Gain of new family member	39
Business readjustment	39
Change in financial state	38
Death of close friend	37
Change to different line of work	36
Change in number of arguments with spouse	35
Mortgage or loan for major purchase	31
Foreclosure of mortgage or loan	30
Change in responsibilities at work	29
Son or daughter leaving home	29
Trouble with in-laws	29
Outstanding personal achievement	28
Wife begins or stops work	26
Begin or end school	26
Change in living conditions	25
Revision of personal habits	24
Trouble with boss	23
Change in work hours or conditions	20
Change in residence	20
Change in schools	20
Change in recreation	19
Change in church activities	19
Change in social activities	18
Mortgage or loan for lesser purchase (car, TV, etc.)	17
Change in sleeping habits	16
Change in number of family get-togethers	15
Change in eating habits	15
Vacation	13
Christmas	12
Minor violations of the law	11

Adapted with permission from T. H. Holmes and R. H. Rahe. The social readjustment rating scale. *Journal of Psychosomatic Research,* vol. 11. Copyright © 1967, Pergamon Press, Ltd. See the original text for complete wording of the items.

Some have argued that individual ratings of events is important and that the many different aspects of life events should be considered. For example, Pilkonis, Imber, and Rubinsky (1985) reported a study that used both life events checklists and interviews to identify the characteristics of life events that are most important. They found three general factors: desirability of an event, control, and required readjustment. How positive an event was, how much control subjects felt that they had over an event, and how much effort was required to cope with the event were also important factors. Problems associated with recall ability, memory biases, reliability of measurement, and the frequent causal relationships among stressful life events must be considered (Hudgens, 1974; Rose, Hurst, and Jenkins, 1979).

The interaction of specific life events is a particularly important factor that is rarely considered. According to the values in Table 3.1, a divorce is rated 73 life change units and remarriage counts an additional 50 units. As a result, we could assume that an individual who is divorced and remarried within a year or so would have experienced substantial life change. However, for many people a quick remarriage may reduce the change or disruption caused by the divorce, canceling out some stress and making life less stressful. For others, the 123 life change unit sum might be more meaningful. Without assessment of individual perceptions and qualitative ratings of these kinds of events, problems like this will persist.

Debate over appropriate outcome measures has also characterized research on life events. The degree to which health measures are really that and not other stress measures will affect this kind of research since if a "health measure" is nothing more than a symptom of stress, predictive power is high and spurious (Schroeder and Costa, 1984). For example, one could interpret some of the life events listed in the table as effects of life events rather than events themselves. Are changes in sleeping or eating symptoms of stress or stressors? However, studies using a variety of measures have reinforced the belief that life events and health are linked. A study of naval submarine students examined the relationships between life events and both self-report and medically documented indices of health. Using a cross-lagged panel design, life events for two different periods of time were correlated with measures of health. Negative life events were associated with measures of health as self-report and medical record measures showed significant correlations with occurrence of events (Antoni, 1985).

Another study of the relationships between stress and illnesses was reported by Engel (1968). He found that illness was usually preceded by a stressful incident or other psychological disturbance. This was not true of all subjects, and illness was most likely to follow stress if the individual felt unable to cope successfully. Like Selye's state of exhaustion, failure to cope effectively can lead to complex "giving up–given up" symptoms. These include (1) helplessness, (2) reduced self-esteem, (3) a sense of isolation or loss of gratification from social relationships, (4) disruption, and (5) reactivation of memories so that the individual can retreat into the past. These fairly dramatic consequences of failure to cope are probably associated with long-term or major stressors that can exhaust our ability to cope. But they are seen as precursors to illness, contributors to the body's general susceptibility to disease. According to Engel (1968), this syndrome has led to disease in better than seven of every ten cases and has been noted by other researchers as a condition that reduces ability to cope with illness (see Schmale, 1958, 1972; Thurlow, 1967).

This research also suggests that failure to cope with stress and the helplessness that results from failure may have something to do with death. Although research has been inconsistent, it now appears that psychological stress does contribute to predisease and illness states such as coronary artery disease, hypertension, and gastrointestinal problems, and that disease may also be more likely when stress or conditioning impairs functioning of the immune system (Ader, 1981). Researchers are now trying to determine why some people are more resistant to the effects of stress than others and how specific illnesses are related to stress.

SUMMARY

Stress has been a topic of concern for centuries, and was formalized in the early twentieth century by Cannon (1914, 1928, 1929). The scientific study of stress was given further impetus by the work of Selye (1956, 1976). Additional theoretical refinements were provided by researchers such as Mason (1975, 1976) and Frankenhaeuser (1972), who emphasized psychological factors as important determinants of the experience of and response to stress.

The physiological stress response is rather well documented. Two different systems appear to be operative. In the first, stimulation of the sympathetic nervous system causes the adrenal medullae to secrete large quantities of catecholamines, neurotransmitter hormones that increase heart rate and other coronary activity, constrict blood vessels, inhibit gastrointestinal activity, and increase a number of other bodily functions. In the second, the pituitary gland secretes a hormone (ACTH) that stimulates the adrenal cortex to produce corticosteroids, particularly cortisol. Cortisol affects carbohydrate metabolism and is an antiinflammatory agent.

Sources of stress, or stressors, have been studied by many disciplines (particularly psychologists, epidemiologists, and sociologists). Lazarus and Cohen (1978) have considered three general classes of stressors: (1) cataclysmic phenomena; (2) powerful events that challenge adaptive abilities in the same way as cataclysmic events but affect fewer people; and (3) "daily hassles." On another level, the appraisal or interpretation of stressors has been considered, primarily by psychologists. The key issue at this level is whether or not the stressor will be perceived as threatening. Responses to stressors are determined by the extent to which the stressors are perceived as harmful, rather than by the objective danger (Lazarus, 1966). Lazarus and Launier (1978) have specified the following types of interpretations:

1. Harm or loss assessments involving analysis of damage that has already occurred.

2. Threat appraisals concerned with future dangers.

3. Challenge appraisals focused on the possibility of overcoming the stressor.

The final determination of the degree of harm or threat presented by a stressor will be affected by several mediating variables, such as attitudes toward the stressor, availability and extent of social support systems, and certain dispositional variables such as perceived control and coping styles.

The physiological response to stress is accompanied by behavioral responses as well. As noted by Lazarus, individuals may respond to stress with action directed toward the source of stress, or they may respond by palliative coping methods. Behavioral and psychological responses will be affected by factors such as the accuracy of expectations and individual susceptibility to stress (i.e., the "stress-prone personality") and can be accompanied by consequences such as anxiety, depression, increased symptom reporting, decreases in problem-solving abilities, and heightened aggressiveness.

Several points can be emphasized in relation to the organization of stress into source, transmission, and recipient levels. First, the three components are interactive. So, for example, recipients may engage in direct action to modify a stressful situation they perceived as threatening, or they may reappraise the nature of the situation such that it does not seem to be dangerous. Second, some stressors may be intense enough to override the recipients' coping mechanisms and produce a debilitating response despite resistance. Third, the influence of variables such as appraisal and coping is not limited solely to the time during which the stressor is actually present. For example, evaluation processes may begin well in advance, may be affected by the recipients' prior experience, and may influence evaluation of future stressors. Many of the effects of stress, particularly physiological ones, are similar whether the source of stress is psychological or physical. Although there are subtle differences in endocrine response among stressors, response to stress is, for the most part, nonspecific. Finally, it is not always possible to accurately identify the source of stress. In fact, some types of psychological anxiety may be viewed as psychological stress where the source cannot be clearly identified.

Stress and behavioral response to it can affect health and facilitate, if not cause, some illnesses. Stress has direct physiological effects on the body, and the cumulative wear and tear on the system caused by recurring stress can eventually cause damage to the system. Lifestyle and coping style are also important, partly because they help to determine the impact of stress and partly because they lead people to adopt habits which may predispose them to illness. Finally, the way in which people react to being ill is important.

RECOMMENDED READINGS

Baum, A., and Singer, J. E. (Eds.) *Handbook of psychology and health,* vol. 5, *Stress.* Hillsdale, N.J.: Erlbaum, 1987.

Cohen, S., and Syme, L. (Eds.) *Social Support and health.* New York: Academic Press, 1985.

Frankenhaeuser, M. Sympathetic-adrenomedullary activity, behaviour and the psychosocial environment. In P. H. Venables and M. J. Christie (Eds.), *Research in psychophysiology.* New York: Wiley, 1975.

Glass, D. C., and Singer, J. E. *Urban stress.* New York: Academic Press, 1972.

Selye, H. *The stress of life.* New York: McGraw-Hill, 1976.

4 CONTROL AND LEARNED HELPLESSNESS

||||||||||||||||||||||||||||||||||||||||||||||||||||||||||||||||||||||||||||||||||||||||||||||||||||||||||||||||||||||||||||||||

Control is an important mediator of stress. Research on both human and animal populations has clearly shown that being able to control a noxious event, believing that one can control the event, or perceiving that one can control other aspects of the environment can reduce the impact of a stressor. In this chapter we will consider control primarily as it relates to health and stress.

WHAT IS CONTROL?

On a general level, control means being able to determine what we do or what others do to us. Most of us will agree that it is important to have control and keep it. But why is control such an important motivator and such an influential determinant of our mood and behavior?

Control is one of the most basic processes in our daily interaction with our environment and other people. Kelley (1967) noted that people may spend a great deal of time and energy trying to explain how and why things happen as they do. This is done, according to Kelley, to achieve control over one's surroundings. White (1959) wrote about control as an intrinsically reinforcing goal that directs much of our behavior toward being able to predict and manipulate our surroundings. Having control is rewarding, regardless of whether it will make any difference in what happens. White (1959) referred to the desire for control as "effectance motivation" and thought of it as an innate need. Achievement of "efficacy"—a sense of control over the environment—was a pleasant state and therefore reinforcing. Bandura (1977) also implied some inherent gratification accompanying a sense of control. He describes self-efficacy as the belief that one can do what is necessary to get desired outcomes. Rodin, Rennert, and Solomon (1980) have indicated that control may be an inherent motivator not in all situations, but only in those where it *will actually make a difference*. If control will not really have much of an effect on what happens in a given situation, it will not be terribly important.

Regardless of whether control is inherently reinforcing, whether it is a primary or secondary drive, or whether it is valued solely for its instrumental value (i.e., value in helping achieve goals), it appears to be important to people. The desire to believe that we have control over things that happen and know how we will be affected by them, along with the tendency to interpret events as being under our control, is pervasive in our culture.

To some extent, these tendencies may cause us incorrectly to assume responsibility for events over which we actually have none. Most of us have, at one time or another, believed that our luck in a game of Monopoly was actually due to our skill at rolling the dice, or that something we did or did not do caused our favorite football team to lose. Mistakenly believing that an outcome was directly determined by us rather than by chance or other factors has been called the **illusion of control** (Langer, 1975). This illusion provides us with a sense of control (perceived control) when actual, objective control does not exist.

The illusion of control was noted in a study by Wortman (1975). Subjects were awarded prizes as a result of drawing marbles—different prizes were associated with different marbles. Some of the subjects were allowed to draw the marbles themselves, while others were not (the experimenter picked them). Despite the fact that the drawing was determined by chance in both cases, when subjects could link their behavior (drawing the marbles) to the prize they received, they reported more control over the situation. Langer (1975) found that in a lottery, the outcomes of which were clearly due to chance, subjects reported a greater sense of control when they had picked the ticket themselves or when they had been given information about the odds of winning.

Langer and Roth (1975) studied another chance-determined task: coin-tossing. They varied feedback to subjects as to their success in predicting the outcomes. All subjects experienced "wins"—they were told they were correct in their predictions—exactly half of the time. However, one group was given more success feedback during early trials and another group was given more failure feedback during early trials. A third group received random feedback, with no bias in early or late trials. Subjects who predicted many of the initial trials correctly felt that they had some ability for predicting each toss and that they therefore had some control over the situation.

These and other studies suggest that people tend to overestimate how much control they really have. There are a number of reasons for this. Most real-world events are complex and outcomes are usually determined jointly by chance and ability (Langer, 1975). As a result, it is often difficult to determine the real causes of an event. Reasons for attributing outcomes to chance (they are negative) or to ourselves (they are good) may determine attributions as much as the actual event does. If we can shift blame for something bad or accept responsibility for a desirable event and thereby bolster our self-esteem, we are likely to do so.

In addition, most of us believe that we exert control over the world around us. The extent of this perceived control may vary, but generally we all expect to be able to control some things. Often, attributing an outcome to one's ability rather than to external forces will reinforce this expectation. We may therefore overestimate our control over events in order to confirm our expectations and self-image (Einhorn and Hogarth, 1978).

This is not always the case, however. When people have had experience with an uncontrollable event, they may judge their ability to control events in the future more realistically. This appears to be true even if there is something to be gained from believing that one could control future outcomes. Parker, Brewer, and Spencer (1980) reported a study of residents in a California area that had been devastated by a brush fire. A year later, victims who had decided to rebuild rather than relocate reported that they would have less control over the outcome of another fire than did a group of people who had not been affected by the fire.

Corah and Boffa (1970) examined another aspect of control—*choice*—as it affects stress reduction among human subjects. Subjects were exposed to loud bursts of noise. Members of one group were told how they could, if they desired, escape the noise. The others were also given either escape or no-escape instructions, but they were not told that they could choose between escaping and not escaping. Several measures were used to assess the stress response in the subjects. Overall, subjects who were given a choice showed somewhat less stress—less discomfort and lower skin conductance readings—than did no-choice subjects. Corah and Boffa suggest that the perception of control provided by having been given a choice influenced appraisal of threat and reduced arousal associated with stress.

Geer, Davison, and Gatchel (1970) also found that the perception of control over aversive events reduces stress whether or not control is real. During the first part of a study, subjects performed a reaction time task in which they received shocks. During the second half of the session, half the subjects were told that if they could reduce their reaction time (improve performance on the task), the length of each shock would be halved. These subjects, then, were given a way of reducing (controlling) the shock. The others were told only that during the second part of the study, all shock durations would be halved. No control was suggested. Thus *all* subjects were given the same shock reductions, regardless of performance. Those who believed that they had earned these reductions and that their performance had reduced the shocks showed less arousal (less skin conductance and fewer spontaneous skin conductance fluctuations) than did the no-control group. The perception of control over aversive events, even when outcomes were the same, reduced arousal.

Control, then, refers to our *real* or *perceived* ability to determine outcomes of an event. When our behavior is perceived as causally linked to outcomes—there is response-outcome contingency—perceptions of control are possible. When outcomes cannot be tied to behavior—they are noncontingent—it is more difficult to believe that we are in control.

Much of the recent interest in control has dealt with two issues: (1) the effects of believing that one has control and that outcomes are contingent on responses and (2) the effects of believing that outcomes are not contingent on behavior and are therefore not controllable. The first has been concerned most directly with the mediating effects of perceived control on response to aversive stimulation and stress. The second has been concerned with learned helplessness and the debilitating effects of believing that one cannot control what happens.

CONTROL AND STRESS

Control appears to be an effective mediator of exposure to aversive stimulation. Whether it is perceived or real, useful or not, it seems to make a difference in the ways people respond to stress. A number of studies on both human and animal subjects have demonstrated this pattern.

THE EXECUTIVE MONKEY

One of the first major studies considering the impact of control on health-relevant outcomes found evidence contrary to the view that control reduces the impact of stress. Brady and his associates (see Brady, 1958; Porter et al., 1958) found that shock delivered over a fairly long period of time was associated with increased incidence of gastric ulcer in monkeys. The pattern of their data suggested that much of the lesioning of the gastrointestinal tract occurred during rest, when shocks were not being delivered. This indicated to them that human executives who are responsible for serious decisions—who have control *and* responsibility—might also show increased incidence of ulcers. In order to test this notion, Brady et al. (1958) designed a study that placed monkeys in situations analogous to those experienced by executives—hence the popular reference to the study as the "executive monkey" study.

As part of an avoidance task, pairs of monkeys were exposed to shock. One monkey in each pair, designated as "executive," was able to avoid the shock for both in the pair. The other monkey was yoked to the executive and could do nothing to affect the shock. Both received shock in the same intensities and frequencies; the only difference between them was in ability to avoid (control) the shock.

The executives were quite good at learning to avoid the shock, and the number received by the animals was thus kept low. Yet, within two months of their having been studied, all of the executives had either died or become so incapacitated that they had to be sacrificed. Equally surprising was the finding that these executives had developed extensive gastric ulceration. Autopsies of sacrificed monkeys who had no control but who had received the same shock showed little if any lesioning. Apparently the control and responsibility associated with the executive role *increased* rather than decreased stress-related illness. One interpretation of this result was that the need to be constantly vigilant increased stress for the executives.

Subsequent work by Weiss (1968; 1971) suggested that the results obtained by Brady et al. were artifactual—caused by sampling error rather than by control or hypervigilance. The executive for each pair in the study was initially selected on a speed-of-learning basis. The monkey that learned the avoidance response first was made executive, and its slower colleague was placed in the uncontrollable condition. Unfortunately, research suggests that more emotional monkeys learn this response fastest, and as a result, the executive group was also a more emotional group (see Weiss, 1968; Weiss and Miller, 1971). Since heightened emotional reactivity can be linked to increased susceptibility to stress and therefore the development of ulcers, control may not have been responsible for the executives' demise.

Research by Weiss (1968) has provided evidence that control reduces the impact of stress. In a situation similar to the one employed with monkeys, Weiss used rats in a three-group design to provide an additional control condition. Rats were considered in threes—one was the executive and could avoid the shock; a second was yoked to the executive and received equivalent shock with no ability to avoid it; and a third was not exposed to shock at all. The sampling error was eliminated and results were directly opposite those obtained with the monkeys. Rats who received shock over which they had no control suffered more severe somatic consequences of stress than did the executives. Both groups, however, showed more deterioration than did the no-shock controls. The ability to avoid the shocks did not completely neutralize stress in this setting.

These results indicated that the opportunity to control an aversive event is an important determinant of the response to a stressful situation. Predictability, a form of control, has been shown to have similar effects on stress in animals. Again using a three-group design, Weiss exposed rats to unpredictable, predictable, or no-shock conditions and found that unpredictable shock was associated with increased corticosteroid production and gastric ulceration as compared with predictable or no-shock treatments.

CONTROL AND PHYSIOLOGICAL RESPONSE

The effects of control in stressful occupational settings have also been addressed by several studies conducted by Frankenhaeuser and her colleagues at the University of Stockholm (see Frankenhaeuser and Gardell 1976; Frankenhaeuser and Johansson, 1982). Those workers whose jobs were self-paced—that is, those who could determine how fast and/or when they did their assigned tasks—showed fewer symptoms of stress than did workers whose jobs were machine-paced or otherwise determined for them. The degree to which the job was under workers' control was related to excretion of catecholamines and self-reported distress. Other evidence of control-related psychoendocrine response patterns has been reported in studies of monkey and human subjects (see Mason, 1975; Mason, Brady, and Tolson, 1966; Mason et al., 1965). Situations involving uncertainty, unpredictability, and/or ambiguity were associated with different patterns of catecholamine and corticosteroid excretion. The Pattern II response, apparently generated by uncertainty, involved increased excretion of epinephrine, norepinephrine, and cortisol, while the Pattern I response, associated with greater predictability, showed no change in epinephrine levels but increases in the other two hormones.

The controllability of a stressor also affects corticosteroid release during stress. Studies have suggested that corticosteroid elevations during stress are greater when the stressor is uncontrollable or inescapable than when it can be avoided or terminated, but these differences do not appear to be very large (see, Maier, Laudenslager, and Ryan, 1985). In addition, it has been reported that corticosteroid levels decline more slowly after inescapable or uncontrollable shock than after shock that is controllable (Swenson and Vogel, 1983).

Another endocrine response during stress that appears to be influenced by control is the release of endogenous opioid peptides such as beta-endorphin. As Maier and his colleagues (1985) note, the major finding regarding these relationships is that learning that one has no control over a situation leads to opioid release.

Inescapable shock produced an opiate-based analgesia while escapable shock did not (Jackson, Loon, and Maier, 1979). Further, while both controllable and uncontrollable stressors appear to produce brief poststressor analgesia, only that produced by inescapable stressors can be eliminated by administering opiate antagonists such as naloxone (see Hyson et al., 1982). Thus there appear to be two different types of analgesia after stress experience; only one is based on endogenous opiate activity, and that type is more likely to be produced by uncontrollable stressors (Maier, et al., 1983).

Control also appears to be important in the effects of stress on immunity. One study found that rats exposed to escapable shock exhibited a stronger immune response to mitogen stimulation than did rats exposed to inescapable shock (Laudenslager et al., 1983). In another study by Maier, Laudenslager, and Ryan (1985), natural killer cell activity was evaluated in light of the controllability of stress. Rats were exposed to escapable or inescapable shock, and the ability of natural killer cells to kill targets was measured. Both stressor conditions reduced the cytotoxicity of natural killer cells, but inescapable stress resulted in greater suppression than did escapable stress.

PERCEIVED CONTROL OVER AVERSIVE STIMULATION

A number of studies have examined the effects of perceived control over delivery of electric shock or negative outcomes. Early studies with both human and animal subjects suggested that self-administration of shock was associated with fewer symptoms of arousal or disruption than was shock administered by others (see Haggard, 1946; Mower and Viek, 1948). Pervin (1963) also found evidence of this by measuring subject preferences for self-delivered versus experimenter-delivered shocks. Not surprisingly, self-administered shock was preferred even though the intensity and duration of shocks to be delivered were the same. Similar evidence of preference for, or reduced arousal under, self-administration of shock has been provided by other studies (see Le Panto, Moroney, and Zenhausem, 1965; Staub, Tursky, and Schwartz, 1971).

These studies are interesting because the perception of control offered by self-administration appears to be illusory. Regardless of who administered shock, in most of these studies shock was experienced. Escape was not possible. Other studies deal with less imaginary forms of perceived control. Ability to terminate an aversive situation or to control the way in which it occurs also appears to reduce the negative effects of aversive conditions (see Corah and Boffa, 1970; Stotland and Blumenthal, 1964).

Against this backdrop, a number of investigators have, during the past decade, studied the effects of perceived control on mood and the consequences of stress (see Glass and Levy, 1982). Among the first programmatic investigations of this subject was the research conducted by David C. Glass and Jerome E. Singer during the late 1960s and early 1970s. Initially interested in noise as a stressor, Glass and Singer (1972) set out to document the physiological and behavioral consequences of exposure to bursts of loud, unwanted sound. Two noise tapes were used in most of their experiments. One, with fixed intermittent bursts, presented noise to subjects at the same point in every minute. Thus a subject listening to the fixed intermittent tape heard nine-second bursts of noise about sixty seconds apart. The occurrence of each burst was predictable. The second basic tape used varying intervals between bursts of noise and also varied the length of each burst. This random, intermittent delivery of noise was not easily predicted—noise was heard at different times throughout each of the twenty to twenty-five minutes of the study, and each burst varied. The noise used was recorded at 108 decibels, about what one would hear "if operating a riveting machine." No-noise conditions were measured at approximately 40 decibels.

In an early study, Glass and Singer measured autonomic reactivity to exposure to noise as well as effects of the noise on task performance. Subjects reported to a laboratory and were exposed to either loud (108 dBA), soft (50 dBA), or no-noise (40 dBA) conditions. In the noise conditions, half of the subjects were exposed to the predictable fixed intermittent tape and half to the unpredictable noise tape.

Skin conductance readings showed that initially loud noise was associated with greater arousal than soft or no noise regardless of its predictability. However, as the experiment wore on, these differences disappeared; apparently subjects habituated quite quickly to the noise. By the end of the experimental session, there were no differences in skin conductance among the five treatment conditions. These findings were replicated, extended to other measures (e.g., constriction of peripheral blood vessels), and found for different age groups. They clearly indicated that physiological response to the noise diminished as the session progressed. In one of these studies, however, physiological response was greater for subjects exposed to loud, uncontrollable noise than for any others. This difference held through the end of the session, indicating that not all effects habituate so quickly.

Glass and Singer also considered the effects of noise on task performance. Three standardized tests were administered during exposure to the noise. Subjects worked on fairly simple tasks that required concentration. As with physiological measures, whatever performance effects of noise appeared early in the session (and these effects were small) had disappeared by the end. Noise did not produce task performance deficits. A subsequent study (Finkelman and Glass, 1970) indicated that when overloaded by a second task during noise exposure, subjects exposed to unpredictable noise showed poorer performance than did subjects exposed to predictable noise. By and large, however, initial investigations suggested that noise by itself did not appear to have major effects on physiological responding or task performance.

This pattern of results was very different when aftereffects were examined. As you will recall from Chapter 3, aftereffects refer to changes in behavior or performance that appear after the termination of a stressor. Glass and Singer found few effects of noise during its administration, but when performance on tasks *after* the noise exposure was considered, more consistent effects appeared. Two types of postnoise tasks were administered. In one, subjects' tolerance for frustration and persistence was measured by asking subjects to solve unsolvable puzzles. In the other, concentration abilities were tapped by having subjects work on a proofreading task—reading a passage to find errors that had been inserted.

Several studies were conducted, comparing loud and soft noise and predictable and unpredictable noise to no-noise conditions. Results of these studies indicated that performance after termination of the noise was affected by the predictability of the noise. When it was delivered in varying length bursts and at random times, the noise had greater consequences for task performance than when it was predictable. This held for both tasks: subjects in unpredictable noise conditions were less persistent (spent less time on the unsolvable puzzles) than were subjects in predictable noise or no-noise conditions, and proofreading errors increased for unpredictable noise subjects relative to the predictable noise or no-noise controls.

Generally, the intensity of the noise did not affect these results. Soft, unpredictable noise produced effects much like those of the loud, unpredictable noise and quite different from those of the other conditions. It appeared, therefore, that the effects produced after termination of noise delivery were primarily related to the degree to which bursts could be predicted accurately.

In order to understand their results more adequately, Glass and Singer also examined the effects of a more direct manipulation of perceived control. In a study reported by Glass, Singer, and Friedman (1969), subjects were exposed only to unpredictable noise. Half were given the same treatments as before, while the others were led to believe that they could shut the noise off if they so desired. The subjects in this perceived control group were told about a switch on the arm of their chair that, if thrown, would stop the noise for the remainder of the session. Subjects were urged not to end the noise unless it was absolutely necessary, but were told that they could terminate the noise if they wished. The perception of control over the noise was successful in reducing performance decrements following the noise. The belief that subjects could terminate the noise was associated with more persistence on the unsolvable puzzles and better proofreading scores than was exposure to the noise without perceived control (see Figure 4.1).

In an elegant series of replications, Glass and Singer consistently found the same results. In explaining these findings, they referred to the fact that a lack of control

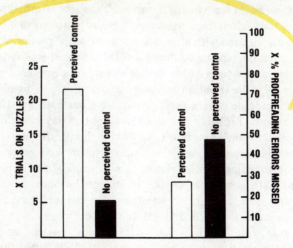

Figure 4.1   Perceived control over noise resulted in more persistence on the puzzles and in fewer proofreading errors than did the absence of control.

Based on D. C. Glass and J. E. Singer. *Urban Stress.* New York: Academic Press, 1972. Copyright © 1972 by Academic Press, Inc., and adapted with permission.

over stress could induce a form of helplessness that suppressed performance. Exposure to uncontrollable and unpredictable noise appeared to induce helplessness, reduce effort on subsequent tasks, and cause poorer performance relative to exposure to controllable noise.

Among the replications of this effect were variations in the stressor. Electric shock that was controllable or uncontrollable produced effects similar to those associated with noise. Further, social stressors appeared to cause the same problems. One study examined a bureaucratic encounter—subjects reporting for the experiment were sent first to the Psychology Department's administrative assistant to complete some forms. Upon arriving, subjects were told that each subject in psychology experiments was required to complete a demographic questionnaire. In one condition—no harassment—subjects were given a questionnaire with all but a few items crossed out. In the other conditions, subjects were given a longer questionnaire. Many of the questions on this lengthier version were repetitious, and inadequate space for answers made completion of the form difficult.

In both conditions involving the longer questionnaire, subjects were told that they had to redo their questionnaires after they had completed them. Further, when they had completed them a second time, they were delayed by a phone call that kept the administrative assistant busy for several minutes. Half of these subjects, however, were given a "regulations responsible" reason for having to redo the forms (the rules of the department required it), while the other half were led to believe that they had to redo the forms because the assistant "did not like the way they had done them." In addition, the nature of the phone call varied; subjects who were told that regulations required redoing the forms overheard a business call, while the others overheard a personal call.

In this way, a no-harassment condition was compared with harassment attributable either to the personal whims of the administrative assistant or to "red tape." After the questionnaires were finally completed, subjects returned to the laboratory and worked on three aftereffects measures. Results indicated that both harassment conditions were associated with aftereffects relative to the no-harassment condition, but that the pattern of responses differed according to the perceived cause of harassment. In the regulations-responsible condition, subjects discovered quickly that they had no control over the situation and showed more signs of helplessness than did others. In the condition where the subjects were harassed by the administrative assistant, control was probably perceived initially but was lost through ineffectual dealings with the assistant. As a result, subjects in this condition were more negative and made attempts to gain control in postharassment settings.

Loss of control has also been viewed as a determinant of stress resulting from social conditions. In a series of studies in college dormitories, Baum and Valins (1977) found that some dormitory designs placed students in residential settings that made control over social contact difficult. In these environments, small local groups did not form readily, interaction with neighbors was frequent, and residents complained about a great deal of unwanted contact. Apparently these students experienced difficulty in regulating when, where, and with whom they interacted. This loss of control over social experience was associated with withdrawal, negative affect, and a limited form of learned helplessness. The effects of prolonged exposure to uncontrollable events on the motivation to assume control over situations outside of the dormitories reflect the consequences of loss of control.

The importance of control in mediating between environmental threats and demands on the one hand and our health on the other is also suggested by research linking controllability of stressors to diseases such as cancer. As we shall see in Chapter 6, a number of behavioral factors appear to be related to cancer, and as Visintainer and Seligman (1983) note, there is substantial anecdotal evidence linking cancer with lack of control. In a study reported in Seligman and Visintainer (1985), rats were injected with live tumor cells and then put through procedures similar to Weiss' (1968) studies (one escapable stress group; one yoked, inescapable group; and one no-shock control group). With the type of cancer cells used, rats who developed the tumor should have died within two months. Rats exposed to the inescapable condition were more likely to develop tumors and die than were rats in the other two conditions. These differences were not small, as about 73 percent of those in the inescapable condition developed tumors while only half of the animals in the other conditions succumbed.

In order to examine long-term loss of control and the effects of early and adult experience with controllable and uncontrollable stress, a study was done that exposed animals to escapable, inescapable, or no-shock conditions at an early age and/or later in life (Seligman and Visintainer, 1985). Within one month of birth, rats were exposed to one of the three conditions, using shock as a stressor. Each animal received four sessions of training, with escapable-condition animals yoked to inescapable-condition animals to assure comparable numbers of shocks. Then, when the rats were ninety days old, all were injected with tumor cells and then randomly assigned to "retraining" as adults: a third of each previous group (escapable, inescapable, no shock as young rats) was given adult experience with escapable, inescapable, or no-shock. In this way, the effects of helplessness training during childhood, as adults, or both together were evaluated.

Table 4.1 presents the percentage of animals that rejected tumors or inhibited their growth in each combination of conditions. Early helplessness training alone seemed to have little effect on adult tumor rejection, as about half of each group receiving no adult shock training did not develop tumors. Escapable shock during early experience appeared to enhance immune defense against tumors regardless of adult experience. Inescapable shock was associated with poorer results. When young rats were exposed to uncontrollable shock and then to either escapable or inescapable shock as adults, the rejection rate was much lower than for other animals. This was also true for animals given no shocks during early experience but inescapable shocks as adults.

Thus early helplessness is important in determining tumor growth when uncontrollable events also occur during adulthood, and it seems to affect tumor growth when controllable events are experienced by adults as well. Only when no shocks were encountered as adults were the effects of early exposure to uncontrollable shock eliminated. Conversely, early experience with controllable shock seemed to protect the animals later—when these animals were exposed to either controllable or uncontrollable shock as adults, tumor rejection was higher than in any other conditions. Childhood experience that suggests that the world is controllable appears to "immu-

TABLE 4.1 Childhood and Adult Experience with Controllable and Uncontrollable Stress Affected Tumor Rejection

		EARLY EXPERIENCE		
		Escapable shock (%)	Inescapable shock (%)	No shock (%)
ADULT EXPERIENCE	Escapable shock (%)	65	30	52
	Inescapable shock (%)	70	26	27
	No shock (%)	48	57	51

From M. E. P. Seligman and M. A. Visintainer. Tumor rejection and early experience of uncontrollable shock in the rat. In F. R. Brush and J. B. Overmier (Eds.), *Affect Conditioning and Cognition: Essays on the Determinants of Behavior.* Hillsdale, N.J.: Erlbaum, 1985.

nize" animals to the effects of adult stress but has no effects when adult experience is stress-free (Seligman and Visintainer, 1985).

LEARNED HELPLESSNESS

What happens when control is not available—when we cannot, under any conditions, gain some sense of control over what happens to us? Work by Seligman (1975) and others suggests that if this response-outcome independence is prolonged, we may learn that we cannot affect outcomes and cease trying to do so. Repeated exposure to uncontrollable events "conditions" us to expect responses and outcomes to be noncontingent, and the reaction that this produces has been called **learned helplessness.**

We all know what helplessness is—the feeling that we cannot do anything, that everything we try to do ends up as failure. This state of low motivation and negative feelings is not new. Psychologists have long been aware that when an individual repeatedly fails to accomplish a goal or exert control effectively over something, he or she not only may stop trying in that setting but also may become unresponsive in new environments where success might be more readily achieved. Beyond the helplessness present in the setting where failure occurred, Seligman (1975) posited that people can *learn to be helpless*—that is, learn that their attempts to control or succeed will not be successful.

According to Seligman (1975), the primary cause of learned helplessness is the recognition that response and outcome are independent—that the probability of achieving a given outcome is the same whether or not responses are made. Once repeated exposure to uncontrollable events has caused the organism to learn that the outcomes cannot be affected, responding ceases.

As an example, consider a common procedure used for experimentally inducing learned helplessness. You are in a situation in which aversive stimulation (e.g., noise, electric shock) is being administered. The stimulation is completely unavoidable; although there are a number of buttons and levers for you to push, nothing you do prevents the noise or shock from being delivered. After several trials, you learn that there is nothing you can do to change the outcomes of each trial and you stop trying. For the remainder of the session, you passively accept the noxious stimulation.

It is not surprising that you would stop trying to control the noise or shock in such a situation. What is surprising, and of potentially greater harm, is the fact that this passivity tends to generalize to other settings. One experience with uncontrollable events appears to affect motivation and cognitive ability in other settings as well as in the situation in which it was first learned.

EFFECTS OF LEARNED HELPLESSNESS

Seligman and his associates have conducted a great deal of research on the learned helplessness phenomenon. Early work with animals showed that trauma or lack of control can have serious behavioral consequences. Defined as a noncontingent relationship between response and outcome (the outcome does not depend upon the response—the chances of something happening are independent of what the subject does), loss or lack of control was associated with passivity in dogs (see Overmier and Seligman, 1967; Seligman, Maier, and Geer, 1968). Typical of these studies was a situation in which a dog was given unavoidable electric shocks while confined in a harness. This uncontrollable trauma was followed by a test phase in which the dog was placed in a two-chambered cell and electric shocks were again administered. In this second phase, however, the dog could control the trauma, since it could escape the shock by jumping into the other chamber. Usually dogs exposed to uncontrollable shock did not learn this escape behavior, remaining passive and continuing to endure the shock.

This kind of helplessness conditioning, where learning of an inability to affect outcomes occurs, has also been explored with human subjects. These studies have largely been conducted in the laboratory and, as a result, may not be indicative of true helplessness conditioning. However, research has demonstrated that real-world helplessness conditioning may occur in crowded situations (Baum, Aiello, and Calesnick, 1978; Rodin, 1976). These studies have found evidence of motivational loss, emotional disturbance, and cognitive impairment as a function of repeated exposure to an uncontrollable situation. Hiroto and Seligman (1975) and Krantz, Glass, and Snyder (1974) conducted studies in which human subjects were placed in settings analogous to the training situations used to study dogs. Subjects were exposed to controllable or uncontrollable noise. In subsequent test phases, where all subjects could control the noise, those who had been exposed to controllable noise in the first part of the study quickly learned to control it in the second. Subjects exposed to uncontrollable noise initially were unable to solve the situation and learn to control the noise; most of them sat passively while the noise continued (Seligman,

1975). Glass and Singer (1972) also reported evidence of helplessness as a result of exposure to uncontrollable noise. Subjects were less persistent on unsolvable puzzles when they had been exposed to uncontrollable or unpredictable noise.

A number of studies have addressed whether effects of noncontingencies are similar for animals and humans. Fosco and Geer (1971) studied subjects who experienced varying amounts of helplessness training. They were exposed to zero, three, six, or nine unsolvable button-pushing problems. When they made an error, they received a shock; when they were correct, they avoided shock. Clearly shock was unavoidable, since there could be no correct solutions. If helplessness affected people as it did animals, exposure to increasing numbers of uncontrollable (unsolvable tasks) would be associated with poorer performance. Results indicated more errors on subsequent tasks as prior experience with uncontrollable aversive stimuli increased.

In order to study learned helplessness in humans, Hiroto (1974) used a triadic design similar to those used with animal subjects. Subjects were exposed first to inescapable noise and then to situations in which escape was possible. Results of the experiment indicated that subjects exposed to inescapable noise took longer to respond, failed to escape more often, and took longer to learn how to escape noise in the second task than did escapable-noise and no-noise groups. In addition, the inescapable-noise subjects who had been told that the second task was random showed greater deficits than did those who had been told that the second task was a skill task.

Hiroto (1974) also considered the differences in response to uncontrollable events between subjects with internal and external locus of control. Externals, who believe that they do not generally control what happens to them, appeared to be more helpless than internals, whose expectations of control were stronger. Cohen, Rothbart, and Phillips (1976) also studied the relation of locus of control and sought to determine the degree to which learned helplessness generalized to a variety of cognitive tasks. Internals and externals were asked to work on solvable or unsolvable tasks; then they were moved to another room and asked to work on a "test" task requiring concentration rather than solution. A persistence-frustration tolerance task was also administered.

Cohen et al. did not find any differences for locus of control in this experiment, but subjects given unsolvable pretreatment puzzles (they were exposed to uncontrollable events) appeared to be more helpless than those exposed to solvable pretreatment. They did not persist as long on the frustration task and took longer to solve those tasks that could be solved.

Other studies have shown that conditioned helplessness can undermine response initiation and cause cognitive deficits or interference with subsequent learning. Findings indicating impaired performance on problem-solving tasks (see Miller and Seligman, 1975; Hiroto and Seligman, 1975) suggest that exposure to noncontingent outcomes makes determining new responses more difficult and learning more lengthy and less successful.

Most of these studies considered fairly unimportant aspects of people's lives. Games, puzzles, and problems presented in the laboratory are the kinds of measures typically used to assess helplessness. The fact that a person does not try to solve a puzzle in the laboratory does not mean that he or she is truly helpless. Perhaps he or she is simply more discriminating. As a result of exposure to an uncontrollable situation, a subject may decide that he or she has better things on which to expend energy. This problem is further highlighted by a finding reported by Hiroto and Seligman (1975). When the test-phase task was described as important (a test of skill), subjects exposed to noise were less helpless than when the task was described as unimportant (chance-determined). More research needs to be conducted to determine whether helplessness can have serious effects on people in real settings. There are case studies that suggest that helplessness can have serious consequences (see boxes in this chapter), and data collected by Baum, Aiello, and Davis (1979) indicate that helplessness may interfere with consulting of physicians and may heighten sensitivity to symptoms. Research at the Los Angeles International Airport has similarly suggested that aircraft noise is associated with helplessness and health among children (see Cohen et al., 1986).

Research on relocation of the elderly has begun to show some real effects of control and helplessness. When older people are moved from familiar surroundings to unfamiliar ones, especially institutions, negative consequences are common. The more similar the old and new environments are, the less severe these consequences tend to be. Research suggests, for example, that patients live longer when the new environments are like the old ones (Schulz and Akerman, 1973; Shrut, 1965).

One of the biggest problems in putting elderly patients into nursing homes or hospitals is that they lose their sense of control over their surroundings. If the new environment is similar to the old one, it will be more predictable and, as a result, will seem more controllable (Schulz and Brenner, 1977). Further, if steps are taken to provide a greater sense of control over a new environment, such as making people responsible for some aspect of it or providing them with information about it, helplessness appears to be minimized and health improved (see Krantz and Schulz, 1980; Langer and Rodin, 1976; Rodin and Langer, 1977).

Seligman has argued that learned helplessness may also be associated with depression. He draws a number of parallels between helplessness and depression and argues that since the kinds of events that produce depression are similar to those that cause helplessness, the two may be linked. Both are characterized by *passive behavior, negative expectations* ("I won't be able to do this"), and *hopelessness.* Seligman believes that helplessness may, in fact, be one basis for depression. Generally depressed people have failed on a number of occasions—they may have lost a job, experienced rejection, or lost control over their lives. This kind of learning history could easily result in a conditioned helplessness as well as a depressed mood. Thus helplessness training may contribute to the development of depression.

Although links between helplessness and depression do appear to exist, the relationship is far more complex than research initially suggested. A great deal of work by Seligman (1975) and others (Beck, 1976; Cohen and Tennen, 1985; Peterson, Rosenbaum, and Conn, 1985; Rizley, 1978) has indicated some degree of relatedness, and a number of reformulations of helplessness theory have appeared to allow incorporation of some of the known cognitive determinants of depression. Klein and Seligman (1976) compared depressed subjects with nondepressed subjects. Subjects were pretreated with escapable-, inescapable-, or no-noise conditions. Following experience with noise, they were presented with solvable problems. Performance on the second task was poorer for nondepressed subjects when noise was

‖‖

CASE EXAMPLE: HOPELESSNESS AND DEATH

When, in early 1973, medical army officer Major F. Harold Kushner returned from five and a half years as a prisoner of war in South Vietnam, he told me a stark and chilling tale. His story represents one of the few cases on record in which a trained medical observer witnessed from start to finish what I can only call death from helplessness.

Major Kushner was shot down in a helicopter in North Vietnam in November 1967. He was captured, seriously wounded, by the Viet Cong. He spent the next three years in a hell called First Camp. Through the camp passed 27 Americans: 5 were released by the Viet Cong, 10 died in the camp, and 12 survived to be released from Hanoi in 1973. The camp's conditions beggar description. At any time there were about eleven men who lived in a bamboo hut, sleeping on one crowded bamboo bed about sixteen feet across. The basic diet was three small cups of red, rotten, vermin-infested rice a day. Within the first year the average prisoner lost 40 to 50 percent of his body weight, and acquired running sores and atrophied muscles. There were two prominent killers: malnutrition and helplessness. When Kushner was first captured, he was asked to make antiwar statements. He said that he would rather die, and his captor responded with words Kushner remembered every day of his captivity: "Dying is easy; it's living that's hard." The will to live, and the catastrophic consequences of the loss of hope, are the theme of Kushner's story. . . .

When Major Kushner arrived at First Camp in January 1968, Robert had already been captive for two years. He was a rugged and intelligent corporal from a crack marine unit, austere, stoic, and oblivious to pain and suffering. He was 24 years old and had been trained as a parachutist and a scuba diver. Like the rest of the men, he was down to a weight of ninety pounds and was forced to make long, shoeless treks daily with ninety pounds of manioc root on his back. He never griped. "Grit your teeth and tighten your belt," he used to repeat. Despite malnutrition and a terrible skin disease, he remained in very good physical and mental health. The cause of his relatively fine shape was clear to Kushner. Robert was convinced that he would soon be released. The Viet Cong had made it a practice to release, as examples, a few men who had co-operated with them and adopted the correct attitudes. Robert had done so, and the camp commander had indicated that he was next in line for release, to come in six months.

As expected, six months later, the event occurred that had preceded these token releases in the past. A very high-ranking Viet Cong cadre appeared to give the prisoners a political course; it was understood that the outstanding pupil would be released. Robert was chosen as leader of the thought-reform group. He made the statements required and was told to expect release within the month.

The month came and went, and he began to sense a change in the guards' attitude toward him. Finally it dawned on him that he had been deceived—that he had already served his captors' purpose, and he wasn't going to be released. He stopped working and showed signs of severe depression: he refused food and lay on his bed in a fetal position, sucking his thumb. His fellow prisoners tried to bring him around. They hugged him, babied him, and, when this didn't work, tried to bring him out of his stupor with their fists. He defecated and urinated in the bed. After a few weeks, it was apparent to Kushner that Robert was moribund: although otherwise his gross physical shape was still better than most of the others, he was dusky and cyanotic.

In the early hours of a November morning he lay dying in Kushner's arms. For the first time in days his eyes focused and he spoke: "Doc, Post Office Box 161, Texarkana, Texas. Mom, Dad, I love you very much. Barbara, I forgive you." Within seconds, he was dead.

Robert's was typical of a number of such deaths that Major Kushner saw. What killed him? Kushner could not perform an autopsy, since the Viet Cong allowed him no surgical tools. To Kushner's eyes the immediate cause was "gross electrolyte imbalance." But given Robert's relatively good physical state, psychological precursors rather than physiological state seem a more specifiable cause of death. Hope of release sustained Robert. When he gave up hope, when he believed that all his efforts had failed and would continue to fail, he died.

From M. E. P. Seligman. *Helplessness: On Depression, Development and Death.* San Francisco: W. H. Freeman, 1975. Copyright © 1975. Reprinted with the permission of W. H. Freeman and Company.

inescapable. Depressed subjects given no helplessness training performed equally poorly. Both depressed subjects and nondepressed subjects given helplessness training showed performance decrements relative to escapable- or no-noise subjects.

Gatchel and Proctor (1976) studied psychophysiological correlates of learned helplessness in human subjects. Subjects were given either escapable, inescapable, or no noise during pretreatment, and heart rate and skin conductance were measured. The results provided little insight into the physiological characteristics of learned helplessness, as no differences were found during a subsequent test task for heart rate. Skin conductance showed some differences between groups—subjects exposed to inescapable noise exhibited more arousal (higher conductance). These skin conductance levels were similar to those found in depressed and anxious patients, suggesting another link to depressed affect.

Somewhat weaker evidence of similarities between helplessness and depression was provided by Gatchel, McKinney, and Koebernick (1977). They considered depressed and nondepressed subjects who were exposed to uncontrollable, controllable, or no pretreatments. In no-pretreatment conditions, depressed subjects exhibited poorer performance on a subsequent anagram task than did nondepressed subjects. In fact, performance by untreated, depressed subjects was similar to that of nondepressed subjects experiencing helplessness training. In contrast to this performance parallel between depressed and helpless subjects, however, Gatchel et al. observed reduction of phasic skin conductance among helpless subjects and increased phasic skin conductance among depressed subjects. They concluded that, despite behavioral similarities between helplessness and depression, there may be different underlying processes and deficits for each. Studies of noncollege populations have provided mixed results; some suggest that depression and helplesslike behavior are not related while others provide evidence of such a link (see Greer and Calhoun, 1983; O'Leary, Donovan, Krueger, and Cysewski, 1978).

It has also been argued that personality may affect an individual's susceptibility

|||||||||||||||||||||||||||||||||||||||||||||||||||||||||||||||||||||||||||||||||||||||||||||||||||||||||||||||||||||||||||||||||||||||||||||||||||||||||||||||||||||||||

CASE EXAMPLE #2

A 76-year-old former horse trader, gambler, and adventurer had been admitted to the hospital in 1957 in a state of severe emaciation and with signs of taboparesis. His physical condition improved with treatment, but he remained confined to a chair or to a walker. He also had a chronic urinary infection, which proved resistant to treatment. His peevish, complaining attitude, constant demands, competition with and provocation of other patients, and cunning attempts to test the personnel made him a management problem. At the same time, several members of the team had a certain liking for this unusual patient. He showed strong, though ambivalent, attachment to the nurse, the charge aide, and the physician. It was possible to handle him only by a well-coordinated, rigid system of privileges and controls.

After the fire, this patient was transferred to the neurological ward where his former special privileges (such as providing him with cartons of milk at certain hours each day) and controls could not be maintained. The patient appeared dejected and sad. He did not express his bitter anger as usual and usually answered when addressed. Two weeks after the fire, he was found dead and the diagnosis was probably myocardial infarction. Autopsy was not performed.

Although the patient had been undernourished and feeble, there was nothing to indicate a critical condition and his death came as a complete surprise. Death was classified as "unexpected."

Reprinted with permission from the *Bulletin of the Menninger Clinic.* Volume 25, No. 1, p. 25. Copyright © 1961, The Menninger Foundation.

to learned helplessness. In other words, some people may react more strongly to exposure to uncontrollable events while others may not react at all. Studies of locus of control and helplessness conditioning discussed earlier were based on the idea that external locus of control and an overriding belief that one is influenced by external factors would be associated with more helplessness in the face of uncontrollable stimuli (see Hiroto, 1974). Other personality variables thought to affect response to controllable and uncontrollable situations include the Type A behavior pattern and attribution style (see Glass and Carver, 1980).

Some studies have since found evidence of helplessness conditioning following exposure to uncontrollable *positive* events, suggesting that contingency is an important determinant of learned helplessness (see Tennen and Eller, 1977). One study found that noncontingent feedback while playing a video game generated symptoms of learned helplessness among college students (Fox and Oakes, 1984). However, research on helplessness has not always conformed closely with Seligman's (1975) initial formulations. For example, Roth and Bootzin (1974) observed performance on a test task after subjects had been pretreated with contingent, noncontingent (random), or no reinforcement of their responses. Unexpectedly, those receiving noncontingent reinforcement exhibited better performance on the second task and reported greater feelings of control than did the other subjects. Roth and Bootzin concluded that they had violated subjects' expectations of being able to control the situation by providing random feedback and may have aroused reactance (Brehm, 1966) rather than conditioned helplessness. Since reactance is a purposive, control-seeking response to threats to one's freedom and sense of control, such an interpretation has persisted and been incorporated into a number of investigations.

Wortman and Brehm (1975) formalized this notion when they proposed that helplessness is mediated by *expectations* for control. Initial exposure to uncontrollable outcomes will arouse reactance as long as an individual expects to be able to control the outcomes. Reactance is often a highly aroused state, where control or regaining freedom is an overriding concern and affect is likely to be angry and hostile. Thus, as long as we expect to control things in the situation, we will be reactant. However, with repeated exposure to uncontrollable outcomes, we may come to believe that we will not be able to control things in the situation and our expectations for control decrease. At this point, helplessness is more likely. As reactance fades with waning expectations for control, purposeful behavior fades into more helpless behavior.

According to this model, people first resist loss of control and become helpless only when they have exhausted their ability to regain control. Our use of "resist" and "exhaust" here is not coincidental, since Wortman and Brehm's description of helplessness is similar to Selye's description of stress. The similarity between these processes suggests that loss of control may serve as a stressor under some conditions and that helplessness may be an outcome of stress.

Research has been generally supportive of this model of developing helplessness. Pittman and Pittman (1979) found that expectations for control were related to whether subjects were reactant or helpless, and Baum et al. (1978) found that naturalistically caused helplessness in college dormitories developed in ways closely approximating Wortman and Brehm's description. Initial experience with uncontrollable events in the dormitories was associated with a facilitative, reactancelike response. This persisted for several weeks. However, after seven weeks of residence, cumulative experience with uncontrollable social outcomes led to diminishing expectations for control and more helplesslike responding.

Additional evidence of this kind of developing learned helplessness was provided by Roth and Kubal (1975). They found that pretreatment with only a small amount of noncontingency resulted in reactancelike behavior but that pretreatment with a great deal of experience with noncontingent outcomes resulted in learned helplessness. Subjects with only minimal experience with loss or lack of control were more persistent and successful on subsequent tasks than were subjects experiencing more of this pretreatment.

ATTRIBUTION AND LEARNED HELPLESSNESS

Other changes have also occurred in the way in which helplessness is viewed. For example, Abramson, Seligman, and Teasdale (1978) introduced a number of cognitive elements into the sequelae surrounding helplessness conditioning. They suggested that when helplessness is being conditioned, people attribute their lack of control or their inability to solve a problem to one or more of a number of causes. They emphasized, for example, the degree to which helplessness is perceived to be personal (caused by one's own failings or lack of skill) or universal (caused by external factors such as the environment or the task itself). Attributing lack of control to one's own failings and assuming personal responsibility may cause more damage to self-esteem than placing blame on other people or on the environment. None of us can control everything. There are many things, such as immortality, that do not condition a generalized helplessness among most people because they are beyond everyone's control. Thus, although specific responding will cease with either personal or universal helplessness, personal helplessness, according to Abramson, Seligman, and Teasdale, may be more costly.

Abramson, Seligman, and Teasdale also suggest that people distinguish between global and specific causes of helplessness—whether uncontrollable events persist in a number of situations or are limited to only one or two. Global helplessness may be more debilitating, as its effects will generalize and characterize a number of settings. Judgments of *stability* are also made. The degree to which failure or lack of control is due to lack of ability (a stable characteristic that is difficult to change) or to lack of effort (an unstable, more easily changed characteristic) will affect helplessness. Stable character or environmental attributions will lead to more persistent helplessness, since loss of control is expected to occur in more different places. The evidence suggests that cognitive factors are important in the conditioning of helplessness at least some of the time. The notion that people have different tendencies or styles of making attributions is appealing because it helps to explain response to ambiguous situations in which control is not available (Seligman, Abramson, Semmel, and Von Baeyer, 1979). When faced with a situation in which there are no clear causes, some people may tend to attribute events to internal causes, while others may be predisposed toward external attributions. Similarly, people may exhibit tendencies to attribute causes to global or to specific events. Subsequent studies have shown that this individual difference variable affects generalization of helplessness to new situations (Alloy, Peterson, Abramson, and Seligman, 1984; Mikulineer, 1986). Other studies of the role of attributions in helplessness indicate that varying likely causes of failure to control a situation can have different effects on subsequent efforts to exert control and that attributional style is associated with symptoms of depression and with school achievement among children (Donovan and Leavitt, 1985; Nolen-Hoeksema, Girgns, and Seligman, 1986).

Research has not fully documented this reformulation, and it has received some criticism (see Wortman and Dintzer, 1978). The framework is appealingly logical, however, and in all likelihood will form the basis for newer descriptions of helplessness. It has been suggested, for example, that personal helplessness may be better thought of as a phase in a Wortman and Brehm (1975) type description of helplessness (Baum and Gatchel, 1981).

The same reactance-helplessness sequence of response to uncontrollable events in college dormitories as was studied by Baum et al. (1978) was considered in light of attributions for the lack of control. During the first month of residence, when students appeared to be more reactant than helpless, attributions for control problems were almost universally personal. At about the same time that expectations for control diminished and behavior became more helplesslike, however, attributions changed and became more external. By the end of the first semester of residence, attributions for control problems were primarily external and behavior was less control-oriented.

Baum and Gatchel interpreted these results in terms of defensive or strategic attributions. As long as one expected to regain control eventually, attributing the problem to oneself was not damaging to self-esteem. However, when these expectations waned and students were ready to give up, it was more "face-saving" to attribute problems to the environment. They also proposed that increased exposure to lack of control sensitizes people to noncontingency and leads to reduced expectations and shortened reactance periods during future encounters with challenging or uncontrollable situations. This is consistent with the finding that helplessness conditioning does not necessarily result in lower perceived control but instead may lead to higher and in some cases more accurate judgments of control during the helplessness training (Ford and Neale, 1985). Research has further suggested that personally attributed loss of control or failure has facilitating effects rather than helpless effects and that the dimensions of locus of attribution, stability, and specificity may be inextricably linked (see Baum et al., 1981; Hanusa and Schulz, 1977; Wortman et al., 1976).

REVERSING HELPLESSNESS

In his original formulations of learned helplessness, Seligman raised the possibility of reversing the effects of learning that responses and outcomes are independent. In a study by Seligman, Maier, and Geer (1968), for example, helplessness in dogs exposed to uncontrollable aversive stimulation was found to be reversible, but reversal usually required a great deal of effort. The difficulties involved in teaching someone that he or she *can* control things that have previously been uncontrollable are obvious. People who have stopped trying may never see that they can control something because they rarely, if ever, make the responses that accomplish it. Seligman was able to undo some of the helplessness learning in dogs by dragging them into escape areas so that they could see for themselves that they could escape shock. With people, however, this process is more complicated.

Dweck and Repucci (1973) studied the effects of low expectancies for reinforcement and control among fifth-grade children using block design tasks similar to those associated with intelligence testing. Children were shown a picture of a design, given some multicolored blocks, and asked to form the design using the blocks. The designs children were asked to work on could not be made with the blocks provided. For children who blamed the problem on the environment, performance was worse than for those who took personal responsibility for their failure. The former group of children believed that their failure was due to external factors, while the latter— whose task performance did not deteriorate—were more likely to attribute their failure to lack of effort. Thus, when children thought that failure was their own fault (e.g., because they had not tried hard enough), they continued to work on subsequent tasks.

These findings are interesting. They suggest ways of undoing or reversing the effects of helplessness conditioning. If (1) expectancies affect response to failure, and

(2) a greater sense of personal responsibility leads to more persistent behavior, then training people to assume that their performance is determined largely by effort and ability could make them more resistant to the effects of lack of control. A child who believes that what he or she gets from the world is determined by personal factors such as effort and ability may be less likely to give up when confronted with failure.

Dweck (1975) tested this possibility by selecting "extremely helpless" children (children showing clear symptoms of helplessness) and providing half with a training procedure that taught them to take responsibility for failure. The other children were given a series of tasks on which they were always successful. Her findings provided support for the idea that personal responsibility for failure will increase resistance to helplessness. Those children given training over a three-week period showed increased persistence, while those exposed to success continued to show helpless behavior. Exposure to success or demonstration of ability to control events was not sufficient to reverse the effects of failure. Helplessness continued unless the causes of it were identified as being under the child's control.

To some extent, these expectancies must reflect reality. Expectations about control may be just as debilitating as helplessness if they are exaggerated or underestimated. Dweck and Gilliard (1975) had children make statements about whether they thought they would be able to solve the tasks they were given. Some were asked to make these statements prior to each task trial, some were asked to make statements before the first and last trials, and the rest were asked to state their expectation before only the last trial. By doing this, they made explicit their feelings about how they would do on each trial and thus their awareness of their expectancies was increased. Discrepancies between expectations and what actually occurred were emphasized for some subjects. When they were, performance was worse than when discrepancies were not emphasized.

Dweck and her associates demonstrated that the perceived inability to control outcomes usually associated with learned helplessness is more likely when attributions for lack of control are due to stable rather than controllable or variant factors (see Diener and Dweck, 1978, Dweck and Bush, 1976). For example, Diener and Dweck (1978) compared performance on a discrimination task by mastery-oriented children and by helpless children. Classification was done on the basis of tendency to attribute positive and negative outcomes to ability, effort, or external factors (e.g., someone else). Those who were prone to blaming effort for outcomes were considered mastery-oriented, while those who did not tend to attribute outcomes to effort were considered to be helpless. During subsequent experience with failure, mastery-oriented children focused on ways of remedying the situation and solving the task while helpless children attributed their failure to ability and did not change strategies in an attempt to overcome the problems.

Another approach to blocking or reversing the effects of exposure to noncontingent situations has been called learned resourcefulness (Meichenbaum, 1977). As you will recall from the last chapter, coping with stress can be divided into two general categories, including direct action taken to change the situation and emotion-focused coping designed to regulate feelings of distress and make one feel better (see Lazarus and Folkman, 1984). "Learned resourcefulness" refers to teaching people to regulate their feelings when confronted with stressors or uncontrollable events (Rosenbaum and Jaffe, 1983). Thus people can acquire skills that allow them to control internal responses such as pain and to perceive uncontrollable situations in alternative ways. In a study of college students rated as high or low in learned resourcefulness, Rosenbaum and Jaffe (1983) found that exposure to inescapable noise produced symptoms of learned helplessness only among those rated as low in resourcefulness; highly resourceful students did not exhibit adverse effects of experience with an uncontrollable situation. This suggests that coping skills and perceptions of self-efficacy may be important in helping people overcome the effects of helplessness conditioning.

Given the complexities in reversing helplessness once it is conditioned, interest has also focused on preventing or "immunizing" people against the effects of exposure to uncontrollable events. Seligman (1976) suggested that prior experience with success and failure might immunize a subject against learned helplessness, and some research has addressed this hypothesis. In one study Jones, Nation, and Massad (1977) found that prior experience with success and failure could immunize subjects against the effects of helplessness. They found that a 50 percent schedule of success on a task immediately before helplessness training was effective in preventing performance deficits. This group performed better than a no-immunization group, a group given only failure experience before helplessness training, and a group given only success experience before training. In another study Thornton and Powell (1974) studied the effect of immunization (previous success/failure experiences) on performance deficits following helplessness training. They reported that immunized subjects performed at an intermediate level on the test task, falling between those of nonimmunized subjects receiving controllable or uncontrollable pretreatments. However, they also found that nonimmunized subjects also performed at an intermediate level if they were made aware of the fact that control was no longer possible. Thus evidence for a real immunization effect was limited. Douglas and Anisman (1975) found that immunization did not reduce helplessness when subjects were immunized on a task that was unlike the one affected by helplessness training. Only when subjects were immunized on a task similar to the one involved in helplessness conditioning was subsequent performance affected.

The term immunization means prior treatment that protects or makes one immune to the effects of something. Thus, giving people vaccines that generate antibodies to an illness helps the body develop defenses to disease, and giving people experience with success and failure experiences before helplessness training helps to protect them from the negative effects of the training. However, it is not necessary to use failure and success as the "vaccine" as other forms of intervention also appear to be effective. Altmaier and Happ (1985) tested the effectiveness of prior training in coping skills to prevent the negative effects of learned helplessness. In this pretraining, subjects were provided with rationale for the notion of reducing arousal during problem solving and were trained in relaxation techniques and coping skills. Performance by "immunized" subjects was then compared with control subjects in a helplessness induction procedure based on Hiroto and Seligman's (1975) procedure. Some support for the predicted effects of prior training were found: after helplessness conditioning, those who received the pretraining performed better than those who did not. However, there were no differences between these groups in attributions for performance, and pretrained subjects were more pessimistic about future performance than were nontrained participants.

Like reversal strategies, immunization is not necessarily useful in the prevention of helplessness. Since all of us have extensive experience with both success and failure, it is difficult to explain why we are not all immunized already. The fact that scheduling of successes with tasks similar to those encountered in uncontrollable situations appears to be effective in preventing performance deficits suggests that situation-specific immunization may be most effective in reducing the effects of helplessness training.

SUMMARY

The role of perceived control as a determinant of stress is important in considering the effects of stress on health and well-being. The consistent finding that perceived control is associated with fewer or less severe consequences of exposure to stressors suggests that uncontrollable stressors are more likely to affect health adversely. The related findings that loss or lack of control can be a cause of stress further highlights the importance of considering control. Some studies have begun to identify instances in which control influences health outcomes.

Research on learned helplessness suggests a number of links to health and illness. Prolonged or repeated exposure to settings or situations in which people have little or no control appears to be associated with reduced motivation, emotional disturbance, and cognitive impairment. Although the reasons for this are not clear and the ways in which helplessness is conditioned have not been clearly established, there is some evidence that helplessness occurs in natural settings as well as in the laboratory. When helplessness is minimized by enhancing an individual's sense of control, health outcomes appear to improve.

RECOMMENDED READINGS

Abramson, L. Y., Seligman, M. E. P., and Teasdale, J. Learned helplessness in humans: Critique and reformulation. *Journal of Abnormal Psychology,* 1978, *87,* 49–74.

Baum, A., and Singer, J. E. (Eds.) *Advances in environmental psychology,* vol. 2. Hillsdale, N.J.: Erlbaum, 1980.

Perlmuter, L., and Monty, R. (Eds.) *Choice and perceived control.* Hillsdale, N.J.: Erlbaum, 1979.

Seligman, M. E. P. *Helplessness: On depression, development, and death.* San Francisco: Freeman, 1975.

Wortman, C. B., and Brehm, J. W. Responses to uncontrollable outcomes: An integration of reactance theory and the learned helplessness model. In L. Berkowitz (Ed.), *Advances in experimental social psychology,* vol. 8. New York: Academic Press, 1975.

5 CARDIOVASCULAR DISORDERS AND BEHAVIOR

||||||||||||||||||||||||||||||||||||||||||||||||||||||||||||||||||||||||||||||||||||||||||||||||||||||||||||||||||||||||||||||||||||||||

Cardiovascular disorders, including coronary heart disease, high blood pressure, and stroke, are widely studied topics in health psychology (Krantz, Grunberg, and Baum, 1985) because there are many physiological, environmental, and behavioral variables that interact in their development (Kannel, 1979). For example, **coronary heart disease** (or **CHD**) is a disorder that is a result of the individual's lifestyle; many of the causal agents can be modified, relate to habits of living, and are under the individual's control.

Diseases of the heart and blood vessels are a major public health problem, accounting for almost as many deaths in the United States as all other diseases combined (U.S. Department of Health, Education, and Welfare, 1979). In the past twenty years, however, death rates from heart disease have been decreasing (NHLBI, 1979). These changes are due partly to developments of drugs and improvements in medical technology, but also to public awareness of behaviors that are risk factors and to attempts by individuals to modify those lifestyle components that constitute risk factors for heart disease.

CORONARY HEART DISEASE

As noted in Chapter 2, the heart muscle, like other organs, needs its supply of blood. Blood to the heart is delivered through the coronary arteries, which can become narrowed by fatty deposits, a condition that is called **atherosclerosis,** popularly known as "hardening of the arteries." (See Figure 5.1.)

Coronary heart disease refers to a set of conditions thought to result from coronary atherosclerosis. As the buildup on the inner coronary artery walls becomes hard and thick, it is more difficult for the blood to move through the narrowed vessels. If a complete blockage occurs, the result may be **myocardial infarction (MI),** a form of heart attack that results when part of the heart does not get enough oxygen and other nutrients and begins to die. Sometimes the nar-

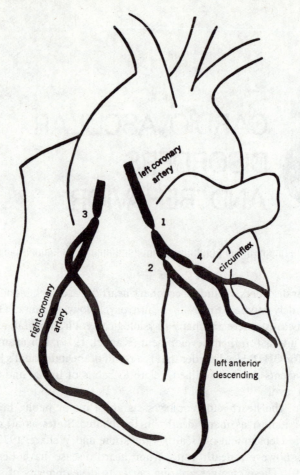

Figure 5.1   The coronary arteries: four points of narrowing due to atherosclerosis.
Adapted from M. Franklin, M. Krauthamer, A. R. Tai, and A. Pinchot. *The Heart Doctors' Heart Book.*
New York: Grosset and Dunlap, 1974. Reprinted with permission.

rowing is not complete and some oxygen, but not enough, is supplied to the heart and the result is chest pain—a conditioned called **angina pectoris.** Under some conditions, angina may lead to MI.

PHYSICAL RISK FACTORS FOR HEART DISEASE

A coronary risk factor is a characteristic of the population or of the environment that increases an individual's likelihood of developing cardiovascular disease. Numerous studies by epidemiologists over the past forty years have established a set of physical risk factors for coronary heart disease (see Table 5.1). The more risk factors that individuals have, the greater is their likelihood of developing heart disease, and individuals who are likely to develop CHD can be identified with a moderate degree of accuracy.

TABLE 5.1   Risk Factors for Coronary Heart Disease

NONMODIFIABLE	MODIFIABLE
• Age	• Hypertension
• Sex	• High low-density lipoprotein levels and low high-density lipoprotein levels
• Family history	• Cigarette smoking
	• Diabetes
	• Obesity
	• Sedentary lifestyle
	• Stress and Type A behavior

Nonmodifiable Factors

Several of the coronary risk factors cannot be controlled. These include chronological age, sex, race, and family history. Unfortunately, the longer people live, the greater their likelihood of developing heart disease because there is more time for plaque to accumulate in arteries. Nearly half of all coronary victims are over the age of sixty-five. Throughout most of their lives, and especially at younger ages, males are at greater CHD risk than females. The reason younger women have lower risk probably has much to do with a protective effect of female sex hormones (Lerner and Kannel, 1986). Also, in the United States, blacks are more prone to CHD than whites; this may be related to the fact that they are much more susceptible to high blood pressure than are white Americans, and high blood pressure is a major CHD risk factor. Last but not least among nonmodifiable risk factors is family history. Susceptibility to CHD can be transmitted genetically, and certain families are at higher risk than others.

Modifiable Factors

It is important to note, however, that even if individuals fall into the higher risk groups because they possess these noncontrollable factors, they can still minimize their risk by modifying certain habits. For example, cigarette smoking is a preventable behavior. The death rate from heart attack is higher among people who smoke than among people who do not smoke. However, for those who give up the habit, the death rate begins to decrease almost to the level of those who have never smoked (AHA, 1982), probably because the pathophysiologic effects of smoking are no longer bombarding the system.

High salt intake and obesity are behaviorally related factors that can contribute to high blood pressure in some individuals. Physicians have incorporated this information into their treatment of hypertensive patients by recommending that people with mild blood pressure elevations begin a program of dietary salt restriction or weight reduction before undergoing treatment with blood pressure–reducing drugs. High blood cholesterol is a major CHD risk factor that is related to dietary behavior. The body manufactures cholesterol, but also gets it from what we eat. Therefore, a diet that is low in cholesterol and saturated fats will help lower the level of blood cholesterol.

Despite extensive research on the epidemiology of heart disease, there is still controversy as to the importance of such factors as diet and exercise in its development. For example, some studies have not found that dietary patterns within the population are predictive of later development of heart disease (Mann, 1977). Generally, the least controversial and most widely accepted risk factors are considered to be smoking, levels of cholesterol in the blood, and high blood pressure (Kannel, 1979).

PSYCHOSOCIAL RISK FACTORS

Behavioral scientists have become interested in coronary heart disease for at least two reasons. First, as noted earlier, many of the standard risk factors involve behavioral components. For example, smoking is a potentially modifiable behavior, and high blood pressure and blood cholesterol levels can be influenced by dietary factors. Second, despite extensive research into the standard physiological risk factors, the best combinations of these factors still do not account for the occurrence of heart disease in many individuals. The search has therefore been broadened to examine potential new risk factors (Jenkins, 1983; Krantz, Baum, and Singer, 1983), including social, psychological, and environmental characteristics. This chapter will discuss three very active areas of research on cardiovascular disorders: stress, Type A behavior and related traits, and physiologic reactivity.

STRESS AND CORONARY HEART DISEASE

Researchers have examined the relationship of several stress-related environmental characteristics to the development and worsening of cardiovascular disease (Ostfeld and Eaker, 1985). Some of this research deals with the influence of acute or short-term stressful life events, utilizing the life change unit methodology described in Chapter 3. These studies collect information about stressful life events or changes in peoples' lives and relate them to measures of heart disease. Unfortunately, these studies have not shown a conclusive ability to predict the occurrence of heart disease (Wells, 1985). One or a few stressful events may not contribute measurably to CHD since it is a chronic disease that progresses over time. Therefore, studying the effects of chronic life situations, such as psychological and social conditions at work and in other life domains (e.g., home and family), has proven more productive.

In humans and animals, researchers have studied chronic stress arising from work and social situations. This research reveals that the effects of most stressful situations on physiology and behavior depend on psychological factors. As described in Chapter 3, if situations are not viewed or interpreted as harmful, threatening, or challenging, they can produce smaller and even opposite physiologic responses (Lazarus and Folkman, 1984). Therefore, the relationship of various psychological and social stresses (e.g., occupational conditions) to CHD seems to depend on the meaning of the situation to the individual and the way individuals perceive their life situations (see Cohen, Evans, Stokols, and Krantz, 1986).

Occupational Stress and Heart Disease
Much of the research in the area of occupational stress and health has attempted to determine which occupations are more stressful or which conditions within a

single work setting are associated with heart disease. The attempt has been to describe the characteristics of particular occupations that lead to high coronary risk (see Tyroler et al., 1987). This research is very promising because it suggests psychological dimensions of settings or individuals that potentially can be modified in order to reduce stress.

Several broad types of working conditions have been associated with CHD risk. These include the psychological demands of the job, autonomy on the job (how much input people have in making decisions), and satisfaction on the job. Job demands refer to job conditions that tax or interfere with the worker's performance abilities, such as workload and work responsibilities. Level of job autonomy refers to the ability of the worker to control the speed, nature, and conditions of work. Job satisfactions include gratifications of the worker's needs and aspirations derived from employment (Wells, 1985).

Low levels of control over one's job and excessive workload seem to be a particularly important combination in heightening job-related stress. The idea that personal control can lessen the negative effects of stress (see Chapter 4) has been applied to workplace effects on CHD by Karasek and colleagues (1982). They have proposed that conditions of high work demands combined with few opportunities to control the job situation (low decisional latitude) are associated with increased coronary disease risk.

Conditions of high demand and low control are called high-strain situations. The Karasek "job-demand/control" hypothesis has been tested in several populations by applying a Job Characteristics Scoring System based on responses to several national surveys of workers. These job characteristic scores can distinguish between occupations along the dimensions comprising job strain, as illustrated in Figure 5.2. Occupations in the lower right quadrant of the figure—those characterized by high demands and low decisional control—are associated with increased coronary risk. The job strain model has predicted cardiovascular disease and mortality in two studies of male Swedish workers and in studies of men and women in the United States (Karasek et al., 1981; Tyroler and Haynes, in press).

Another interesting study of occupational stress and CHD among women also indicates that the relationship of job conditions to coronary disease depends on the individual's work and family demands and her control over these situations. Haynes and Feinleib (1980) analyzed data from the Framingham Heart Study, a major epidemiologic study of heart disease conducted by the National Institutes of Health. They asked whether the increasing employment of women outside the home has adversely affected their cardiovascular health. In the mid-1960s, middle-aged women were examined for the development of CHD for the ensuing eight years. Working women—that is, women who had been employed outside the home for more than half their adult years—were compared to housewives and to men. Results indicated that working women in general were *not* at significantly higher risk of subsequent coronary disease than housewives. However, clerical workers (who perhaps have low job control) and working women with children (who have high family demands) were more likely to develop CHD, as were women whose bosses were nonsupportive. Interestingly, likelihood of CHD increased linearly with the number

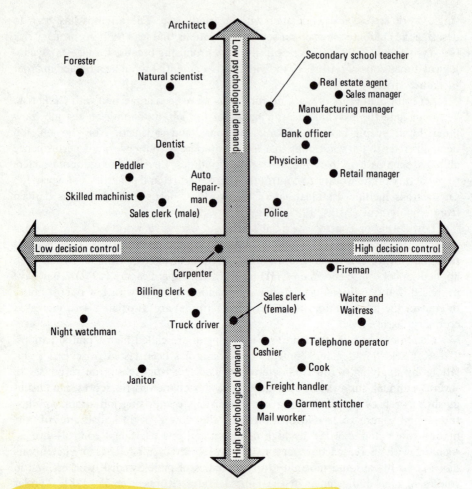

Figure 5.2   The dimensions of job strain, with corresponding job categories.
Reprinted with permission from B. Nelson. Bosses face less risk than the bossed. *New York Times,* April 3, 1983. Copyright © 1983 by The New York Times Company.

of children for working women, but not for housewives (Haynes and Feinleib, 1980). (See Figure 5.3.)

ANIMAL STUDIES OF STRESS AND CORONARY DISEASE

Experimental studies of several animal species have shown that when animals are exposed to conditions that disrupt the social environment, coronary artery disease pathology can result (Manuck, Kaplan, and Matthews, 1986). In recent years a particularly important series of studies in this area have been conducted at the Bowman-Gray School of Medicine (Kaplan et al., 1982). The researchers used cynomolgous monkeys, which are a particularly good species for studying the influence of behavior on atherosclerosis for two reasons. First, in these animals coronary

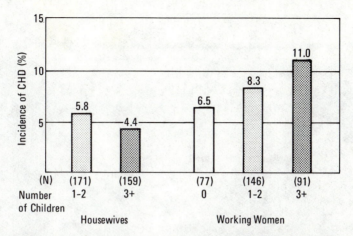

Figure 5.3 Eight-year incidence of coronary heart disease by number of children among women aged 45–64 years.
Reprinted with permission from S. G. Haynes, M. Feinlieb, and W. B. Kannel. Women, work, and coronary heart disease. *American Journal of Public Health,* 1980, *70,* 133–141.

disease pathology closely resembles that of the human condition. Second, many of the prominent aspects of these animals' behavior, such as forming a social hierarchy, friendship and isolation, competition, and aggression, are salient aspects of human behavior analogous to those that have been implicated as potential contributors to coronary disease in humans (see Figure 5.4). The social organization of these monkeys involves the establishment of stable hierarchies of social dominance, and dominant and submissive animals can be identified within a given group based on the animals' overt behavior.

Observations of these animals' social behavior showed that the introduction of unfamiliar monkeys into an established social group is a powerful social stressor, leading to increased aggressive behavior as group members attempt to reestablish a social dominance hierarchy (Manuck et al., 1986). In recent studies these stressful conditions were created by periodically reorganizing social groups (called the *unstable* condition). Groups composed of five monkeys each were, at intervals, newly exposed to three to four different monkeys. Unstressed animals in *stable* social conditions were assigned to similarly sized groups having fixed memberships over the duration of the study (Kaplan et al., 1982). Based on the patterns of their behaviors in the groups, monkeys were categorized as either dominant or subordinate.

In one study of male monkeys, the dominant animals in the *unstable* social condition developed more extensive coronary atherosclerosis than their subordinate counterparts, but differences were also evident between dominants and subordinates in the *stable* social condition. Under stable social conditions, dominants were slightly *less* affected than subordinates. Providing a clue as to the possible behavioral reasons for the development of disease, dominant animals in the *unstable* condition showed the most aggression toward other animals and a disruption of positive social interactions. The psychological influences on development of atherosclerosis in this

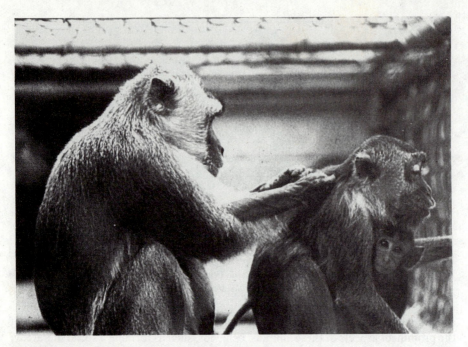

Figure 5.4   **Cynomolgous monkeys during social interaction.**
Photo courtesy of Jay Kaplan.

study were apparently independent of levels of physical risk factors (e.g., cholesterol, blood pressure, etc.). This is similar to what is found in studies of Type A or "coronary-prone behavior" (to be discussed later) in humans. However, all animals had relatively high cholesterol levels because they were maintained on a diet high in saturated fat and cholesterol.

A second study examined whether social stress would show similar effects for animals with certain "personalities" if monkeys were maintained on a low-cholesterol, low-fat diet (the American Heart Association's "prudent" diet). With the same social conditions, dominant animals in the unstable condition again developed the most severe disease. However, comparing the extent of atherosclerosis across the two studies, results indicated that social influences on coronary disease development were greatly magnified in the presence of high cholesterol levels induced by diet (Manuck et al., 1986).

In a third study conducted with female monkeys, subordinate animals developed *greater* coronary artery disease than dominants (Kaplan et al., 1984). As in the other studies with male animals, these effects could not be attributed to the physical risk factors. Reproductive function in many of the subordinate animals was also disrupted, and these behaviorally induced reproductive problems may have lessened the animals' "protection" against coronary disease.

These experiments demonstrate the effects of psychosocial stress in the development of coronary artery disease. Interestingly, the specific effects of stress depend on individual characteristics (e.g., level of dominance) that determine how objective conditions will affect each animal's behavior. Thus we might conclude that these studies are similar to the occupational stress findings indicating that the effects of stress depend on psychological processes such as the perception and/or interpretation of demands on the individual. The aggressive behaviors observed in male monkeys who developed the most coronary disease also resemble some of the characteristics of Type A behaviors and hostility observed to predict CHD in humans.

TYPE A BEHAVIOR PATTERN AND CHD

One of the most researched aspects of the stress-heart disease link is the **Type A** or **coronary-prone behavior** pattern. The concept of a coronary-prone personality—that is, a set of emotions, behaviors, and personality attributes that characterize people who are likely to develop CHD—dates back to the last century. For example, noted physician Sir William Osler (1892) described the typical coronary patient as "not the delicate, neurotic person . . . but the robust, the vigorous in mind and body, the keen and ambitious man, the indicator of whose engine is always at full speed ahead." (Dembroski, MacDougall, Herd, and Shields, 1983, p. 59). In the twentieth century, the Menningers (1936) focused their attention on the trait of *aggressiveness* associated with those who developed CHD.

However, during the 1950s two cardiologists, Rosenman and Friedman (1959), described the Type A behavior pattern (TABP) and developed a reliable technique for its assessment (Rosenman, 1978). Type A is characterized by excessive competitive drive, impatience, hostility, and vigorous speech characteristics. A contrasting behavior pattern, called **Type B**, consists of the relative lack of these characteristics and a more easygoing style of coping. Rosenman and Friedman considered Type A to consist of patterns of behavior brought out by certain environmental challenges, and a **Structured Interview (SI)** was developed that focused on observable behavior. Assessments in the SI are based primarily on speech characteristics and the *manner* in which subjects respond to questions, rather than relying on whether subjects describe themselves as impatient, competitive, and so on. (See Chapter 9 for sample questions and criteria.) In contrast to the SI, several questionnaire measures developed to assess Type A behavior, such as the **Jenkins Activity Survey**, or **JAS** (Jenkins, Zyzanski, and Rosenman, 1971), rely solely on subjects' self-reports of their own behavior (Matthews and Haynes, 1986).

Early studies by Friedman and Rosenman showed that Type A traits could be related to certain coronary risk factors. In one interesting study, accountants were tested for their levels of serum cholesterol every two weeks over a six-month time period. (See Figure 5.5.) It was found that cholesterol levels rose as the April 15 tax preparation period approached. The changes in cholesterol in this study could not be explained by dietary factors, suggesting that the intense feelings of time pressure produced by occupational deadlines could raise cholesterol levels.

In the 1960s and 1970s, numerous studies examined the relationship of Type A behavior to heart disease. The results of these epidemiologic studies were almost all uniform in showing a positive correlation between TABP and risk of CHD in men and women, comparable to and independent of the effects of risk factors such as

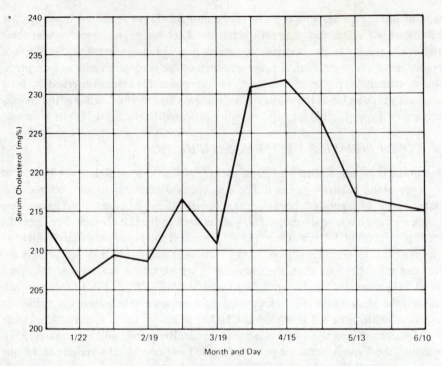

Figure 5.5   Impact of socioeconomic and psychological stress factors on serum cholesterol levels is evident in sharply increasing values recorded in a group of tax accountants as April 15 deadline neared for filing tax returns. Values promptly declined as pressure eased.
Reprinted with permission from R. H. Rosenman, and M. Friedman. The central nervous system and coronary heart disease. In P. M. Insel and R. H. Moos (Eds.), *Health and the Social Environment.* Lexington, Mass.: D. C. Heath, 1974.

smoking and hypertension. However, in the last five years several major studies have failed to find a relationship between Type A behavior and coronary disease (see Matthews and Haynes, 1986).

Evidence supportive of Type A behavior as a risk factor included two major studies of initially healthy individuals. The Western Collaborative Group Study (WCGS) began in 1960 and examined over three thousand men for eight and one-half years. At the end of the study, those men assessed as Type A by interview and questionnaire were more likely to have developed heart disease than Type B men (Jenkins et al., 1974; Rosenman et al., 1975). In the Framingham Heart Study, Type A behavior was a predictor of CHD among men in white-collar occupations and women working outside the home (Haynes et al., 1980).

Yet the results of several recent studies have not always found consistent relationships between Type A behavior and coronary heart disease. For example, the **Multiple Risk Factor Intervention Trial,** or **MRFIT,** was a study conducted to determine whether interventions to modify coronary risk factors such as smoking, high cholesterol levels, and high blood pressure in high-risk men would lessen their likelihood of coronary disease. Measures of Type A behavior were obtained for over three thousand MRFIT subjects, who were followed for seven years. In this high-risk group, Type A behavior, as assessed by the SI and by the JAS, was unrelated to incidence of a first heart attack (Shekelle et al., 1985). This study, then, failed to support a link between Type A behavior and heart disease.

The reasons for these inconsistent findings for Type A behavior are not entirely clear, and some researchers have suggested that Type A behavior might not be a risk factor for certain high-risk groups (as were tested in the MRFIT study; see box). Nevertheless, it appears that certain components of Type A behavior—particularly hostility and vigorous speech characteristics—are correlated with coronary disease even in studies where overall or "global" Type A behavior has not been related to CHD.

DO TYPE A CORONARY PATIENTS FARE BETTER OR WORSE?

As we noted in the text, the Western Collaborative Group Study (WCGS) established that initially healthy Type A men were about twice as likely to develop coronary heart disease. Recently, this study was extended to examine the relationship of Type A behavior to survival in the 257 men who had developed coronary heart disease (Ragland and Brand, 1988). Surprisingly, among those individuals with heart disease who did survive their first heart attack, the coronary death rate was *higher* among Type B patients than among Type As.

How might these unexpected findings be explained? One possibility is that Type A patients respond to heart disease differently from Type B subjects. The Type As may have a better ability to cope and would comply better with medical treatments or lifestyle changes. Another possibility not fully accounted for in the study is that Type A patients were more likely to seek treatments for symptoms than Type B patients, thereby leading to a better prognosis. A third possibility concerns the fact that in this study, the classifications as Type A or Type B occurred an average of four years before the patients' initial heart attack. It is not clear how much the behavior type was altered in these individuals either spontaneously or due to heart disease during the twenty-two years of follow-up included in the study.

The Ragland and Brand (1988) findings certainly question the notion that the presence of Type A behavior is a risk factor in patients with known coronary disease. (Because the same WCGS study found that Type A predicted initial CHD, the findings seem less relevant to healthy individuals.) These results also seem to conflict with those obtained in the *Recurrent Coronary Prevention Project* (Friedman et al., 1986), a study that demonstrated that cognitive-social learning interventions to lessen Type A behavior can decrease the rate of recurrent heart attacks in CHD patients (see text). Perhaps the RCPP interventions were effective because they also resulted in increased social support, environmental modification, and/or general stress reduction. However, we are currently unable to resolve this controversy concerning Type A behavior, which has led at least one commentator to "wonder whether the 'A' in Type A behavior stands for 'acrimony' " (Dimsdale, 1988, p. 110).

Type A Behavior Pattern and Reactions to Uncontrollable Stress

The psychological processes underlying the Type A behavior pattern have been the subject of some research. For example, Glass (1977) focused on the Type A pattern as a coping style that individuals use to establish and maintain control over stressful situations. Glass (1977) noted that Type A individuals appear to respond to stress or challenge by accelerating the pace at which they work, by assuming competitive orientations, or by becoming aggressive or hostile.

Several studies were directed at the notion that the attempt to control potentially stressful situations is central to the Type A behavior pattern. The bulk of research on this topic has focused on reactions to controllable and uncontrollable stressors. These studies show that Type A individuals work harder and/or faster following exposure to uncontrollable stress than do Type B individuals or Type As exposed to controllable stress (Glass, 1977). Type A individuals seem to perceive challenges to their control as more threatening than do Type B individuals (Krantz, Glass, and Snyder, 1974).

When Type As are exposed to uncontrollable stress, the time-urgent, competitive, and hostile aspects of the behavior pattern are aroused. As we shall describe later, these behaviors appear to be associated with greater physiological response to challenge. Therefore, just as uncontrollable stress produces increased sympathetic arousal and secretion of epinephrine and norepinephrine by the adrenal system (see Chapter 3), it appears that uncontrollable stress evokes even greater increases in physiological arousal in Type As (see below). This is illustrated by a study of Type A behavior in the occupational setting. Type A workers who described their work environments as not encouraging autonomy (i.e., low in worker control) had higher blood pressures than Type As who felt the work setting was high in control. The opposite was found for Type Bs: for them, blood pressure was higher in settings rated as high in autonomy (Chesney et al., 1981).

Anger, Hostility, and Other Type A Components

As noted earlier, Type A behavior consists of several behaviors, including competitiveness, time urgency, and hostility, yet it is possible that not all of these behaviors contribute equally to coronary risk. Recent studies have tried to identify the components of TABP that are most strongly associated with coronary disease. What have consistently emerged as correlates of CHD in these studies are characteristics relating to hostility, certain speech characteristics derived from the Structured Interview, and the characteristic of not expressing anger or irritation, or "anger-in." For example, a reanalysis of data from the WCGS study just described showed that "potential-for-hostility," vigorous speech, and reports of frequent anger and irritation were the strongest predictors of CHD (Matthews et al., 1977).

The Cook and Medley Hostility Inventory (Cook and Medley, 1954), a scale derived from the Minnesota Multiphasic Personality Inventory, or MMPI (see Chapter 9), has been shown in two studies to be related to occurrence of coronary disease. This scale appears to measure attitudes such as cynicism and mistrust of others (Costa, 1986). In one study involving a twenty-five-year follow-up of physicians who completed the MMPI while in medical school, high Cook-Medley scores predicted incidence of CHD as well as mortality from all causes, and the relationship was independent of the individual effects of smoking, age, and presence of high blood pressure (Barefoot et al., 1983).

Psychophysiologic Reactivity and Coronary Disease

It has long been known that wide individual differences exist in physiologic reactions to stress, and these reactions have been of interest to psychosomatic practitioners and researchers. A body of research now suggests that physiological responses (reactivity) to emotional stress may be involved in the development of coronary heart disease and/or high blood pressure (Krantz and Manuck, 1984; Matthews et al., 1986).

To measure reactivity, cardiovascular and/or hormonal *changes* in response to stress are assessed—not just resting levels of physiologic variables. For example, one commonly used task used for determining reactivity is a competitive video game such as Pong or Pack-Man. Subjects are hooked up to a blood pressure and heart-rate monitor and are challenged to perform as well as possible on the game. Resting levels of heart rate and blood pressure are taken before the instructions are given, and these measurements are repeated throughout the time the subjects perform the task. It turns out that there are wide individual differences in the magnitude of physiological responses shown during such a task, with some people (so-called hot reactors) showing sizable increases to the challenging task and others showing little or no increases. An underlying assumption in measuring reactivity in such a manner is that changes over resting levels in response to real-life or laboratory stresses give an index of how the body is responding during the challenges of everyday life and/or during exposure to environmental stress.

It is thought that psychological factors such as stress and Type A behavior contribute to the development of CHD because they are related to activity of the sympathetic nervous system and to activity of the adrenal cortex (which secretes corticosteroids) (Krantz and Manuck, 1984; Schneiderman, 1983). Certain types of cardiovascular and endocrine reactions are thought to promote the development of coronary atherosclerosis and/or heart attack. Particular attention has been directed to the role of catecholamines in leading to cardiovascular pathology. Apparently, high levels of catecholamines and repeated rapid increases in cardiovascular responding facilitate injury or damage to arteries, increasing the likelihood of plaque accumulation (see Ross and Glomset, 1976). Catecholamine elevation may also contribute to blood clot formation, thereby leading to heart attack (Schneiderman, 1983).

Because Type A behavior appears to be related to CHD even after controlling for the physical risk factors (Review Panel, 1981), it has been suggested that behaviors evidenced by Type A persons are accompanied by the same kinds of cardiovascular and neuroendocrine responses thought to link psychosocial stress to CHD. Studies demonstrate that Type A persons, compared to Type Bs, display larger increases in blood pressure, heart rate, and stress hormones when confronted by challenging or stressful tasks (Matthews, 1982). Type As seem not to differ much physiologically from Type Bs when they are at rest and not psychologically challenged.

It is also worth noting that at least in coronary patients, some evidence exists that there may be an inherited or acquired psychobiological basis for Type A behavior. In two studies of patients under general anesthesia for coronary bypass surgery—a situation where patients' consciousness is certainly minimized—Type A patients showed increased systolic blood pressure responses during the surgical procedure (Kahn, et al., 1980; Krantz, Arabian, Davia, and Parker, 1982). These results suggest that at least among coronary patients, there may be an underlying psychobiological or constitutional basis for Type A behavior, and that certain overt behaviors exhibited by Type A patients could *reflect* an underlying sympathetic nervous system hyperreactivity (Krantz and Durel, 1983).

Research has also examined the possibility that excessive reactivity to stress may itself be a risk factor for coronary disease. In one study of initially healthy men followed for twenty-three years. (Keys et al., 1971), the magnitude of their diastolic blood pressure reactions to a cold pressor test (which involves immersing the hand in cold water) predicted later heart disease. In fact, this physiologic response was a stronger predictor than many of the standard risk factors assessed in the study.

Additional evidence of a relationship between cardiovascular reactions to stress and coronary disease was obtained in the Bowman-Gray monkeys described earlier. In studies of male and female cynomolgous monkeys fed a cholesterol-rich diet, animals were exposed to a standard laboratory stress (threat of capture) that produced large heart-rate elevations (Manuck, Kaplan, and Clarkson, 1983; Manuck et al., 1986). There were large individual differences in heart-rate reactions to stress, and animals were categorized as either high or low heart rate reactive. At the end of the study, high heart rate reactors had nearly twice the amount of coronary atherosclerosis than did low heart rate reactors. (See Figure 5.6.) Interestingly, the heart-rate responses correlated with the animals' behavioral characteristics, with high heart rate reactivity being correlated with aggressiveness in male monkeys and submissiveness in female monkeys.

There is also great interest in behavioral methods for reducing reactivity. Among the behavioral techniques used for this purpose are cognitive techniques, relaxation training, biofeedback, and aerobic exercise (Jacob and Chesney, 1986; Matthews et al., 1986). (See Chapter 8.)

The Development of Type A Behavior

Because coronary atherosclerosis is a lifelong process that apparently begins in the first or second decade of life, attention has been directed to whether Type A behavior is present in middle childhood. For example, Mathews and Siegel (1982) note that behaviors such as achievement, anger-arousal, and impulsiveness are stable from around ages six to ten to adulthood, and there is also evidence that Type A children, like their adult counterparts, show elevations in heart rate and blood pressure in response to psychological challenges (Matthews and Jennings, 1984).

Matthews and her associates (see Matthews, 1980; Matthews and Angulo, 1980) have developed a measure of Type A behavior in children, the **Matthews Youth Test for Health (MYTH)**. This scale is completed by an observer familiar with the child's behavior, and has been used in studies of children as young as age five. Recently an adolescent Structured Interview has also been developed and validated, and has been used in children as young as age nine to classify them as either Type A or Type B.

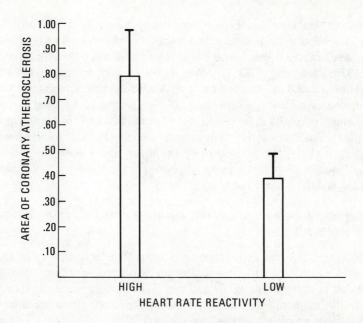

Figure 5.6 **Amount of coronary atherosclerosis in high heart rate and low heart rate reactors.**
Adapted with permission from S. B. Manuck, J. R. Kaplan, and T. B. Clarkson. Behaviorally-induced
heart rate reactivity and atherosclerosis in cynomolgous monkeys. *Psychosomatic Medicine,* 1983, *45,*
95–108.

The development of ways to measure Type A behavior in children is important
because it provides standardized measurement techniques that allow researchers to
study factors that could lead to such behavior. There is some evidence from studies of
twins that only certain components of Type A—speech characteristics and hostility—
are inherited (Matthews et al., 1984). At present, definitive answers to the environmental origins of Type A behavior are lacking, but there are some hints of likely social
origins. In particular, learning experiences in the family and parental influences
appear to play a significant role in the modeling of Type A behavior. Available studies
show that parents use unique child-rearing practices with Type A children compared
with Type Bs. For example, when children are asked to complete a set of tasks while
their mothers observe, Type A boys are given fewer remarks of praise, such as "that
was very good" and more comments seeking to bring out improvement, such as "that
was fine, but next time try harder" than Type B boys (Matthews and Siegel, 1982).
What is interesting about these maternal behaviors is that they are precisely those that
indicate that current performance is never satisfactory, irrespective of the child's
actual accomplishment. This implies that Type A children must strive after ever-
increasing goals, one of the hallmarks of Type A behavior.

No doubt there are other conditions that promote the development of Type A
behavior in males, females, and in various ethnic and cultural groups. Such factors
may include cultural and social role expectations. For example, Friedman and
Rosenman (1974) suggest that American society today rewards people who can
think, work, and even play more aggressively than their peers.

What is the evidence that Type A behavior is culture-bound? Type A has been shown to be related to heart disease in a number of western nations, including the United States, France, Belgium, and Poland (Belgian-French Pooling Project, 1984; Jenkins, 1978; Zyzanski, 1978). However, fewer than 15 percent of Japanese men living in Hawaii could be classified as Type A according to criteria used to classify subjects in western societies. (Cohen et al., 1975). The data also suggest that westernization of subjects results in increased risk of heart disease. That is, Japanese who move to the United States and become acculturated to American society have higher CHD rates. Similarly, the differences between men and women in both behavior pattern and incidence of heart disease suggest that cultural factors could play a role in this relationship (Waldron et al., 1977).

TREATMENT AND PREVENTIVE IMPLICATIONS OF BEHAVIORAL RISK FACTORS

Since there is evidence that Type A behavior, traits of anger and hostility, and habits of living such as smoking and high-fat diet are associated—perhaps causally—with heart disease, is there anything we can do? Type A behavior and other lifestyle factors are the result of long learning histories, and changes in these factors are difficult for most people to achieve (see Chapter 13).

Modifying Type A Behavior

A variety of clinical interventions have attempted to decrease Type A behavior either in persons with elevated levels of other CHD risk factors or in samples of coronary patients. Most of these studies have demonstrated that elements of Type A behavior can be decreased to some extent in subjects who are motivated to change (Suinn, 1982). Unfortunately, in these studies changes were primarily measured by self-reports, and it is unknown whether changes in self-perception correspond to actual changes in Type A behavior. Besides measuring changes in Type A behavior, some studies also measured changes in traditional CHD risk factors such as cholesterol or blood pressure. The findings from these studies are inconsistent (Suinn, 1982). These results are not surprising considering that the therapeutic regimens are not typically directed at decreasing risk factor levels other than Type A behavior, and also since Type A behavior is not usually related to resting levels of other risk factors (Review Panel, 1981).

Thorough studies comparing the effects of different interventions to reduce Type A behavior have been conducted in healthy individuals (see Roskies et al., 1986). However, the most important and ambitious Type A intervention study to date is the **Recurrent Coronary Prevention Project**, or **RCPP** (Friedman et al., 1986). The major purpose of this project was to determine whether Type A behavior could be modified in a large group of heart attack patients, and whether such behavior changes would lower the recurrence of heart attacks and deaths from CHD. Beginning in 1979, over one thousand patients were recruited for a five-year intervention study.

Patients were assigned to one of three groups: a cardiology counseling treatment group, a combined cardiology counseling and Type A modification group, or a no-treatment control group. The cardiology counseling included encouragement to comply with dietary, exercise, and drug regimens prescribed by the participants' personal physicians; education about CHD and its treatment; and counseling about psychological problems, other than Type A behaviors, associated with the postcoronary experience. The Type A counseling included drills to change specific Type A behaviors (see Table 5.2), focused discussions of beliefs and values underlying Type A behavior, rearrangements of home and work demands, and relaxation training to decrease physiologic arousal.

In the final results of the study after four and one-half years, the rate of heart attack recurrence for the Type A behavioral counseling group was significantly lower than for the cardiology counseling and control groups (Friedman et al., 1986). These results are unique in demonstrating, within a controlled experimental design, that cognitive and behavioral interventions that have the effect of altering Type A behavior may reduce coronary disease recurrence in post–heart attack patients. However, in light of some recent surprising results (Ragland and Brand, 1988) suggesting that Type A post–heart attack patients may survive longer, the status of Type A as a risk factor for adverse health outcomes among patients who have already manifested evidence of coronary disease is controversial (see Box, this chapter). Since the interventions in the RCPP project were effective in preventing recur-

TABLE 5.2   **Example from the Recurrent Coronary Prevention Project's** *Drill Book* **Used in the Type A Behavioral Group Treatment**

	OCTOBER
Monday:	Set aside 30 minutes for yourself
Tuesday:	Practice smiling
Wednesday:	Practice removing your grimaces
Thursday:	Eat more slowly
Friday:	Recall memories for 10 minutes
Saturday:	Verbalize affection to spouse/children
Sunday:	Linger at table

1.* "The only future we can conceive is built upon the forward shadow of our past"—Proust.
2. "If you make the organization your life, you are defenseless against the inevitable disappointments"—Peter Drucker.
3. "The moment numeration ceases to be your servant, it becomes your tyrant"—Anonymous.
4. "Habit is the hardiest of all the plants in human growth"—Anonymous.

*Reflect on the first quote daily for the first week; the second daily for the second week, and so on.

From C. E. Thoresen, et al. Altering the Type A behavior pattern in post-infarction patients. In D. S. Krantz and J. A. Blumenthal (Eds.), *Behavioral Assessment and Management of Cardiovascular Disorders.* Sarasota, Fla.: Professional Resource Exchange, 1987, pp. 97–116.

rent heart attacks, they may have worked because of the social support, environmental modification, and/or general stress reduction fostered by the Type A cognitive-behavioral interventions. On the other hand, Ragland and Brand's (1988) findings have other possible explanations than that Type A is not a risk factor after a patient has already had a heart attack.

BIOBEHAVIORAL FACTORS IN HYPERTENSION

Essential hypertension refers to a condition in which the blood pressure is chronically elevated and for which no single cause has been identified. The frequency of this condition in the United States is estimated at about 15 percent of the population, or more than 35 million people. The prevalence of this disorder increases with age, is more common among blacks than among whites, and below the age of fifty is less frequent among women than men (Weiner, 1977). Hypertension is considered to be asymptomatic—no particular symptoms are associated with it. People with hypertension are not usually aware of changes in their temperament or in bodily sensations. However, it is a serious and potentially lethal disease, and untreated hypertension increases the risk of stroke, heart attack, and kidney and vascular disease. Fortunately, because of recent strides in the medical treatment of hypertension, the disease can be controlled. However, because it has no observable symptoms and the drugs used to treat it may have unpleasant side effects, patients often do not comply with drug treatment regimens, and the problem of maintaining adherence to treatments is considerable. (See Chapter 8.)

A number of factors have been associated with risk for hypertension, including age, race, family history of hypertension, "borderline" high blood pressure, dietary intake of salt, and obesity. Like coronary heart disease, there are numerous social, environmental, and cultural factors that interact with genetic background in predisposing individuals to hypertension, and considerable attention has been paid to studying the role of stress and personality factors in the development of this disorder. Many findings in the area of hypertension risk factors are controversial because of the complex interactions among behavioral, physiological, and genetic factors, and also because essential hypertension is probably not a single homogeneous disease. Instead, blood pressure is thought to progress over a period of years from moderately elevated or "borderline" levels to more appreciably elevated levels, called established hypertension.

Several different pathogenic mechanisms can bring about blood pressure elevations, and different physiologic and/or behavioral mechanisms are implicated at different stages of the disorder. For example, individuals with borderline hypertension are commonly observed to have an elevated output of blood from the heart but little evidence of increased resistance to the flow of blood in the body's vasculature (Julius and Esler, 1975). This physiological pattern is consistent with an increased activation of the sympathetic nervous system (see Chapter 2), which is the body's initial reaction to psychological stress. Indeed, high levels of blood and tissue catecholamines—such as those produced by stress—have been found in some hypertensive humans and animals (Julius and Esler, 1975). However, in older individuals with more established hypertension, the heart's output of blood is normal or even decreased and resistance to flow of blood is elevated.

GENETIC–ENVIRONMENTAL INTERACTIONS

Evidence from animal research and from studies of human twins indicates that genetic factors are important in the development of hypertension (Pickering, 1977). In humans, however, it is likely that sustained hypertension is produced by an interaction of environmental and genetic factors. Population studies reveal a difference in the prevalence of hypertension among various social and cultural groups, a difference that cannot be accounted for by genetic factors alone (Henry and Cassel, 1969). For example, even though blacks in the United States experience more hypertension, prevalence of this disease is more common among poor than middle-class black Americans (Harburg et al., 1973). Animal research similarly reveals examples where environmental factors, such as dietary salt intake or stress, can lead to sustained blood pressure elevations—but only in certain genetic strains (Dahl et al., 1962).

BEHAVIORAL FACTORS AND HYPERTENSION

Sociocultural and psychological studies of humans, in conjunction with research on animals, have identified some factors related to behavior that might play a role in the development of hypertension. These factors include dietary intake of salt, obesity, and psychological stress.

Salt Intake
There has been much written about the role of salt in essential hypertension, largely because excessive intake of sodium has the physiological effect of acting on the kidneys to increase the volume of blood. However, studies indicate that high salt intake may be related to high blood pressure levels in some cultures and population groups. For example, among people who live in underdeveloped tribal societies, sodium intake is often low, as is the prevalence of hypertension (Page et al., 1970). As individuals move or become acculturated to modern societies, the prevalence of hypertension increases. This phenomenon has been discussed in terms of increasing stress with acculturation, but it has also been argued that acculturation is also associated with increased salt intake, which plays an equally important role in the development of hypertension (Page et al., 1970). Clearly, both the salt and stress explanations for the increased prevalence of hypertension in modern societies have merit.

There is also evidence that decreasing sodium intake in the diet of hypertensives will lower blood pressure and that, in healthy people, progressively greater salt intakes will result in a proportional blood pressure rise (Luft et al., 1978; Parjis et al., 1973). Therefore, reduction of salt intake has become an important part of the nonpharmacological treatment of hypertension. In accord with our prior discussion of genetic-environmental interactions, we should note that high salt intake is correlated with increased prevalence of hypertension only in certain populations or groups and that animal studies reveal that excessive salt intake results in sustained hypertension only in certain genetic strains (Dahl et al., 1962).

Obesity

Obesity is another social and cultural phenomenon that plays an important role in hypertension. There is an increased prevalence of hypertension in obese persons, although the precise reasons for this remain to be determined (Shapiro, 1983). Some have thought that it is merely that obese patients consume more sodium, but recent studies have demonstrated that weight loss without salt restriction can result in significant decreases in blood pressure (Reisen et al., 1978). For this reason, weight loss is an important behavioral method for managing high blood pressure.

STRESS, SOCIOCULTURAL FACTORS, AND ESSENTIAL HYPERTENSION

As noted earlier, there is an increased risk for hypertension among blacks compared to whites in the United States and among persons of lower socioeconomic status compared to those of higher socioeconomic status. Although these relationships have long been observed, there is still no universally accepted explanation for these differences. Possible explanations include differences in dietary patterns, exercise habits, or the social and physical characteristics of the environments in which these individuals live and work (Krantz et al., 1985). Some studies have suggested that exposure to environments (e.g., urban high-crime settings) that require sustained vigilance as well as recurrent mobilization of coping resources to ward off harm may raise blood pressure (Guttman and Benson, 1971; Henry and Cassel, 1969), and it is well documented that poorer people are overrepresented in such environments.

Related anthropological studies show that "primitive" or underdeveloped rural populations living in small, cohesive societies (e.g., nomadic tribes in Africa, Australian Aborigines, etc.) have low blood pressures that do not increase with age. However, when members of such societies migrated to areas where they are suddenly exposed to western culture, they were found to have high blood pressure levels that did increase as they got older (Henry and Cassel, 1969). This result suggested that the new living conditions had some stressful effects that became evident over the course of the life span. Another study supporting the role of stress in hypertension is one of residents of Detroit (Harburg et al., 1973). Four areas were categorized as "high stress" or "low stress" based on socioeconomic status, crime rate, population density, residential mobility, and marital breakup rates. Blood pressure levels were highest among black high-stress males, while white areas and black low-stress areas did not differ in blood pressure levels.

Research has also shown that people engaged in highly stressful occupations, such as air traffic controllers, have more than four times the prevalence of hypertension when stress is high (see Figure 5.7) than individuals of similar age in other professions (Cobb and Rose, 1973). Current studies of urban bus drivers in several places in the world suggest that they also have higher rates of hypertension than demographically comparable groups of employed persons. The high rates of hypertension observed in these occupational groups is consistent with the job-demand/control hypothesis advanced to explain the relationship between occupational stress and coronary heart disease (Karasek et al., 1982). Specifically, hypertension may

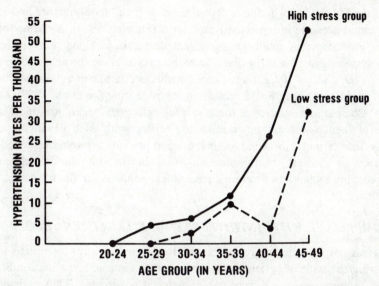

Figure 5.7 Incidence of hypertension as a function of stress. High-stress air traffic controllers (men working at high-traffic towers) show greater prevalence of diagnosed hypertension than do low-stress controllers (men working at low-traffic towers).

Adapted from S. Cobb and R. M. Rose. Hypertension, peptic ulcer, and diabetes in air traffic controllers. *Journal of the American Medical Association,* 1973, *224* (4), 489–492. Copyright © 1973 by the American Medical Association and adapted with permission.

occur more frequently in jobs that are demanding but in which there is little opportunity or flexibility to deal with these demands. (See Figure 5.2.)

Experimental studies with animals further demonstrate that social or behavioral stress can produce hypertension in predisposed individuals. Classic studies by J. P. Henry and associates (Henry and Stephens, 1977) have shown that psychosocial stimuli can cause hypertension in mice. In an early study, mice that had been kept in isolation were housed in a specially designed cage setting. There they were forced to interact with a number of other animals in a common space designed to facilitate contact between mice when they went to obtain food or water. Those animals that were previously isolated showed chronic elevation of blood pressure in response to frequent contact with others. Other studies demonstrate that hypertension can be induced in animals exposed to environmental stressors such as fear or shock and experimentally produced conflict (Campbell and Henry, 1983). However, unlike the human condition, blood pressure tends to normalize when the stress is removed unless the animals are genetically predisposed to hypertension. Consistent with the notion that genetic-environment interactions are important in the development of hypertension, studies have demonstrated that strains of animals that are susceptible to hypertension are also likely to show stress-induced blood pressure elevations (Friedman and Iwai, 1976).

The idea that emotional and behavioral stimuli affect the development and/or maintenance of high blood pressure receives additional support from human studies indicating that techniques such as biofeedback and relaxation training can be used to modify the stress-induced components of high blood pressure and thereby reduce blood pressure in hypertensive patients (Shapiro, 1983). A variety of studies have indicated that small but significant decreases in blood pressure (e.g., 15 mmHg systolic and 10 mmHg diastolic blood pressure) can be achieved in hypertensives after a series of training sessions with biofeedback or relaxation methods such as meditation, progressive relaxation, or yoga (Shapiro et al., 1977); see Figure 5.8. Comparative studies of these various behavioral techniques indicate that no one of them is clearly superior to the others, with each producing modest declines. Interestingly, these reductions in blood pressure are achieved without any side effects or medical contraindications, thus heightening the attractiveness of stress-reducing techniques as nonpharmacologic adjuncts for the treatment of hypertension.

COMPLIANCE WITH ANTIHYPERTENSIVE TREATMENT REGIMENS

Any discussion of behavioral factors and hypertension is not complete without considering the issue of patient compliance with regimens. Hypertension is a progressive, asymptomatic, and irreversible disease if not treated. Thus patients must be persuaded to undertake treatment, perhaps for a lifetime, and become susceptible to side effects and considerable inconvenience. If treatment is adhered to and blood pressure reduced, there is good evidence that the negative health effects of hyperten-

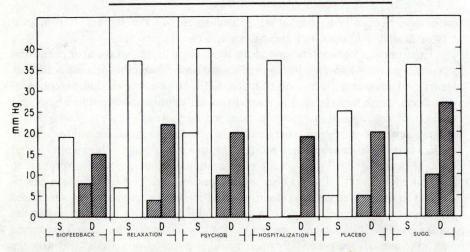

Figure 5.8 Comparison of nondrug techniques in reducing blood pressure levels, with means derived from a review of the literature (PSYCHOR = psychotherapy; SUGG. = suggestion). The white bars indicate the lowest and highest falls in systolic (S) and the striped bars the lowest and highest falls in diastolic (D).

Adapted with permission from A. P. Shapiro. The non-pharmacologic treatment of hypertension. In D. S. Krantz, A. Baum, and J. E. Singer (Eds.), *Handbook of Psychology and Health (Volume 3): Cardiovascular Disorders and Behavior.* Hillsdale, N.J.: Erlbaum, 1983.

sion can be avoided. As we have noted, the asymptomatic nature of the disease and the side effects that often result from drug treatments often result in poor compliance with medication taking. As will be described in Chapter 8, good communication between doctor and patient is important, and the patient must be effectively educated as to the benefits of treatment. In addition, by making other lifestyle changes such as modifying diet, losing weight, and exercising, drug dosages can be reduced. In some patients with mild blood pressure elevations, the necessity of taking drugs can even be avoided.

SUMMARY

There are many environmental, behavioral, and physiological variables that interact in the development of cardiovascular disorders. The risk factors for coronary heart disease (CHD) include nonmodifiable factors such as aging, male sex, and a family history, as well as controllable factors such as serum cholesterol, smoking, and hypertension.

Psychosocial risk factors for CHD have also been identified. These include occupational and social stress, Type A behavior, hostility, and physiologic reactivity to stress. With regard to occupational stress, low levels of control over the job combined with high job demands seem to heighten job stress and to increase risk of CHD. An interesting primate animal model has demonstrated that dominant animals placed in an unstable social environment develop more extensive athero-sclerosis than dominant animals in stable environments or than socially subordinate animals.

The Type A behavior pattern, characterized by excessive competitiveness, impatience, hostility, and vigorous speech, has been linked to increased risk of developing coronary disease, but recent studies suggest that the hostility component of Type A behavior is most pathogenic. In addition, there is some evidence that individuals who are physiologically reactive to stress may also be more likely to develop CHD, although further research is needed before reactivity can be regarded as an established risk factor. Recent studies have explored developmental antecedents of Type A behavior as well as techniques for modifying such behavior and reducing coronary risk.

In this chapter, we have also discussed biobehavioral influences on essential hypertension, a condition in which the blood pressure is chronically elevated. These include excessive salt intake, obesity, and stress. Evidence indicates that genetic and environmental factors interact in the development of hypertension. There is evidence that societies characterized by rapid cultural change and individuals in certain high-stress occupations are more prone to hypertension. Animal studies also indicate that stress can result in hypertension, although unlike the human condition, blood pressure tends to normalize when the stress is removed. The effectiveness of behavioral stress-reducing techniques such as relaxation training, biofeedback, and meditation in lowering blood pressure also is consistent with the role of stress in the development of this disorder.

RECOMMENDED READINGS

Kaplan, N. M., and Stamler, J. *Prevention of coronary heart disease.* Philadelphia: W. B. Saunders, 1983.

Krantz, D. S., Contrada, R. J., Hill, D. R., and Friedler, E. Environmental stress and biobehavioral antecedents of coronary disease. *Journal of Consulting and Clinical Psychology,* 1988.

Krantz, D. S., Baum, A., and Singer, J. E. (Eds.). *Handbook of psychology and health, vol. 3: Cardiovascular disorders and behavior.* Hillsdale, N. J.: Erlbaum, 1983.

Shepard, J. T., and Weiss, S. M. (Eds.). Conference on behavioral medicine and cardiovascular disease. *Circulation, 76* (Suppl. 1, Monograph #6), 1987.

Steptoe, A. *Psychological factors in cardiovascular disorders.* London: Academic Press, 1981.

6 PSYCHONEURO-IMMUNOLOGY, CANCER, AND AIDS

||||||||||||||||||||||||||||||||||||||||||||||||||||||||||||||||||||||||||||||||||||||||||||||||||||||||||||||||||||||||||||||||||||||

Knowledge about the immune system and how it works has expanded rapidly in the past decade, partly because of the introduction of new technologies that can be used to examine and assess immune system status and function. As was discussed in Chapter 2, we now know that there are many different cells that participate in immune responses and that these cells undergo transformations and evolutions through their lifetime. We also know that they are not autonomous cells operating independently of other bodily systems. Both nervous system influence and endocrine involvement in immune system activity have been noted, and there is reason to believe that the influence works both ways—that the immune system may also affect the nervous and endocrine systems. A field of study has recently grown up around these ideas, called neuroimmodulation or **psychoneuroimmunology**.

PSYCHONEUROIMMUNOLOGY

The name tells us a lot about this area of study. It includes three areas of bodily functioning formerly thought to be relatively independent. Psychological influences and the function of the nervous system have long been seen as interrelated, but the association of both with the immune system is a new and important development. Research on the effects of psychological and central nervous system (CNS) influences on the mutual influences of the immune, nervous, and endocrine systems has grown rapidly and clearly indicates that these systems are interrelated. The notion of an autonomous immune system has been discredited, and the ways in which the immune system interacts with other bodily systems have begun to be made clear. In this chapter we shall examine some of this research, considering conditioning of the immune system as well as evidence that stress can influence responsiveness of this system. We shall then turn our attention to two diseases that are closely related to immune system function—cancer and AIDS.

CONDITIONING AND IMMUNITY

One way to demonstrate that the immune system is not autonomous is to show that it can be conditioned—for example, that it can be made to respond to neutral stimuli paired with agents that affect it directly. We know from research on biofeedback (see Chapter 10) and from other studies that a number of bodily systems can be altered by operant and classical conditioning techniques. Miller (1969) and others have shown that physiological responses previously thought to be involuntary, such as heart rate, can be conditioned or shaped by instrumental procedures. Drug effects have also been found to be conditionable, as the effects of opiates may be elicited by neutral stimuli (such as the setting in which one takes drugs) in much the same way as by the drugs themselves (see Siegel, 1977b).

Ader's research on conditioning of the immune system function was based on a particularly powerful form of conditioning, learned taste aversion. Garcia et al. (1974) discovered that animals for whom illness and novel, neutral taste stimuli are paired develop an aversion to the previously neutral taste. Thus if an animal is given a sweet-tasting fluid and then made ill (by injection or by exposing it to radiation), it will avoid drinking the sweet-tasting liquid after this encounter. The strength of this paradigm is underscored by the fact that this learning seems to require only one pairing of neutral and unconditioned stimuli. Once the pairing has been accomplished, the animal will avoid the conditioned stimulus. Anecdotes about people's experiences with illness also give support to the single-trial nature of conditioned taste aversion. People report that there are times when they are ill that they will eat something, vomit later, and develop an aversion to the food they had eaten. However, experience also tells us that this conditioning is not universal and depends on many factors.

Ader and Cohen (1975, 1981) found immune system changes could also be conditioned to neutral taste stimuli. They had been using cyclophosphamide (CY), a drug with immunosuppressive properties, to cause nausea and vomiting. In the course of taste aversion studies, they discovered evidence of conditioned immunosuppressive effects (Ader, 1981). In a series of elegant studies designed to follow up on this possibility, the researchers found that a single pairing of a taste stimulus and CY produced an association between the taste and immune status. Following a single pairing of saccharin-flavored water with CY, subsequent exposure to the saccharin water alone produced effects of CY, including immunosuppression.

In most of these studies, conditioned animals were provided saccharin-flavored water to drink while unconditioned animals received plain water or saccharin that was not paired with the unconditioned stimulus. After allowing fifteen minutes for drinking, the animals were injected with CY. Three days later all animals were injected with an antigen, intended to "set off" an immune response, and subgroups of each conditioning group were again given saccharin or plain water. Thus animals who had received CY after drinking saccharin solution the first time were now exposed to saccharin or plain water. Subsequent injections of CY or saline further divided these groups. (See Table 6.1.)

The results were as predicted: animals exposed to the pairing of saccharin and CY exhibited immunosuppressive effects when reexposed to the saccharin alone. As

TABLE 6.1   Design of Conditioning Studies Showing Conditioned Immunosuppression

| Group | Adaptation | Cond. Day | Sub group | DAYS AFTER CONDITIONING / DAYS AFTER ANTIGEN | | | | |
		0	3	0 (Antigen)	1-2	3	4-5	6
Conditioned	H_2O	SAC + CY	US	H_2O + CY	H_2O	H_2O	H_2O	Sample
				H_2O	H_2O	H_2O + CY	H_2O	Sample
			CS$_0$	H_2O + Sal	H_2O	H_2O	H_2O	Sample
				H_2O	H_2O	H_2O + Sal	H_2O	Sample
			CS$_1$	SAC + Sal	H_2O	H_2O	H_2O	Sample
				H_2O	H_2O	SAC + Sal	H_2O	Sample
			CS$_2$	SAC + Sal	H_2O	SAC	H_2O	Sample
Nonconditioned	H_2O	H_2O + CY	NC	SAC + Sal	H_2O	H_2O	H_2O	Sample
				H_2O	H_2O	SAC + Sal	H_2O	Sample
Placebo	H_2O	H_2O + P	P	H_2O	H_2O	H_2O	H_2O	Sample

From R. Ader, Psychoneuroimmunology. San Diego: Academic Press, 1981, p. 286.

can be seen in Figure 6.1, the placebo group, never exposed to CY, showed the strongest antibody response to the antigen, followed by the nonconditioned animals that had received CY after drinking plain water and had subsequently been given saccharin water. The conditioned groups showed weaker antibody responses, particularly when saccharin was presented immediately after introduction of the antigen. Thus pairing of the two stimuli and subsequent presentation of saccharin produced a weaker antibody response. Animals receiving CY alone showed almost no response to the antigen (Ader and Cohen, 1975).

Various combinations of conditions were used to rule out possible alternative explanations and/or to identify mechanisms by which this conditioned immunosuppression was accomplished. Replications of the basic paradigm produced comparable findings, again showing evidence of conditioned immunosuppression of antibody response to antigens (see Rogers et al., 1979; Wagner et al., 1978). All in all, evidence is fairly strong that immune system responses can be conditioned to neutral stimuli.

The importance of this finding may be seen in several ways. Not only does it

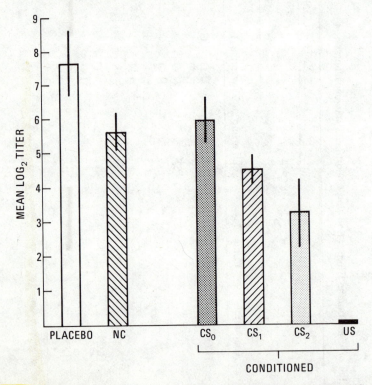

Figure 6.1   Antibody titers (mean ± s.e.) obtained 6 days after injection of antigen. NC, nonconditioned animals provided with saccharin on Day 0 (day of antigen) or Day 3; CS_0, conditioned animals that did not receive saccharin following antigen treatment; CS_1, conditioned animals reexposed to saccharin on Day 0 or Day 3; CS_2, conditioned animals reexposed to saccharin on Days 0 and 3; US, conditioned animals injected with cyclophosphamide following antigenic stimulation.

Reprinted, by permission of the publisher, from R. Ader and N. Cohen. Behaviorally conditioned immunosuppression. *Psychosomatic Medicine,* 1975, *37,* 334–340.

serve as confirmation of earlier conditioning studies and provide new information about how conditioning of autonomic responses occurs, but it also opened up a new area of investigation by demonstrating psychological influence on immunity. The applicability of these studies is potentially important as well. Other studies have shown, for example, that conditioned immunosuppression reduces the graft-versus-host response (see Bovberg et al., 1981), suggesting that rejection of transplanted tissue may be reduced through careful application of a conditioning paradigm. It is also possible that conditioning could be used to reduce the medication doses required in cancer chemotherapy. Presentation of a novel stimulus during initial chemotherapy and subsequent presentation of the now-conditioned stimulus with a smaller dose of whatever drug is being used might produce needed effects and reduce the aversive nature of the procedures. Studies of conditioned nausea in cancer treatment, however, suggest that some of these aversive effects may also become associated with the conditioned stimulus.

STRESS AND IMMUNITY

A number of studies have suggested that stress is associated with suppression of immunocompetence. **Immunocompetence** refers to the ability to recognize and reject that which does not belong in the body. Thus immunocompetence may be defined as the degree to which antigen is identified, destroyed, and disposed of by a host of cells and processes. The occurrence of an infection or the development of a tumor may reflect a deficiency in immunocompetence, which may be temporary or long term. These simple definitions belie the complexity of the immune system but provide scientists with a working notion of what they are seeking to measure. If we wish to determine whether stress increases the likelihood of infectious illness and seek to study immune system response as a means by which this occurs, the notion of immunocompetence provides us with some hint of what we will measure. Many measures of immunocompetence have been used, varying from observation of tumor growth to counts of numbers of lymphocytes and estimates of how active lymphocytes are.

Tumor Growth

Some studies consider tumor growth as an index of immunocompetence. It has been suggested that the immune system serves an **immunosurveillance** function, wherein immune cells scout for signs of tumor growth and help to destroy them while they are small. If stress or some other event interferes with this function, tumors may be allowed to grow to a size that the immune system can no longer deal with easily. At the same time, suppression of various immune system functions leading to generalized reduction of immunocompetence may also allow more rapid growth of tumors. These are among the ways that researchers have suggested that stress may be linked to cancer.

Studies that look at tumor growth as a function of stress have generally found evidence of stress-related changes. Sakakibara (1966) exposed one group of animals to bright, flashing light for eight hours each day, a second group to continuous light, a third to continuous darkness, and a control group to normal lighting conditions. Chemically induced tumor growth was measured over a twenty-week period, and results showed that the first group, exposed to flashing light, developed tumors more rapidly and nearly 80 percent of the animals in the group developed tumors. In the second group, tumor growth took longer and was less common (64 percent); in the third group, tumor growth took still longer and was less likely (24 percent). The control mice showed the same latency in tumor development as the mice kept in darkness and exhibited similar incidence of tumors (36 percent developed tumors).

Other studies of tumor growth are not as clear or consistent with the notion that stress reduces immunocompetence and increases tumor growth. Newberry et al. (1976) found no effects of electric shock on tumor growth in rats, while Henry and his colleagues (1975) found that isolation was associated with more rapid development of tumors in mice. Other studies report evidence of reduced tumor growth due to stress (see Marsh et al., 1959; Nieburgs et al., 1979). In an extensive series of studies, Riley and his colleagues found evidence of stress effects on tumor development and some of the conditions that affect host resistance to the tumors. Using a number of stressors, this research group found associations between increases in corticosteroid secretion and decreases in time required for development of tumors (Riley, Fitzmaurice, and Spackman, 1981). Stress was associated with dramatic differences in mortality following implantation of tumors in female mice; twenty days after tumor implant, more than 40 percent of mice that had been stressed prior to receiving the tumor had died, compared with about 20 percent of animals exposed to low-stress conditions. By the twenty-fifth day after implant, more than 80 percent of stressed animals and 40 percent of low-stress animals had died.

Other studies suggested mechanisms by which these effects are generated. Riley and colleagues were able to demonstrate rapid decreases in numbers of circulating white blood cells following stress and damage to thymus tissue associated with elevations in corticosterone after stress (Riley et al., 1981; Spackman and Riley, 1974). Administration of corticosterone independent of stress was also found to be associated with enhanced tumor growth. Though other changes have also been noted, the role of corticosteroids in stress effects on tumor growth appear to be important.

Lymphocyte Responsiveness
Another index of immune function is how reactive a cell is when it is called into action. If lymphocytes are very responsive, they will do their work well; if they are slow, weak, or inactive, they will not. As a result, many studies have used measures that tap how large a response is made by T- and B-cells to challenges or stimulation by antigen. Blood is drawn, prepared, and challenged *in vitro* by any of a number of stimulating **mitogens** including concanavalin A (ConA), phytohemagglutinin (PHA), and pokeweed. Many of these studies have used these mitogens, substances that cause lymphocytes to multiply, to stimulate cells and mark cell activity. The resulting value from this test yields an estimate of how strong a response is being made by lymphocytes. Proliferation of lymphocytes in the presence of mitogens, called **blastogenesis**, is thus studied. If exposure to a mitogen results in large increases in cells, the immune system is considered strong.

Several studies have considered stress due to bereavement as a factor in immune function. Bartrop et al. (1977), for example, studied both T- and B-cells following death of a spouse, and found that lymphocyte response to PHA and ConA was reduced during the two months after the death compared to response by a control group. (See Figure 6.2.) Numbers of T- and B-cells were comparable across time and group. Stein and colleagues have reported several studies of immune changes associated with depression and bereavement (see Schleifer et al., 1983; Schleifer et al., 1984). Schleifer, Keller, McKegney, and Stein (1980) studied a small group of men whose wives were dying, assessing immune function before the spouse's death as well as five to seven weeks after. Again, numbers of cells did not appear to change, but responsiveness of cells to mitogens was sig-

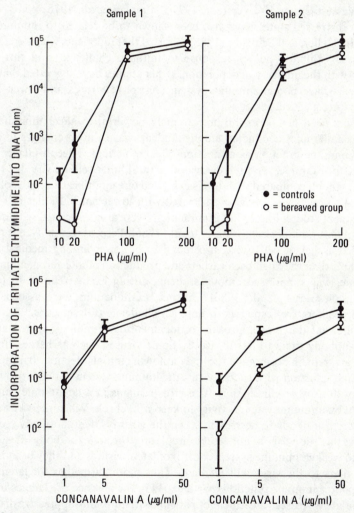

Figure 6.2   **The effect of bereavement on lymphocyte proliferation after challenge with phytohemagglutinin (PHA) and concanavalin A *in vitro*. Sample 1 was obtained shortly after and sample 2 about 8 weeks after bereavement.**

Reprinted, by permission of the publisher, from R. W. Bartrop, et al. Depressed lymphocyte function after bereavement. *Lancet* 1977, *I*, 834–836.

nificantly different from pre- to postbereavement samplings. Control group subjects showed no changes over time.

A study relating the occurrence of life events to changes in immune status also showed effects of stress on immunity (Locke, Hurst, Williams, and Heisel, 1978). When life changes were frequent and reported distress was high as well, measures of natural killer cell activity were lowest. This finding is similar to that reported by Greene, Betts, and Ochitill (1978) indicating that high stress and poor coping were related to proper immune function. Other studies have reported poorer lymphocyte response to mitogens among people subjected to two days of sleep deprivation and among astronauts following return to earth (see Fisher et al., 1972; Palmblad, Petrini, Wasserman, and Ackerstedt, 1979; Palmblad et al., 1976.

Other distressed states have also been shown to be related to immunocompetence. Stein, Keller, and Schleifer (1985) reported that inpatients who were classified as depressed exhibited poorer response to mitogen challenge, and this may be correlated with the intensity of depression. Other studies have suggested that psychiatric patients have poorer immune system control of viruses and fewer T-helper lymphocytes (e.g., Krueger et al., 1984).

Stressors need not be exotic or extremely powerful to affect immune system status. Several studies conducted among students have shown changes in different indices of immune function as a function of examinations. Kiecolt-Glaser and her colleagues, for example, reported decreased natural killer cell activity due to exams in medical school, compared with levels exhibited one month earlier (Kiecolt-Glaser et al., 1984). Loneliness was also associated with lower natural killer cell activity, and subsequent studies found that examinations were also associated with decreased numbers of natural killer cells (Glaser, et al., 1986). Percentages of T-cells that may be classified as helper cells were also found to be lower among medical students during exams than they had been earlier, and production of interferon, an important lymphokine, was suppressed among students during exams relative to pre-exam levels (Kiecolt-Glaser et al., 1986). Further, examinations were associated with decreased proliferative responses to mitogen challenge (Glaser et al., 1985).

A somewhat different approach to documenting immune system status is to examine antibody titers to latent viruses. Some viruses, such as herpes simplex or Epstein-Barr, remain dormant in the body following initial infection. In other words, after the first infection with such a virus, the immune system may control the virus but cannot destroy or eliminate it. The virus remains in a latent state, sufficiently suppressed by immune system activity to keep it in check. When the virus is active, B-cells secrete antibody to destroy it; when the virus is latent, antibody secretion is much lower as the virus is not freely circulating through the body. If something happens to weaken immune system control of latent viruses and they become active, antibody titers to the virus will *increase.* Thus more antibodies for latent viruses suggests poorer immune function, particularly in the absence of changes in antibodies to nonlatent viruses. Treatment of patients with immunosuppressive drugs, such as in chemotherapy, has been shown to increase antibodies to latent viruses (Kiecolt-Glaser and Glaser, 1987). Results of studies measuring antibody titers to latent viruses have also provided evidence of stress-related changes in immune function. Loneliness and examination stress were found to be associated with elevated antibody titers to Epstein-Bar virus among medical students (see Glaser, Kiecolt-Glaser, Speicher, and Holliday, 1985).

Given this acute stress-related immunosuppression, is it possible to reverse this pattern, prevent stress-related decreases in immune function, and/or increase function among stressed individuals to "normal" levels? A study by Kiecolt-Glaser and associates (1985) suggests that the answer is affirmative. In a study of residents of old-age homes, subjects were given one of three treatments. In one, they were trained to relax; in another, they were provided with enhanced social contact; and in the third, no intervention was applied. Subjects in the first treatment group were the only ones to show changes, but these changes were important. Relative to baseline and to the other groups, subjects given relaxation training exhibited heightened natural killer cell activity and lower antibody titers to latent viruses and reported fewer stress-related symptoms. Similar findings have been noted with medical students, among whom most frequent relaxation practice was associated with higher levels of T-lymphocytes, and among undergraduates taught different ways to relax (e.g., Kiecolt-Glaser et al., 1986).

Chronic Stress and Immunity

While these and other studies provide reasonably clear evidence that acute stress is associated with transient immunological changes, the nature of these changes makes it less clear whether chronic stress has longer-term effects. Monjan (1981) suggests that chronic stress may have the opposite effects that acute stress has—that is, chronic stress may *enhance* immune system function. Earlier studies of rats exposed to crowding for one or five weeks prior to immunization produced fewer circulating antibodies in crowded animals than in uncrowded animals, while after five weeks crowded animals showed an enhanced effect to immunization (Joasoo and McKenzie, 1976; Solomon, 1969). Similarly, Monjan and Collector (1977) varied the duration of noise stress in a study of mice and found differences in immune system effects depending on the length of noise exposure. All mice were exposed to fifteen minutes of noise per day, spread out evenly over a three-hour period. Duration was varied by comparing mice exposed to the noise for different numbers of days. Findings suggested that acute noise exposure (fewer days) was associated with suppression of immune responsiveness while longer-term stress was associated with enhancement of immune function. (See Figure 6.3.) Consistent with this, results of a study by Sklar and Anisman (1979) showed that a single day of noise stress reduced resistance to tumor growth while ten days of noise stress resulted in enhancement of resistance and diminished tumor growth.

A likely explanation for the enhancing and suppressing effects of stress is that adaptation or habituation of stress responding is responsible for different effects. Recall from Chapter 3 that organisms adapt to stressful experiences; after repetitive exposure to the same stressor, response to it decreases and may disappear entirely. This appears to occur as a result of psychological adaptation, such as successful coping, rather than as a result of changes in physiological systems. In other words, as people or animals deal with a stressor or "get used to it," biological responses return to normal. In the studies of stress and immune system function just discussed, it is possible that the animals adapted to the stressor when it was chronic and were

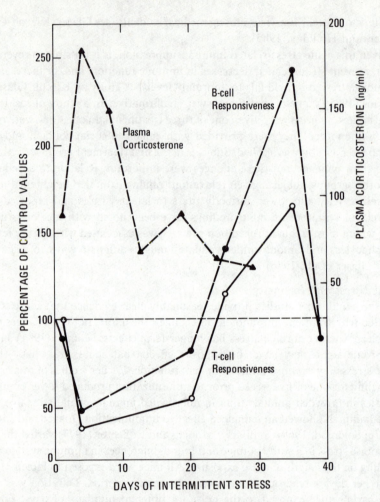

Figure 6.3   Immunosuppression is followed by immunoenhancement during a chronic stress experiment. Plasma corticosterone levels were elevated during the period of immunosuppression, but dropped as the animals apparently became adapted to the chronic stress.
Adapted from Monjan and Collector (1977). Adapted by V. Riley, M. Fitzmaurice, and D. Spackman. Psychoneuroimmunologic factors in neoplasia: Studies in animals. In R. Ader, *Psychoneuroimmunology.* New York: Academic Press, 1981, p. 82.

therefore exhibiting fewer stress responses after ten days than they were after one or two days. If so, one could expect that immune system function would return to normal or exceed baseline levels over time (many physiological systems show a rebound effect when a suppressing force is removed, actually exceeding basal levels for a short time). This has been used to explain initial suppression and subsequent recovery or enhancement of immune function during chronic stress in animals (see Riley et al., 1981). A recent study, however, found a delayed but persistent suppression of natural killer cell function among mice following exposure to a stressor (Kandil and Borysenko, 1987).

Studies of chronic stress and immune response in humans have provided some support for the notion that adaptation is an important factor in the course of immune system activity. Kiecolt-Glaser and colleagues (in press) have argued that findings showing adaptation and/or enhancement of immune system function during chronic stress may have been due to the nature of the stressor. Physical stressors, such as noise, that were used in the studies just discussed may be more easily adapted to than are the complex chronic stressors that people encounter. They reported a study of family caregivers for patients with Alzheimer's disease, a progressively debilitating disease that places great demands on those responsible for patient care. Arguing that people should adapt less readily to such a stressor, they studied a group of thirty-four caregivers and compared them to a control group of matched, noncaregiving subjects. The length of care provided among the caregivers from diagnosis ranged from new diagnosis to eleven years, with a mean of more than thirty-three months. The results of a battery of immunological assessments suggested that caregivers had suppressed immune systems; cellular immune system control of latent viruses was poorer, percentages of T-lymphocytes and T-helper lymphocytes were lower, and the helper/suppressor ratio was smaller among caregivers than among controls. These data were interpreted as indicating that chronic stress can give rise to persistent changes in immunity.

Another study of humans exposed to chronic stress, comparing people living near the Three Mile Island nuclear power plant with a control sample, also suggests that long-term stress can result in immune system change in an apparently negative direction. A very small sample of people living near the power plant who continued to exhibit symptoms of stress were studied more than six years after the accident there; comparable measures were collected among similar control subjects. Results showed an increased number of circulating neutrophils and decreased numbers of B-cells, natural killer cells, and T-suppressor lymphocytes among the Three Mile Island area residents (McKinnon, et al. 1986). Data also suggested poorer cellular control over latent viruses among TMI subjects than among controls.

Stress appears to have direct psychophysiological effects on immunity—stress is associated with bodily changes such as increased levels of cortisol, which can destroy immune tissue and alter the system's ability to function. However, there is another way in which stress can effect immunity, and that is a more indirect pathway through behavioral change. Stress can result in increases in drug use, smoking, drinking, and so on, which could contribute to chronic effects on immunity. Do these behaviors have any implications for the immune system?

SMOKING AND IMMUNE SYSTEM FUNCTION

One way that cigarette smoking is influential in immunity is straightforward enough: tobacco and its products (e.g., smoke, tar) are antigens, interacting with the immune system in ways that result in production of specific antibodies. Some studies have shown that animals can be shown to experience allergic reactions to tobacco products and have argued that this allergy may be relevant to understanding coronary heart disease and hypertension (see Fontana et al., 1959). Among humans, allergic reactions to tobacco extracts have also been found (Kreis et al., 1970; Panayotopoulos et al., 1974).

Cigarette smoking, independent of its role as an antigen, appears to affect immune status as well. Chronic smoking damages the respiratory tract mucus, reducing the number and function of cilia that normally trap invading microorganisms, dust, and other particles (see Ballenger, 1960; Regland et al., 1976). Impairment of this resistance increases the work that must be done by other agents of immunity. However, studies have also shown wide variation in effects of smoking on mucosa, with some smokers showing evidence of damage and others showing little change or even enhanced resistance (Cameron et al., 1970; Yeats et al., 1975).

However, the consequences of smoking extend beyond mucociliary damage and include effects on macrophages and lymphocytes. Smoking appears to increase the number of macrophages in the lungs (see Holt and Keast, 1974). It has also been reported that the composition of macrophages is different in smokers than in nonsmokers (Pratt et al., 1969) and that macrophages are capable of adapting to the effects of cigarette smoke (Holt and Keast, 1974). However, macrophage function appears to be harmed by smoking; the ability of macrophages to engulf and destroy foreign material was reduced by cigarette smoke (Green and Carolin, 1967; Maxwell et al., 1967). Some studies have found no differences in macrophage function among smokers and nonsmokers, suggesting that this effect may be more common among animals than among humans.

The numbers and function of T-lymphocytes are also affected by smoking. In animals, initial exposure to cigarette smoke appears to enhance proliferation of lymphocytes to mitogen stimulation, while prolonged exposure decreases proliferation (Carlens, 1976; Thomas et al., 1973). In humans, the picture is more complex. Increased numbers of T-cells were found in young smokers, mirroring the findings with initial exposure of mice (Silverman et al., 1975). However, for older smokers or for those with a history of heavy, chronic smoking, there were no differences in numbers of T-cells between smokers and nonsmokers. Several other studies in humans have revealed few differences in T-cell numbers or function among smokers and nonsmokers, and the importance of smoking for cellular-based immunity has not been clearly established.

These findings, many based on animal studies, do not provide much information about whether smoking actually affects the immune system's illness-fighting activity. Other studies do suggest that smoking increases incidence of infectious illnesses such as influenza. In one, those smoking more than ten cigarettes a day showed increased risk for the flu, and in another, incidence of clinical and subclinical influenza among smokers was higher than among nonsmokers (Finklea et al., 1969; Waldman et al., 1969). These studies suggest that smoking has immune system effects that may be associated with enhanced susceptibility to illness.

Overall, smoking affects bodily resistance to infection in several ways. In humans nicotine affects lymphocyte function, and tobacco smoke has stimulatory effects at low levels and inhibitory effects in higher doses, with the overall effect suggesting immunosuppression (Holt and Keast, 1977). It appears that smoking affects lymphocytes and macrophages, and it may well be associated with mucociliary damage and destruction of tissue that helps protect us from bacteria and viruses. Much work needs still to be done to determine more clearly how and when cigarette smoking affects immunity and resistance to disease.

ALCOHOL AND IMMUNE FUNCTION

Alcohol has been shown to have a number of effects on immunity. Most of the studies have used animal models of alcohol administration. For example, the ability of macrophages in rabbits to move toward infections was reduced by consumption of alcohol in quantities that approximated a 0.1 percent blood level in humans (Louria, 1963). Recall from Chapter 2 that one mechanism by which macrophages find sites where they are needed is by responding and moving toward chemical signals released by the body. The diminishing of this chemotaxis by macrophages was also observed by Nungester and Klesper (1939) following administration of as little as 100 mg/al of ethanol, and more recent studies show that larger doses also retard the ability of human granulocytes to approach infected areas (Spagnuolo, 1975). In Spagnuolo's (1975) study, continuous oral administration of alcohol (320 ml of 100 percent ethanol daily) for a week reduced chemotaxis by granulocytes, but similar administration of much smaller quantities (less than 100 ml of 100 percent ethanol) did not cause any impairment.

Several studies have addressed the question of whether lymphocytes are affected by alcohol. Monjan and Mandell (1980) examined children of alcoholics and found that their T-cells exhibited poor DNA synthesis and inhibited proliferation; several other studies suggest that alcohol retards the ability of lymphocytes to multiply when they are needed to deal with foreign material (see Atkinson et al., 1977; Johnson et al., 1981; Lundy, 1975). Lymphocyte activity is suppressed among alcoholics and among children with fetal alcohol syndrome (Johnson et al., 1981; Young et al., 1979).

Of more clinical significance, it has been noted that after infusion of alcohol, immune activity against E. coli and H. influenza type B was reduced, but it returned to normal levels five hours after administration (Johnson et al., 1969). The killing ability of lymphocytes also appears to be affected by alcohol, with significant reductions of T-cell cytotoxicity observed following administration of relatively high levels of alcohol (Kemp and Berke, 1987; Stacey, 1984). At lower levels of alcohol, lymphocyte toxicity may be increased or unaffected (Kendall and Targan, 1980).

Research provides some evidence of consequences for immune system function associated with alcohol. Macrophages appear to be inhibited, moving more slowly to sites where they are needed and, perhaps, being produced in smaller numbers. Some lymphocytes also show effects, as T-cell proliferation in the face of challenge and their cytotoxicity appears to be inhibited. However, several aspects of the immune system appear to be unaffected; no inhibition of antibody production has been observed and overall numbers of lymphocytes are not reduced by alcohol (Caizza and Orary, 1976; Conge and Gouche, 1985; Lundy, 1975). The dose and chronicity of alcohol consumption also appears to be important. In most cases, where alcohol is consumed in small or moderate amounts and drinking is irregular, effects are small and/or transient. Among alcoholics, however, effects are substantial and are related to more widespread damage to bodily tissues, including the thymus.

CAFFEINE AND IMMUNITY

People tend to drink more coffee and other caffeine-containing beverages when they are under stress, and research suggests that this may hinder immune function. Studies have shown that high doses of caffeine suppress a range of functions including increased mortality to E. coli bacteria (see Saxena, et al., 1984). At low doses, some evidence of enhanced immune function was observed. Addition of caffeine directly to cultures of spleen cells after antigen stimulation resulted in a reduction of antibody production (Laux and Klesiuns, 1973), but evidence suggests that whatever effects are found may likely be due to caffeine stimulation of cyclic adenosine monophosphate (AMP), which in turn can reduce overall activity of lymphocytes (Borysenko and Borysenko, 1982). In this regard, the immuno-enhancing or suppressing effects of caffeine should be similar to effects of catecholamines released during stress. Drinking coffee while under stress could produce particularly clear effects.

SUMMARY

The importance of research showing direct psychophysiological effects on immune status or function and of behavioral influences on immune system activity lies in several areas. On the one hand, the notion that the immune, nervous, and endocrine systems are interrelated and integrated by the central nervous system opens new possibilities for the study of regulation of internal bodily function and homeostasis. Conditioning studies show that the same processes by which heart rate or other peripheral responses may be regulated by an individual may apply to the immune system as well. Finally, the finding that stress can affect the immune system demands study of how stress may contribute to illness associated with immune system deficiency. Impaired immune system function clearly contributes to the incidence of infectious illness, though available research evidence has not clearly established stress-related immunosuppression as a cause of these illnesses. In another category, however, are more devastating diseases directly related to immune system function—cancer and acquired immune deficiency syndrome (AIDS).

CANCER

Cancer is the second leading cause of death in this country. One reason for the increased incidence of cancer is the growing number of older people, who are more likely than younger people to develop cancer (Krantz et al., 1980). Other factors include smoking, diet, and increased levels of certain suspected carcinogens in our environment—food additives, asbestos, chemical wastes, defoliants, and radiation. Diagnoses of cancer are more likely now as well.

Cancer is actually a set of related diseases in which altered cells of the body—cancer cells—multiply in unrestrained and rapid fashion, generating tumors or clusters of cells whose growth is also uncontrollable. Basic to the growth of cancerous neoplasms is damage to the DNA inside cells. The rapid increases in abnormal cells cause a diversion of nourishment from functional cells and eventual invasion of bodily tissue by the cancerous growth. This proliferation of cancer cells may cause damage or death of organ systems and the organism.

BEHAVIORAL FACTORS AND CANCER

Despite the fact that there are a hundred or more different forms of cancer, some general theories of how cancer begins and develops have been formulated. One belief is that cancer is related to genetic cell defects that are triggered by a number of environmental or physiological factors (see Cohen et al., 1979). Another suggests that breakdown or temporary dysfunction of the immune system, which routinely attacks and kills mutagenic or alien cells or tumors, is responsible for cancer. Basically this theory posits a "surveillance" function in the immune system. By recognizing and killing precancerous cells under conditions of normal functioning, the immune system protects the body from invasion by alien cells. When the surveillance role is suppressed, however, by any of a number of physiological, social, or psychological events, the immune system may fail to detect and kill cancerous cells, allowing tumors to develop unhindered. There is evidence, for example, that natural killer cells are involved in cancer protection (see Herberman and Holden, 1978). If these cells are responsible for surveillance and early destruction of tumors, disruption of their activity as appears to occur during or after stress could have important implications for cancer. Locke and his colleagues (1979), for instance, reported a study of life events and natural killer cell activity that suggested that stress could suppress this activity.

Studies addressing this surveillance notion have been criticized on methodological grounds, so evidence is as yet inconclusive. Research clearly suggests, however, that psychological factors affect the course of the disease once established. These data are largely in the form of correlations, linking personality variables or coping styles with length of survival, recurrence, and the general course of illness (see Derogatis, Abeloff, and Melisaratos, 1979; Rogentine et al., 1979). These studies indicate that the rate at which the disease progresses (rather than the factors that first caused it) is associated with psychological variables.

The search for behavioral factors in the onset of cancer appears largely concerned with two factors: lifestyle variables such as smoking and variables associated with the immune system. Studies have suggested that the loss of a close and important person is associated with reduced immune competence or the onset of cancer (see Bartop et al., 1977; Tache, Selye, and Day, 1979). Recall, for example, that in a study of men who had recently lost their wives, Schleifer et al. (1980) found that their immune systems showed marked depression during bereavement.

Social support can also affect cancer. Studies suggest that a lack of close interpersonal ties is often associated with cancer (Thomas and Duszynski, 1974). In one study almost one thousand medical students were interviewed and then followed for ten to fifteen years. Of the original group, those who had developed cancer after fifteen years reported that they did not have very much family closeness.

Recent studies examining mechanisms by which stress-induced immunosuppression might cause or facilitate cancer have yielded promising results. Sklar and

Anisman (1981) had concluded that stress probably did not cause tumors to appear but rather affects growth of neoplasms. Glaser et al. (1985) found evidence of stress effects in one of the basic bodily defenses against carcinogens: DNA repair within cells was disrupted due to stress-related reductions in the level of an enzyme that helps to repair cellular DNA and minimize damage due to cancer-causing agents. The same link was identified in another study of psychiatric patients varying in reported distress. Those reporting more stress showed poorer DNA repair in lymphocytes than those reporting less stress or than nonpatient controls (Kiecolt-Glaser et al., 1985). These studies begin to show us the ways in which stress may affect immune function and disease states.

Smoking and diet have been established as risk factors for cancer, and the routes by which they exert this influence are varied. Smoking can affect immune system and reduce immunosurveillance, possibly increasing the chances for a tumor to grow. Other immune system functions are also affected by smoking, and direct organ system damage is also possible. Dietary factors have been associated with cancer as well (Levy, 1983). Recent research has also suggested a link between alcohol consumption and cancer (see Heirch et al., 1983). In combination with smoking, alcohol consumption has been found to contribute to risk for several types of cancer (see Flanders and Rothman, 1982; Herity et al., 1982). Dietary variables may be factors in findings relating cultural background with cancer. For example, it was found that Japanese-American women were more likely to develop breast cancer when they lived in the United States; the "Americanization" of these women was associated with increased susceptibility to breast cancer (Wynder, 1963). Because social and cultural differences are so complex and include so many possible causes, it is difficult to determine which variables are responsible for differences in cancer rates. However, the pronounced differences in diet across cultures is one likely agent.

Stress in general appears to be involved in the etiology and progression of cancer. This is not surprising, since lack of support is associated with greater stress impact and the loss of significant others can be extremely stressful. Studies of animals exposed to stress have noted damage to tissues involved in immunity, such as the thymus (which, as you will recall, is part of Selye's triad of responses) and lowered immune functioning (Amkraut and Solomon, 1977). Further studies have reported that crowding or noxious stimulation can increase the incidence of spontaneous cancers (Ader, 1981). Similarly, stressed animals are more susceptible to a range of infectious diseases (see Amkraut and Solomon, 1977; Bartop et al., 1977; Friedman, Glasgow, and Ader, 1969).

The reasons for this relationship are not known. Some have proposed that sympathetic arousal associated with stress or the pituitary-adrenal-cortical responses described by Selye may be responsible. The latter notion is supported by findings showing reduced immune responses in humans following corticosteroid therapy (see Rinehart et al., 1975). These reductions in the ability of the body to combat infection were apparently caused by increased levels of corticosteroids in the body.

Catecholamines, associated with adrenal medullary response to sympathetic arousal, have also been implicated. Gruchow (1979) has reported findings indicating that higher levels of catecholamine excretion in urine were related to onset of infectious illness. Elevated levels were found for two to three days prior to the onset of illness more often than after illness or during a nonillness interval. Gruchow concluded that higher levels of catecholamines increase susceptibility to illnesses that are communicable, suggesting that they suppress immune competence.

PERSONALITY FACTORS AND CANCER

The immune system's role in cancer is still unknown. Despite promising findings and some apparent relationships, much work remains to be done. However, other dimensions are also being explored. Wittkower and Dudek (1973) suggested that psychological factors are involved in the onset of cancer, and some research has suggested the possibility of a cancer-prone personality (see Le Shan, 1959). Several characteristics that seem to be associated with cancer have been identified. The first includes a tendency to keep in resentment and anger rather than express it and a "marked inability to forgive." In addition, research suggests that cancer victims are ineffective in forming and/or maintaining close, long-term relationships with other people. They are more likely to be loners without extensive social support systems. Third, they engage in more self-pity than what might be considered normal. And these people tend to have poor self-images. Thus the cancer-prone individual "puts on a happy face and denies any sense of loss, anger, distress, disappointment, or despair" (Scarf, 1980, p. 37) while living an inner life of self-pity, insecurity, and a certain degree of loneliness. Other research has described the cancer-prone person as pleasant, compliant, and passive, or as extreme expressors or suppressors of anger (Greer and Morris, 1975; Renneker, 1981).

One of the problems in determining whether there is a personality style that predisposes someone to get cancer is causality. If you find that certain types of people develop cancer more often than others, is this sufficient to show a personality cause? The answer, clearly, is no. Most studies of personality factors and cancer have compared cancer patients with healthy control subjects *after* the patients have become ill (Fox, 1976). The inference that is often made is that any differences observed between patient and nonpatient groups were there prior to the onset of illness and were responsible for it. This is difficult to prove, and as Fox (1976) suggests, cancer causes a number of perceptual and cognitive changes that could affect or produce differences between patients and nonpatients. Chemotherapy agents are toxic and may have effects on mood as well. Some studies have shown differences between cancer and noncancer patients that existed before disease status was known, but the data do not clearly support the idea that personality factors contribute to cancer (Fox, 1976; Krasnoff, 1959; Perrin and Pierce, 1959; Stavraky, 1968). It is possible, though, that personality may be related to behaviors that are associated with cancer, such as smoking and poor diet (Fox, 1976).

Personality variables may not be as important in the cause of cancer as in its progression. Research has suggested that personality profiles in which behavior is overly polite and passive are associated with rapid progression of cancer and early death compared with the longer time course of illness exhibited by people who are more aggressive (see Derogatis, et al., 1979). Levy et al. (1985) reported that apathy, depression, and fatiguelike behavior was associated with poorer biological status (lower natural killer cell activity) among women with primary breast cancer. However, this could be true of a number of degenerative or progressive diseases—that combative people live longer (because they "fight" harder). In addition, women who were rated as being "well adjusted" or who reported low levels of social support also showed lower natural killer cell activity. Those who were seen as being better adjusted may have, in fact, been exhibiting symptoms of learned helplessness and as a result appeared more compliant and cooperative (see Chapter 8). The relationship between personality and disease progression requires further study.

It is very difficult to study psychological or behavioral components of cancer, and this limits our ability to determine their roles. The relatively long period of time over which cancer develops (some forms require twenty years or more before they can be detected) is the basic problem. Studies must be retrospective, and recollections may be affected by the knowledge that one has cancer. Also, since we do not know when the disease began, it is difficult to attach significance to psychological events. How does one know, for example, that loss of a spouse affected the disease if one cannot determine whether the disease started around the time of the loss?

AIDS

Since its "discovery," AIDS has quickly become one of the most deadly and feared diseases in history. Like cancer, it involves the immune system, but in different ways. It is caused by infection with **human immunodeficiency virus (HIV)** and has a number of immunologic effects, including decreases in T-lymphocytes, some types of immunoglobins, T-helper lymphocytes, and reduced responsiveness of lymphocytes to antigens (see Coates et al., 1987; Lange et al., 1987). Because the virus attacks helper cells specifically, it disrupts cellular immunity and increases victims' susceptibility to opportunistic infections. Thus many AIDS patients develop other illnesses, which may actually be the cause of their death. Among the opportunistic infections identified in AIDS patients are pneumocystis carinii pneumonia and Kaposi's sarcoma (a rare cancer).

Exposure to HIV is not the same as having AIDS. Once exposed, an individual may develop the disease or a related syndrome, AIDS-related complex (ARC), an intermediate stage in which symptoms are present and immunosuppression detectable but in which the intensity of the illness is more moderate. In some cases ARC may be fatal, and in most cases it precedes AIDS. Some individuals who are exposed do not immediately develop AIDS or ARC; of those who test positive for the AIDS virus (seropositive, i.e., having antibodies for HIV), less than half have developed AIDS (Goedert et al., 1986). The virus may remain dormant for varying periods before becoming active and causing AIDS or ARC. Some researchers believe this is similar to the way in which latent viruses, such as herpes, emerge periodically to cause illness. However, some believe that all or at least a majority of those who are seropositive will develop AIDS. Estimates of deaths from AIDS through 1991 approach 200,000 Americans. And, of course, the disease is not just an American phenomenon; it threatens most of the world's population. In some countries the epidemic has been more destructive than in this country.

TRANSMISSION OF AIDS

HIV is spread by exchange of bodily fluids during sex, sharing of needles or other drug paraphernalia, blood transfusion, and from mother to child prior to delivery (Coates et al., 1987). The disease was initially found in this country among identifiable subgroups (e.g., homosexuals) and was apparently spread within these groups (e.g., by sexual contact in the gay community). Thus homosexuals are one of several high-risk groups; the others include intravenous drug users, bisexual men, and hemophiliacs (who require frequent blood transfusions). Estimates of the percentage of AIDS cases among gay or bisexual men have ranged up to three-quarters of AIDS cases, with intravenous drug users, hemophiliacs, and transfusion recipients behind them in reported incidence of the disease (Centers for Disease Control, 1985). Another "problem group" is pregnant women who test positive for the HIV antibody or young children with HIV infection. The virus does not appear to be communicable by casual contact, but requires intimate contact and substantial exposure to infected blood or semen to be transmitted from one person to another.

Reported cases have increased dramatically since 1978 (e.g., May and Anderson, 1987). In one study of gay men done in San Francisco, the percentage of tested individuals who were seropositive—who showed evidence of infection with HIV—increased from less than 10 percent in 1978 to more than 70 percent in 1985 (Centers for Disease Control, 1986). Similar results have been reported in studies of homosexuals in London and intravenous drug users in Italy (Angarano et al., 1985; Carne et al., 1985). The time needed for reported cases to double has decreased steadily since discovery of the epidemic, and the number of cases of AIDS has risen rapidly (see Figure 6.4) (May and Anderson, 1987).

A number of treatments have been proposed and promising drugs have been developed. As of this writing, one drug, AZT, has been used widely. Early studies indicate that AZT may inhibit spread of the virus, but whether it improves immune function is not clear (Selwyn, 1986). Despite the life-lengthening effects of AZT, its ultimate value remains to be seen as long-term survival and possible side effects are evaluated. However, *there is currently no cure for AIDS or vaccine to prevent infection by HIV.* Because of this, prevention is particularly important, as once an individual develops the disease, the prognosis is not good. Behavioral principles become very important as a result of this situation and because the ways in which the disease is transmitted are largely controllable. In other words, spread of AIDS can, it is believed, be stopped or greatly reduced by getting people to avoid high-risk behaviors and/or to change their behavior so as to minimize risk. Use of condoms during sexual intercourse, for example, greatly reduces the chances of spreading disease in this manner. Thus getting people to adopt safer behaviors appears to be one of the only avenues by which we may be able to deal with AIDS, at least for the present.

It appears that anyone can get AIDS, and predictions suggest that the disease is spreading into the heterosexual community and over the next few years will begin to affect significant numbers of heterosexuals. However, because the initial spread of the disease has occurred in two or three groups, most attempts to change behavior have taken shape therein. There is some evidence, for example, that health education programs have increased knowledge about the disease and how it is spread among

COPING WITH A POSITIVE HIV TEST

When someone tests positive for the virus that causes AIDS, what can be done for him or her? It is not currently known what the likelihood of developing AIDS is once someone has been infected, and we do not know enough about the disease to predict how long it may take for the disease to develop. Studies indicate moderate rates of disease among seropositive people over three- or four-year periods, showing that about one in five people testing positive for the virus actually gets AIDS (Goedert et al., 1987; Kaplan et al., 1987). Further complicating this is the fact that we do not know what factors affect the development of the disease. There appear to be genetic factors involved (Elaes et al., 1987), but stress and other psychosocial variables may be important as well. The need for programs for education and counseling for seropositive individuals is clear.

One such program has been described by Morokoff, Holmes-Johnson, and Weisse (1987). Patients are given a thorough medical screening and evaluation, including retesting for HIV antibodies, laboratory analysis of immune status, and rediagnosis. This is followed by psychosocial evaluation by a social worker, chaplain, and psychiatrists, and patients are assigned to a support group meeting at least once a week. Finally, an educational program is presented, including discussion of the relationships between stress and immune function, medical and legal aspects of HIV-positive status, stress management, safer sex practices, and alcohol and drug abuse.

The support groups focus on management of grief, depression, feelings of helplessness, anger, fear of dying, and related issues. Educational programs are directed primarily at providing information relevant to problems dealt with in the support groups as well as coping and self-management skills that may help people deal with their situation. One lecture deals specifically with the ways in which people react to the knowledge that they are seropositive for HIV. This provides a normative context within which individuals may evaluate and work through their fears and concerns. The stress management instruction is designed to help patients regain a sense of control over their lives and, perhaps, to reinforce immune system response. A lecture about safer sex practices deals with the very mundane but vitally important issue of how to avoid the further spread of the virus.

In attempting to address the information needs and emotional concerns of the individual who is positive for the AIDS virus, this program represents an important example of the kind of treatment program that will not only help those already infected but also contribute to the prevention of further transmission of the disease. The problems that go along with a positive test for the virus are great and difficult to cope with in the isolation that may follow disclosure of the diagnosis. Education about the nature of AIDS, its biological and psychological characteristics, and coping skills may improve the health and well-being of these people as well as help to prevent the spread of the disease.

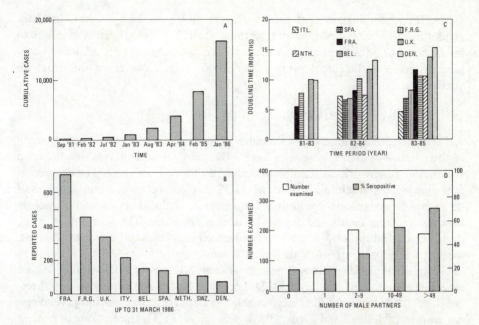

Figure 6.4 *A,* The rise in the number of reported cases of AIDS in the United States, September 1981 to January 1986. *B,* Reported cases of AIDS in nine countries of the European community up to March 31, 1986. *C,* Doubling times in the cumulative incidence of AIDS (t_0) recorded in months for various European countries over various time intervals (1981–83, 1982–84, 1983–85; DEN, Denmark; BEL, Belgium; NTH, Netherlands; FRA, France; F.R.G.. Federal Republic of Germany; SPA, Spain; ITL, Italy; UK, United Kingdom). *D,* The relationship between sexual activity among a sample of homosexual/ bisexual males (from San Francisco) as measured by the number of male partners over a two-year period, and the percentage of each group (based on sex partners) who were seropositive for HIV antibodies. From R. M. May and R. M. Anderson. Transmission dynamics of HIV infection. *Nature,* 1987, *326,* 138.

gay men, and that sexual behavior that appears to have been associated with the spread of AIDS has decreased (see McKusick, Hortsmann, and Coates, 1985; McKusick, et al, 1985). Emphasis has been on **safer sex**, taking precautions such as **condom** use to reduce spread of HIV during sex, and on reducing numbers of sex partners and other aspects of sexual activity that increase transmission of illness. However, these interventions have not been wholly successful; in some reports gay men state they have continued high-risk behavior. College students, regardless of sexual orientation or lifestyle, are at risk because of frequent sexual contact and because they may not engage in "safe" practices due to a sense of invulnerability or the belief that if any of their partners had AIDS, they would let others know (see Hirschorn, 1987). Some allow the belief that only homosexuals and drug users get the disease to dissuade them from taking proper precautions.

Research on interventions and on the risk-taking behavior among drug users suggests that most engage in behavior that can spread the disease. Data show that nearly 90 percent of drug users with AIDS or ARC shared needles and that a majority of drug users share needles regularly (Black et al., 1986; Friedland et al.,

1985). Data also suggest that drug users are aware of the risks but that they engage in risky behaviors anyway (Coates et al., 1987). Complicating attempts to intervene is the addictive nature of the behavior; because drugs are addictive, stopping drug use is difficult, leaving modification of how one takes the drugs an "easier" target.

PSYCHOSOCIAL CONSEQUENCES OF AIDS

AIDS is a frightening illness with a number of consequences other than deterioration of the immune system. Those who have AIDS may find themselves isolated from social support networks as friends and family withdraw from them. The decision of how and when to disclose that one has AIDS may generate social consequences of its own and may require disclosure of a lifestyle or habit that one had previously kept hidden from family and friends (Coates et al., 1987). Thus the nature of the disease and conditions by which it is transmitted may cause people to provide less support for victims just when they need it most.

Psychiatric impairment and emotional complications of AIDS and ARC are relatively common, with estimates that more than half of AIDS patients and three-quarters of ARC patients show diagnosable emotional disturbances and psychological disorders (Holland and Tross, 1985); Selwyn, 1986). The higher rate of distress among ARC patients may reflect the uncertainty of their prognosis, though seropositive but healthy individuals show a lower rate of distress (Selwyn, 1986). The effects of stress among patients with AIDS or ARC may be responsible for some of these disturbances as well as for variations in the progression of the disease due to factors such as immunosuppression, poor diet, smoking, and so on.

Stress and emotional problems are likely among those who test positive for HIV but who are not ill (see box). The knowledge that one has tested positive can generate profound distress and has been associated with psychiatric problems. Several studies have shown that problems such as depression, anxiety, fear, and adjustment problems can occur as a result of testing, though other research has suggested that the testing procedures and knowledge of one's HIV status can have little or even positive effects (Selwyn, 1986).

Neuorological consequences of the disease are also serious and may further complicate psychosocial adjustment. AIDS dementia, which refers to a variety of CNS problems, appears to be common among AIDS patients (Selwyn, 1986). Symptoms of CNS impairment include memory problems, difficulty in concentrating and in coordination of motor skills, balance problems, and severe impairment of impulse control and decision making. These problems further affect attempts to stop the spread of the disease, and may interfere with its management and treatment. Impairment occurs not only among AIDS patients but among those testing positive for the HIV antibody as well. In about 25 percent of cases, dementia-related symptoms are detected before any signs of AIDS or ARC appear (Navia Jordan, and Price, 1986), a fact that suggests parallel CNS and immune effects of the virus and the usefulness of neuropsychological testing in diagnosing and managing the illness.

This discussion of AIDS is necessarily brief and does not approach the complex problems that the epidemic presents. A number of behaviorally based prevention and treatment programs have been developed, and some of these will be discussed in more detail in Chapter 13. The role of psychological variables in the progression of the disease is also important, and some studies have begun to address the effects of psychosocial variables. Research has, for example, suggested that stress may affect the immune system so as to increase immunosuppression and contribute to progression of AIDS (see Coates et al., 1987; Temoshok, Zich, Solomon, and Stiles, 1987). Personality characteristics may also be associated with better or poorer coping and with different prognoses (see Temoshock, Sweet, and Zich, 1987). In cases of victimization, research suggests, for example, that self-blame can enhance coping by reaffirming one's sense of control (see Chapter 8). In the case of ARC, this holds up, but among AIDS patients, self-blame contributes to negative emotional states, suggesting different perceptions and implications (Temoshok et al., 1987). Further research is needed to clarify these issues, to better understand the role of psychological variables in the disease, and to further develop effective preventive and treatment programs.

SUMMARY

The importance of psychological and neural interactions with the immune system has become increasingly clear in the past decade and suggests a number of important things. Immunocompetence appears to be conditionable, providing evidence of psychological mediation of immune responsiveness and suggesting a number of important practical and research issues. Stress appears to affect immunocompetence as well, suggesting the possibility that psychophysiological states do predispose one to a range of infectious illnesses. Tumor growth appears to be affected by stress, expanding more rapidly when growing during stress than immediately after exposure to a stressor. Lymphocytes and other agents of immunity are also weakened by stress. Further research is needed to determine whether these changes are associated with increased susceptibility to illness.

In this chapter we also discussed two diseases that involve the immune system—cancer and AIDS. Both are often fatal and frighten people greatly, but they involve very different processes and are affected by many psychosocial variables. The notion of immunosurveillance was considered and discussed as a possible contributor to cancer, and the role of personality factors in cancer was also considered. Similarly, in the case of AIDS, a number of psychological variables of possible importance to development and/or progression of the disease were presented. The importance of behavioral factors in both diseases is clear, though the lack of effective treatments for AIDS makes behavioral issues involved in treatment and prevention particularly prominent.

RECOMMENDED READINGS:

Ader, R. (Ed.). *Psychoneuroimmunology.* New York: Academic Press, 1981.

Burish, T., Levy, S. and Meyerowitz, B. (Eds.). *Cancer, nutrition, and eating behavior.* Hillsdale, N.J.: Erlbaum, 1984.

Fox, B. (1978). Premorbid psychological factors as related to cancer incidence. *Journal of Behavioral Medicine, 1,* 45–134.

Jemmott, J. B. and Locke, S. E. Psychosocial factors, immunologic mediation, and human susceptibility to infectious diseases. *Psychological Bulletin, 95,* 78–108.

Temoshok, L. and Baum, A. (Eds.). *Psychosocial aspects of AIDS.* Hillsdale, N.J.: Erlbaum, 1988.

7 PSYCHOPHYSIOLOGICAL DISORDERS

||||||||||||||||||||||||||||||||||||||||||||||||||||||||||||||||||||||||||||||||||||||||||||||||||||||||||||||||||||||||||||||||||

Psychophysiological disorders, traditionally called psychosomatic illnesses, are characterized by physical symptoms or dysfunctions in various bodily organs that are intimately linked with psychological factors. The close interplay of psychological and physiological processes involved in these disorders makes their diagnosis and treatment particularly difficult. The symptoms of psychophysiological disorders are often similar to those present in a systemic disease. As a result, distinctions between these types of disorders are usually made on the basis of etiology. For example, in the case of hypertension, renal hypertension is a systemic disease caused by kidney malfunctioning. Essential hypertension (discussed in Chapter 5) is classified as a psychophysiological disorder because it has no known medical cause. In other words, it is **idiopathic.** However, even though psychological factors appear to cause the chronic elevation of blood pressure in the disorder, the physical problem is nevertheless very real.

In many instances, the distinction between psychosomatic and nonpsychosomatic illnesses is difficult to make. Buss (1966) pointed out that psychological factors may be sufficient but not necessary causes of certain somatic disorders so that the line dividing purely psychophysiological from systemic disorders is frequently blurred. Investigating childhood asthma, Rees (1964) isolated three causal factors: allergic, infective, and psychological. These factors, either alone or in any combination, can trigger an asthma attack. Rees suggested that multiple causation is usually the rule, with various sequences and combinations of factors culminating in the attack.

We still do not know enough about the process by which psychological factors produce changes in somatic factors. It should also be noted that in the field of medicine as a whole, the exact causes of many disorders are not totally understood. As a result, the general rule of assessment has been to diagnose a particular case of hypertension, headache, or the like as psychophysiological only after a complete medical evaluation has ruled out organic factors as the primary cause, and only where good evidence exists for emotional factors that are antecedent or coincident to the disorder.

Most medical explanations of disease have been **functional** in nature—that is, they have not explained the antecedents of symptoms of a disorder, but only the functional disturbances they express. Explanations have basically been descriptive in nature, without much predictive power. For example, they tell us about the relationship between high blood pressure and renal dysfunction, but they do not indicate why at a particular point in time the kidneys failed. The contribution of the field of psychosomatic research to medicine has been to provide a historical explanation of a disorder as well, in order to allow the prediction of who might be at risk for a particular disorder and under what conditions the predisposed person is most likely to develop it. Unfortunately, this field initially overemphasized the unitary role of psychological predisposition in the etiological process. A great deal of psychological research was conducted without simultaneously taking into account physiological and genetic factors that interact in predisposing an individual to a particular disorder. Later in this chapter we will again consider the diathesis-stress model of illness, which was proposed to account for all of these variables.

THE DSM-III CLASSIFICATION OF PSYCHOPHYSIOLOGICAL DISORDERS

Until recently the *Diagnostic and Statistical Manual of the American Psychiatric Association* (DSM-II; see Chapter 9) recognized the existence of psychogenic illness (see Table 7.1) but separated such disorders and implied that only certain ailments could have psychological causes. Nine major categories of disorders were delineated, with the major factor being the affected part or system of the body (e.g., cardiovascular disorders such as hypertension or Raynaud's disease; skin disorders such as hives or neurodermatitis). The problem with this scheme is readily apparent; with the increasing recognition that psychological or emotional factors are important in the precipitation and/or exacerbation of most organic illness, a change was needed in this classification system. Research had implicated psychological factors in the etiology and development of a number of illnesses not considered to be psychophysiological, ranging from neurological disorders such as multiple sclerosis to infectious diseases and malignancies such as tuberculosis and leukemia (see Wittkower and Dudek, 1973). The DSM-II could not account for this.

Lipp, Looney, and Spitzer (1977) originally pointed out that the DSM-III would have to take into account the degree to which psychosocial factors can influence any physical condition. In their proposal, which was subsequently adopted and incorporated into the third edition of the manual (DSM-III), they recommended that the separate section on psychophysiological disorders be deleted and a section entitled "Psychological Factors in Physical Conditions" be substituted. (The title was subsequently changed to "Psychological Factors Affecting Physical Condition.") This section includes not only the traditional psychophysiological disorders listed in the old DSM-II, but also any physical

TABLE 7.1   Classification of Psychophysiological Disorders Used in DSM-II

1. **Skin Disorders**
   Acne—Eruption of blemishes on skin, especially facial skin.
   Eczema—Inflammation, itching, and redness of the skin.
   Hives (Urticaria)—Raised edematous patches of skin usually associated with intense itching.
   Neurodermatitis—Skin eruptions, ranging from a chronic rash to running sores.
   Psoriasis—Circumscribed red patches on skin covered by white scales.

2. **Musculoskeletal Disorders**
   Backache—Pain in the muscles of the back produced by chronic tension.
   Muscle tension headache—Headache caused by chronic contraction of the head and neck muscles.

3. **Respiratory Disorders**
   Bronchial asthma—Breathing difficulties including wheezing, gasping, and coughing.
   Hyperventilation—Extremely fast and deep breathing.

4. **Cardiovascular Disorders**
   Essential hypertension—Chronically elevated blood pressure.
   Migraine headache—Headache caused by dilation of cranial vasculature.
   Raynaud's disease—Cold hands and/or feet caused by decrease of blood supply to these limbs.

5. **Hemic and Lymphatic Disorders**

6. **Gastrointestinal Disorders**
   Gastric ulcers—Lesion in the walls of stomach.
   Gastritis—Excessive amount of gas in the digestive tract.
   Mucous colitis—Inflammation of the colon which produces disturbances in bowel functioning.

7. **Genitourinary Disorders**
   Dysmenorrhea—Painful and/or irregular menstrual periods.
   Dyspareunia—Painful intercourse experienced by the female.
   Impotence—Inability of male to achieve or maintain a penile erection.
   Vaginismus—Irregular and involuntary contractions of the vaginal muscles prior to or during intercourse.

8. **Endocrine Disorders**
   Goiter—Enlargement of thyroid gland that is not due to a neoplasm.
   Obesity—Excessive overweight.

9. **Disorders of Organs of Special Sense**
   Ménière's disease—Disorder of the semicircular canals of inner ears, and progressive deafness.

10. **Other Types**

From American Psychiatric Association, *Diagnostic and Statistical Manual of Mental Disorders,* 2nd ed. Washington, D.C.: APA, 1968.

condition in which psychological factors are found to be significant in precipitating, exacerbating, or prolonging the disorder. The new system allows clinicians to avoid considering a given condition exclusively in psychological or organic terms. Most professionals in the field of psychosomatic medicine currently take such a multicausal etiological approach to disease. In describing psychophysiological disorders, they refer not to a distinct group of illnesses but to any physical condition that is precipitated, exacerbated, or prolonged by psychological factors. Thus the

DSM-III and more recent DSM-IIIR embrace the notion that psychological factors are important in many disorders.

MAJOR FORMS OF PSYCHOPHYSIOLOGICAL DISORDERS

In Chapter 5 we considered one of the most common and potentially dangerous forms of psychophysiological disorders—essential hypertension. In this section we will briefly review a few of the other traditional forms of psychophysiological disorders. For a more in-depth review of these as well as other psychophysiological disorders, the reader is referred to Weiner's (1977) comprehensive survey.

BRONCHIAL ASTHMA

Bronchial asthma is a common psychophysiological disorder, occurring in approximately 5 percent of the general population (Mears and Gatchel, 1979). It is an obstructive disease of the bronchial airways characterized by shortness of breath, coughing, wheezing, and a sensation of choking caused by a decrease in the diameter of the bronchi through which air passes to the lungs. These constrictions are produced by swelling of the bronchial mucosa and/or contraction of the bronchial muscles. Asthmatic attacks usually begin suddenly, with the symptoms lasting anywhere from less than an hour to several hours or even days. Between these attacks, no abnormal symptoms are usually detected. Two distinct forms of asthma are frequently referred to: *extrinsic,* in which there is strong evidence of allergy involvement, with patients having a strong family history of allergy, and *intrinsic,* in which there is less evidence for hereditary and allergy factors. Approximately 30 to 50 percent of all cases of asthma are extrinsic (Holman and Muschenheim, 1972).

As we noted earlier, Rees (1964) isolated three causal factors when examining the case histories of children with asthma. The allergy factor reflected situations in which some substance (e.g., an allergen such as pollen or dust) caused a biochemical reaction that constricted the bronchi. The infection factor included microbial or pathogenic etiology, with the most common type of respiratory infection being acute bronchitis. Rees noted that 35 percent of the asthmatic children he studied had their first asthmatic attacks during a respiratory infection. Finally, psychological factors such as anxiety, depression, and other emotional reactions were considered as potential causes of an asthmatic attack.

Other investigators have also isolated the importance of these three factors. For example, Williams et al. (1958), in their study of 487 asthmatic patients of all ages, found that allergy factors played a dominant precipitating role in 29 percent, infection factors in 40 percent, and psychological factors in 30 percent. However, even in the group where psychological factors played a dominant role, asthmatic attacks were also precipitated by allergic factors in 50 percent of these patients. Thus no one factor appears solely responsible for the precipitation of asthmatic attacks. Multiple causations are most common, with the majority of cases involving two or more of these factors in various sequences and combinations.

DYSMENORRHEA

Dysmenorrhea is characterized by irregular or painful menstrual periods. An accurate estimate of the percentage of women who suffer from this disorder is difficult to determine since many women do not seek medical help for menstruation-related problems. Moreover, many physicians still dismiss such problems as purely emotional, merely prescribe painkillers, and may not look thoroughly for organic involvement. As a consequence of these difficulties in evaluating exact frequency of occurrence, estimates of the percentage of American women with dysmenorrhea range from 4 to 62 percent (Santamaria, 1969).

There have been no systematic, large-scale investigations attempting to evaluate the impact of psychological factors in the development of dysmenorrhea. The bulk of evidence suggesting such a relationship has been obtained from uncontrolled clinical observations. For example, many women report that changes in their life situation (e.g., moving away from their families) and the concomitant emotional effects produce changes in the length and level of pain produced by menstruation. Thus clinical accounts suggest that emotional factors are involved in this disorder. However, biofeedback and relaxation have been used effectively in treating this problem and suggest that psychological factors are involved (Bennink, Hulst, and Benthem, 1982). Controlled research is needed to help validate these speculations as well as to delineate the interaction among the biochemistry, physiology, and mood disturbances associated with menstruation. Studies have implicated the role of overproduction of prostaglandins by the uterus in painful menstrual cramps (Kreutner, 1980). Investigations assessing the relationship between psychological factors and this overproduction would be a valuable step in isolating the psychophysiological underpinnings of dysmenorrhea. Indeed, many researchers believe that both psychological and physiological factors are involved in a range of menstrual problems (see Ruble and Brooks-Gunn, 1979).

HEADACHE

Headaches can result from a wide variety of organic causes such as tumors, systemic infections, or concussions. The vast majority of headaches, however, are psychophysiological in nature and can be divided into three major categories: (1) migraine headaches, (2) muscle contraction or tension headache, and (3) a mixed-category headache in which symptoms of both migraine and tension headaches are present. Headache is common in the general population. Migraine headaches occur in about 5 percent of the population, while approximately 30 percent more experience those in the tension and mixed categories.

Migraine headache is a vascular disorder caused by a loss of tone in the major extracranial vessels, leading to painful pulsatile distention. A pain-threshold chemical (bradykinin or neurokinin) is thought to be released at the site of the dilated vessels, causing an inflammatory reaction. Edema develops (i.e., the walls of the blood vessels become filled with fluid), resulting in a sharp, painful, and throbbing sensation in the head. The pain is often unilateral. The headache is often preceded by an aura—a subjective sensation alerting the person that the headache is about to start. Symptoms such as nausea, vomiting, and dizziness may accompany this prodromal or precursory symptom. These headaches usually do not occur during an immediate period of stress, but rather during the poststress period. They can last anywhere from a few hours to several days.

Muscle contraction or tension headaches are quite different from migraine headaches. They are caused by sustained contraction of the head and neck muscles. They often last for days or weeks and usually begin during an immediate stress period. There are no significant prodromal symptoms, and the headache itself consists of a nonthrobbing ache, with a sensation of tightness frequently described as a feeling of having a "tight band" around the head.

Clinical observation frequently reveals an association between emotionally stressful events and the emergence of symptoms in chronic headache sufferers. Wolff conducted a number of studies using an "emotional provocation technique" to precipitate headaches in patients (Dalessio, 1972). The psychological stress produced by this technique, in which patients were criticized and rebuked for their behavior, was found to trigger headache attacks. More recently Bakal (1975) thoroughly reviewed the literature on migraine and muscle contraction headaches and concluded that headache appears to be a psychological reaction to stressful stimulation.

NEURODERMATITIS

Neurodermatitis is a common form of skin disorder characterized by chronic, nonallergic reddening of the skin and by skin eruptions, ranging from rashes to running sores and accompanied by extreme itching. The symptoms are similar to those of other psychophysiological skin disorders such as eczema, psoriasis, and hives. It is often difficult for the untrained eye to differentiate one from another.

Emotional or psychological factors are assumed to be involved in skin disorders such as neurodermatitis because it is readily shown that the skin responds to emotional situations (e.g., facial blushing caused by embarrassment). If chronic, such modification of the blood circulation beneath the skin can be damaging, because the health of the skin is dependent on proper blood circulation. Skin reactions associated with emotional stress usually clear up when the stress situation is alleviated but may be resistant to medical treatment if the stress is not alleviated, both factors suggesting the psychophysiological nature of these disorders.

Although neurodermatitis usually clears up when stress is eliminated, it may leave some residual scars if the skin was especially itchy and continually scratched. It also may leave "psychological scars," since most cases are clearly visible and often unsightly, causing a poor self-concept and possible disruption of interpersonal relationships because of extreme self-consciousness. Even though skin disorders are not the life-threatening type of psychophysiological disorder that hypertension is, they can seriously disrupt an individual's life and level of self-esteem.

PEPTIC ULCER

A peptic ulcer is a lesion or sore in the lining of the stomach or in the upper part of the small intestine or duodenum that lies immediately below the stomach. A basic problem with the term peptic ulcer is that it does not precisely define two different forms of ulcers—gastric ulcers and duodenal ulcers. Although these two forms have certain characteristics in common, there are also significant differences between them. For example, duodenal ulcer is usually associated with an increase in gastric secretion of hydrochloric acid and pepsin, while gastric ulcer is usually characterized by normal, subnormal, or elevated gastric secretion levels. Another important difference is that emotional factors appear to play a more important role in duodenal ulcer than in gastric ulcer (Yaeger and Weiner, 1970). Indeed, gastric and duodenal ulcers are viewed by clinicians as separate disorders that are associated with different predisposition and preadaptation factors (Kirsner, 1968). Thus the general term peptic ulcer can be misleading because it refers to two diseases that differ in their anatomical location, natural history, pathophysiology, and response to treatment.

Ulcers are quite common in the general population, with a prevalence rate of about 2 percent. Of these, the majority are duodenal ulcers, which tend to occur at an earlier age than peptic ulcers (Young, Richter, Bradley, and Anderson, 1987). They are sometimes "quiet," in the sense that they cause no pain or discomfort and remain unnoticed and therefore unreported. More often than not, however, the individual feels discomfort, ranging from a "burning sensation" in the stomach, usually the first sign of an ulcer, to severe pain (caused by enlargement of the lesion) accompanied by nausea and vomiting. Many ulcers heal by themselves, though treatment can reduce the pain and speed up recovery (Welgan, Meshkinpour, and Hoehler, 1985). If the ulcer perforates (blood vessels break in the walls of the stomach), vomiting of blood will occur. If hemorrhaging and internal bleeding are severe, the person may die.

Peptic duodenal ulcers are assumed to be produced by excessively high levels of gastric secretion of hydrochloric acid. The stomach produces this acid to aid in the digestive process; the walls of the duodenum and the stomach have a protective mucous lining that is normally able to resist its mildly corrosive action. However, if the acid is secreted when food is no longer present, it may begin to eat away the protective mucous lining among those individuals who cannot tolerate excessive secretion. When the output of acid is excessive and a particular site is no longer resistant to the acid, an ulcer will develop.

The most popular explanation holds that psychological stress causes the excessive secretion of acid in the absence of food (see Wolf and Wolff, 1947). This viewpoint is based on both animal and human research demonstrating a relationship between stress and secretion activity. There have been numerous examples of patients exposed to emotionally stressful situations showing an increase in the volume and acidity of gastric secretion (see Wolf, 1965). In research with animals, it has been demonstrated that the persistent exposure of rats to stress (unpredictable or uncontrollable electric shock) leads to a significant increase in ulceration rate (see Weiss, 1968, 1982).

Treatments for people suffering from ulcers range from prescription of drugs to stress and anxiety management. Several studies have reported that stress management training, permitting patients to reduce stress and/or discomfort associated with stressful situations, reduces ulcer pain and increases healing (Whitehead and Schuster, 1985). Anxiety management and training people to be assertive have also been shown to reduce pain and need for medication among patients (Brooks and

Richardson, 1980). In the long term, ulcer patients given these skills were far less likely to experience recurrence of symptoms. However, these and other studies did not examine mechanisms by which these changes may have occurred and in some cases do not adequately rule out alternative explanations. Thus, though stress is suggested as a primary mechanism for ulcer formation and stress management a useful treatment, more research is needed.

THE ROLE OF PHYSIOLOGICAL FACTORS IN PSYCHOPHYSIOLOGICAL DISORDERS

Although a great deal of additional work still needs to be done, significant developments in biomedical research have led to an increase in our understanding of the pathogenesis of psychophysiological disorders. Because of the great complexity of these various disorders, there is a trend toward greater specialization within the field of psychophysiological medicine, with a research focus usually on only one disorder. The investigator who is conducting research on essential hypertension, for example, may therefore not be aware of progress being made in understanding peptic ulcer.

Before this move toward specialization, a relatively broad theoretical model was used to conceptualize the physiological contribution to psychophysiological disorders. It was assumed that such disorders occur because of a bodily weakness, either a weak organ such as the stomach (ulcers) or a weak physiological system such as the cardiovascular system (essential hypertension). It was further assumed that this bodily weakness could be inherited or could develop as a result of disease (e.g., respiratory infection predisposing an individual to develop asthma).

An extension of this **weak organ/system theory** was the idea that specific physiological response patterns to situations, including stressful ones, are inherited. The term **specific-response pattern approach** was used to convey the assumption that individuals tend to respond physiologically to stressful situations in their own idiosyncratic ways. It has often been shown that individuals differ in physiological responding to situations (see Lacey, 1967). One person may demonstrate an increase in heart rate and blood pressure level, but little increase in muscle tension; another person in the same situation may display very little increase in heart rate and blood pressure, but a great increase in muscle tension. This difference in response patterns is known as **individual response stereotypy** (i.e., individual differences in the stereotypic way of responding to situations). As an early example of these individual differences in an actual clinical population, Malmo and Shagass (1949) demonstrated that under stress, patients with cardiovascular symptoms showed more cardiovascular response than increase in muscle tension, whereas patients with muscle tension headaches showed an opposite pattern.

It was generally assumed that the particular physiological symptom or organ that is most constantly activated, and therefore most stressed, may be susceptible to a breakdown and the resultant development of a psychophysiological disorder. That is, the person who persistently responds to situations with a greatly elevated blood pressure level may stress the cardiovascular system, causing a disruption of its homeostatic mechanism and, as a result, rendering it more susceptible to hypertension. A major problem with this general model, however, is its lack of predictive validity. It cannot answer the basic question of why all individuals who respond with a significant degree of cardiovascular activation do not eventually develop a cardiovascular disorder such as hypertension. Psychological factors are thus assumed to play an important role in determining who does or does not develop a disease.

THE ROLE OF GENETIC FACTORS IN PSYCHOPHYSIOLOGICAL DISORDERS

It is generally accepted that genetic factors are likely to play an important role in predisposing individuals to various psychophysiological disorders (Weiner, 1977). Mirsky (1958) demonstrated that pepsinogen levels of ulcer patients are significantly higher than those of patients without ulcers. **Pepsinogen,** a gastric secretion, is a good measure of gastric secretion activity. In the stomach, it is converted to the enzyme **pepsin,** which digests proteins and which, together with **hydrochloric acid,** is the primary active agent in gastric digestive juices. Many investigators view an excess of pepsinogen as a cause of ulcers. In an initial study Mirsky assessed significant individual differences in pepsinogen levels in newborn infants. Infants with high pepsinogen levels were found to be likely to be members of families in which there was a high pepsinogen level. In addition, twin studies have shown that pepsinogen levels for identical twins are very similar (Mirsky, Futterman, and Kaplan, 1952; Pilot, Lenoski, Spiro, and Schaefer, 1957). This provided some early evidence that pepsinogen level, which is viewed as an important contributing factor in the development of ulcers, is an inherited characteristic.

In another study, Weiner et al. (1957) sought to evaluate whether oversecretors of pepsinogen were more prone to develop ulcers than undersecretors. From a group of newly inducted soldiers, a group of oversecretors was selected on the basis of a gastrointestinal examination conducted before basic training. Only soldiers who did not have ulcers at the time were chosen for the study. At the end of basic training (approximately four months later), the men were reexamined. It was found that 14 percent of the oversecretors had developed ulcers, whereas none of the undersecretors had. A similar study by Mirsky (1958), conducted with a population of children and adult civilians, showed a similar tendency for ulcers to develop in those individuals with a high pepsinogen level.

Thus the evidence indicates that individuals who develop ulcers may be genetically predisposed because of excessive secretion of gastric acid, which, in turn, produces stomach lesions and ulcerations. Family studies have also suggested the importance of genetic factors. For example, Rosen and Gregory (1965) reported that brothers of ulcer patients are about twice as likely to develop ulcers as comparable members of the general population. There is reason to believe that other disorders are similarly predisposed.

A great deal of additional research, using better methodology such as twin studies, is still needed to delineate more clearly the importance of genetic predispositions in many psychophysiological disorders. Although numerous family studies have shown that patients with various psychophysiological disorders come from families in which there is a high incidence of the same disorder, such findings could be attributed to common factors in learning and experience rather than to a genetic factor. A number of studies, for example, have indicated that certain patterns of disturbed parent-child relationships are common in cases of childhood asthma (see Purcell et al., 1969). Such common family relationship experiences could partly or totally explain the high family-incidence findings. Future research will have to parcel out the relative contributions of such factors to each specific psychophysiological disorder. Moreover, as Weiner (1977) indicates, currently more is known about factors that predispose an individual to the disease than about factors that initiate or sustain it. Research is needed to isolate these latter factors.

PSYCHOLOGICAL FORMULATIONS OF PSYCHOPHYSIOLOGICAL DISORDERS

Dunbar (1943) was among the first to report reliable and consistent associations between specific diseases and particular personality characteristics (assessed in terms of attitudes, behaviors, and traits). Subsequently there were numerous attempts to delineate personality traits that are associated with specific psychophysiological disorders. Indeed, the unsubstantiated view that a disorder such as peptic ulcer is typical of the ambitious, hard-working, high-achieving executive is engrained in popular folklore and language. Research has, for example, reinforced the notion that there may be a specific cancer-prone personality. For example, Dattore, Shontz, and Coyne (1980) have found that certain measures on the **Minnesota Multiphasic Personality Inventory (MMPI),** which were obtained before the development of any cancer symptomatology, differentiated between those who subsequently developed cancer and those who did not. Specifically, it was revealed that the subjects who developed cancer (irrespective of site) were significantly different from noncancer patients in terms of greater repression and less self-report of depression.

The first widely accepted psychological formulation of psychosomatic disorders was the psychoanalytic approach of Franz Alexander (1950). Alexander suggested that each specific psychophysiological disorder was associated with specific unconscious emotional conflicts. His formulation was based to a large extent on clinical observation of patients undergoing psychoanalysis. He believed that repressed psychic energy could be discharged directly to the autonomic nervous system, leading to impairment of visceral functioning. He assumed that specific unconscious emotional conflicts were associated with specific psychophysiological disturbances.

A more recent formulation of psychophysiological disorders centers around the concept of alexithymia. Sifneos (1967) and Nemiah (1973, 1975) contend that the psychophysiological process is often characterized by **alexithymia,** which refers to a cluster of cognitive traits marked mainly by an inability of patients to describe their feelings. According to Nemiah (1975), the alexithymic personality displays the following: (1) an inability to describe feelings verbally, (2) a significant paucity of fantasy, and (3) an inability to make any significant internal psychological changes in the course of psychodynamically oriented psychotherapy.

Nemiah, Freyberger, and Sifneos (1976) have more recently noted that alexithymic patients ". . . are often unable to localize effects in their bodies and appear unaware of any of the common automatic somatic reactions that accompany the experience of a variety of feelings. If there is a somatic component, it is identical with the symptoms of their bodily illness" (p. 431). It is this emotionality deficit that is assumed to be the major underpinning of psychophysiological disorders. Some have assumed that this deficit is associated with exaggerated left-hemisphere response or a functional disconnection between the hemispheres (Taylor, 1984).

Graham and his colleagues conducted a series of classic experiments examining the relationship between specific attitudes toward a distressing life situation and the occurrence of particular psychophysiological disorders (see Graham, 1972). These attitudes, were originally obtained in clinical interviews with patients suffering from various psychophysiological disorders (Grace and Graham 1952). This evaluation indicated that patients with the same disorder showed similarities in describing their attitudes toward events that occurred just before the appearance or worsening of their symptoms. Subsequent and better controlled studies further validated the presence of these attitudes (Graham et al., 1962), leading these investigators to conclude that different psychophysiological disorders were indeed associated with different attitudes. Some of the associations found were:

Asthma: The person feels left out in the cold and wants to shut out another individual or the situation.

Essential hypertension: The person feels threatened by harm by an ever-present danger and, as a result, needs to be on guard, watchful, and prepared.

Migraine: The person feels that something has to be achieved and then relaxes after the effect.

Peptic ulcer: The person feels deprived of what is due him or her and wants to seek revenge or get even.

A significant advantage of the Graham formulation over previous approaches was the more precise operational definition of constructs, the availability of an independent variable that could be experimentally manipulated (the specific attitudes), and dependent measures that could be reliably and objectively measured (physiological responding). According to this line of reasoning, we should be able to predict the type of psychophysiological illness an individual is likely to get by assessing his or her attitudes toward life. However, proof for this is not easily found. In one study, Graham, Stern, and Winokur (1958) hypnotized subjects and provided them with suggestions leading to attitudes specific either to hives (you feel you are taking a beating and feel helpless to do anything about it) or to Raynaud's disease (you want to take hostile physical action, but do not know what the actual act should be). Hives are accompanied by an increase in real skin temperature, while Raynaud's disease is characterized by decreasing skin temperature. If the specific-attitudes notion is useful in predicting these conditions, suggestions related to taking a beating (hives-related attitude) should result in an increase in skin temperature, while suggestions about wanting to take hostile action should lead to a decrease in skin temperature. Findings confirmed the hypothesis—attitudes specific to hives raised skin temperature while attitudes specific to Raynaud's disease lowered it.

Other studies have also provided mixed evidence for this theory, (see Buss, 1966; Graham, Kabler, & Graham, 1962; Peters and Stern, 1971). In spite of the promise of this specific-attitudes theory to understand better psychophysiological disorders, few investigators attempted to pursue and extend it during the 1960s and 1970s. Lang (1979) noted several reasons for this abandonment. One major reason was the difficulty in replicating the results in nonhypnotized patients. The inability to deal adequately with this hypnosis confound presented major problems for subsequent attempts at validating Graham's formulation.

COPING STYLES

Dissatisfied with earlier psychodynamic formulations, many investigators interested in the role of psychological factors in psychophysiological disorders began to shift their attention to the role of more easily and reliably quantified situational variables such as bereavement and separation as precipitating events (see Engel, 1967; Schmale, 1958). This research has established that behavioral and physiological responses to separation and other environmental stressors may be correlated with an important intervening psychological variable—coping mechanisms (Weiner, 1977).

We discussed the topic of coping styles in Chapter 3. We also reviewed research on the Type A behavior pattern, which is the most systematic investigation of a coping style to date. A characteristic of situations shown to have a significant influence on cardiovascular reactivity in humans is the active-passive coping dimension proposed by Obrist et al. (1978). According to these investigators, passive coping is exemplified by a classical aversive conditioning situation in which escape or avoidance from an aversive stimulus such as electric shock is not possible. Active coping, in contrast, is characterized by shock avoidance when the subject can exert some control over the receipt of an aversive stimulus contingent on some aspect of his or her behavior such as performance on a reaction time task. Obrist and colleagues found that during passive coping, beta-adrenergic influences on the heart, as assessed by cardiovascular measures such as heart rate and diastolic and systolic blood pressure, were either minimal or rapidly dissipated. Under active coping conditions, beta-adrenergic effects were more pronounced. Though the terms active and passive may not accurately describe the differences between these situations, this research suggests that the type of coping available to subjects has a significant impact on cardiovascular responding. This is a fruitful area for future systematic research.

Coping style processes may prove to be important variables to consider in any comprehensive model of psychophysiological disorders. However, to date, not enough systematic research has been conducted to determine the predictive validity and utility of such psychological constructs.

THE DIATHESIS–STRESS MODEL OF PSYCHOPHYSIOLOGICAL DISORDERS

In Chapter 3 we introduced the diathesis-stress model of illness (Levi, 1974). Employing this model specifically with psychophysiological disorders, Sternbach (1966) emphasized the importance of considering all factors in any attempt to understand a particular disorder. The diathesis portion of this model postulates the presence of two major factors: (1) individual response stereotypy, which Sternbach sees as a constitutional predisposition to respond in a particular way physiologically to various situations with consistent activation of certain physiological systems or organs; and (2) inadequate homeostatic restraints, which may be caused by stress-induced breakdown, previous accident or infection, or genetic predisposition. The stress portion of the model refers to the persistent exposure of the individual to stressful, activating situations. Situational determinants are very important and must be taken into account. For example, an individual exposed to an emotional stressor in a work situation may respond quite differently than if he or she were at home. Socially accepted methods of dealing with stressors will differ from situation to situation, and thus the physiological consequences must be expected to differ.

Along with exposure to actual external activating/stressful situations, Sternbach also includes in his model the possibility that, in the absence of such objective real-life stressors, an individual may perceive ordinary situations and events as stressors and so react to them with heightened physiological responding. These misperceptions are due to the person's chronic attitudes (e.g., *specific* attitudes) or personality characteristics that significantly affect his or her perception and interpretation of stimuli.

There has been some recent animal research supporting a diathesis-stress model of various psychophysiological disorders. For example, Ader (1963) bred rats for their susceptibility to gastric lesions under conditions of restraint (restraint and immobilization have been found to be significant stressors for rats). These individual differences in susceptibility to gastric lesions are due to individual variations in serum pepsinogen levels. Ader found that ulcer-susceptible rats exposed to restraint conditions were more likely to develop ulceration than other rats. (This relationship was found only when the rats were restrained at the peak of their circadian activity cycle.)

Friedman and Iwai (1976) demonstrated that when rats that were bred to be genetically prone to salt-induced hypertension were clinically exposed to stress (an approach-avoidance conflict), they showed persistent elevation in systolic blood pressure. In contrast, rats that were genetically resistant to salt-induced hypertension did not develop high blood pressure when exposed to the same stressor. These results indicate that stress is selectively effective in producing hypertension-type effects, depending on the animal's genetic predisposition. More recently Lawler et al. (1980) have found similar effects of conflict on tonic levels of blood pressure in the genetically borderline hypertensive rat.

Clearly the investigation of psychophysiological disorders is complex. Many variables—genetic, physiological, situational, behavioral/personality—obviously need to be taken into account in any comprehensive understanding of these disorders. As we have noted, significant progress is also being made in biomedical research in the development of an understanding of the pathogenesis of these disorders. Unfortunately, parallel progress has not yet been made in research on psychological factors. Such research in the past has been sorely inadequate. However, more recent evaluations of specific behavioral characteristics—such as Type A behavior and coping styles—may provide useful avenues for future investigation.

||||||||||||||||||||||||||||||||||||||||||||||||||||||||||||||||||||||||||||||||||||||||||||||||||||||||||||||||||||||||||||||||||

A CASE STUDY OF STRESS IN AN ULCER-GASTROINTESTINAL REACTION

Edward Polowski was examined by a specialist in internal medicine, and then referred to a clinical psychologist for further evaluation. The patient complained of a longstanding problem of severe cramps and diarrhea whenever he ate highly seasoned foods or encountered any type of stressful situation. This problem was diagnosed as an irritable colon when the patient was a child. Since that time, he had been treated by a series of physicians, all of whom confirmed this diagnosis. The patient reported the medications prescribed for him had varied in effectiveness, and he had recently been in severe discomfort.

Edward was 35 years old, married, and the father of a six-year-old boy and a two-year-old girl. He was a college graduate with a degree in library science and had been a librarian in the same city library since he graduated from college. Edward stated that he began having unusually severe gastrointestinal symptoms at the time that a new director was appointed to the library a number of months ago. . . .

Edward related that he had had numerous occurrences of intestinal difficulties ever since childhood. These episodes were associated with circumstances such as his mother or teacher insisting that he do something he did not want to do. He also became ill when he had to make a public appearance such as participating in his First Communion or in a play at school. His mother tended to be quite concerned about making him comfortable when he had intestinal symptoms, although she always told him that it was just a "nervous stomach." She said that she knew how he felt because she was also troubled with a "nervous stomach" when she was anxious or upset.

When Edward was nine years old, his mother took him to her physician because Edward was in severe discomfort. He was in the midst of an episode of cramps and diarrhea that lasted for about a week. The onset of the symptoms was associated with Edward's complaints that his new teacher was too strict and forced him to keep going over material he had already mastered. Edward stayed home from school during the latter part of that week, and the physician prescribed some medication which relieved a great deal of the discomfort. Mrs. Polowski pleaded with the doctor to call the school principal and explain the reason for Edward's symptoms. This was done and Edward reported that his teacher became somewhat more flexible in relation to his school activities. Edward had other occurrences of cramps during that school year, but none as severe as the earlier occasion.

Edward also had periodic intestinal problems while he was growing up, but these attacks usually lasted for just a few hours at a time. In high school, he experienced another prolonged occurrence of intestinal symptoms during a final examination period. Edward generally received good grades in school, but he was always quite anxious before a test because he was afraid that he would not do well. He was very anxious during these particular examinations because he had received lower grades than he had expected on some of his previous tests. He therefore studied a great deal and ignored his mother's assurances that he would do well on the exams.

Edward began having intestinal symptoms during the examination period, and the symptoms did not subside, even with medication, until ten days later when he went to a physician. He was given a complete medical examination, including a number of special tests of the gastrointestinal tract. These tests revealed no structural defects or damage, and the problem was again diagnosed as chronic irritable colon. Edward was given a new medication to take when he felt that the symptoms were about to recur.

From Gloria Rakita Leon. *Case Histories of Deviant Behavior: An Interactional Perspective,* 2nd ed. Boston: Allyn and Bacon, 1977. Copyright © 1977 by Allyn and Bacon, Inc. Reprinted with permission.

TREATMENT OF PSYCHOPHYSIOLOGICAL DISORDERS

The disturbing organic symptoms of some psychophysiological disorders (bleeding ulcers, cardiovascular disease) often demand immediate as well as long-range medical treatment. In such cases, medication and dietary patterns must be prescribed to deal effectively with the physical symptoms of the disorders. Simultaneously, treatment directed at modifying the psychological/behavioral causes and stressors should be administered.

Traditionally a major form of treatment of these disorders has been drug therapy. Minor tranquilizers are commonly prescribed to reduce the anxiety and emotional tension usually associated with such disorders. These tranquilizers can be an effective means for reducing high levels of stress in certain individuals in combination with certain forms of behavioral/psychotherapy. However, the indiscriminant use of minor tranquilizers alone, without an attempt to deal with the situational/interpersonal factors involved, will not bring about any permanent long-term improvement in these disorders. Besides the lack of long-term improvement, certain side effects such as drowsiness usually are associated with such drug usage. Further, individuals may develop tolerance for a particular dosage level, so that the amount of drug must be increased continuously to dangerously high levels to produce the same tranquilizing effects. If the medication is terminated after prolonged and heavy usage, severe withdrawal symptoms such as insomnia, tremors, and hallucinations may occur.

A number of therapeutic techniques have been found to be effective in treating anxiety and stress-related disorders. In Chapter 10 we shall discuss various cognitive-behavioral approaches to treatment.

SUMMARY

Psychophysiological disorders, formerly called psychosomatic illnesses, are characterized by physical symptoms or dysfunctions in various organs of the body that are intimately linked with psychological factors. The relationship between the mind and the body has long been a controversial topic among philosophers, physiologists, and psychologists. Today it is assumed that psychological factors are important in all diseases. The current view of these disorders is that they are the result of many causes—physical, psychological, and sociocultural. It is the search for the unique interaction of these factors that interests investigators of psychophysiological disorders. Common forms of psychophysiological disorders—bronchial asthma, dysmenorrhea, headache, neurodermatitis, and peptic ulcer—demonstrate the role of physiological and genetic factors in these disorders. Major psychological formulations have been proposed to account for them. A review of these various orientations emphasizes the importance of taking into account genetic, physiological, and psychological factors in a comprehensive diathesis-stress model of psychophysiological disorders.

RECOMMENDED READINGS

Gatchel, R. J., Baum, A., and Lang, P. J. Psychosomatic disorders: Basic issues and future research directions. In R. J. Gatchel, A. Baum, and J. E. Singer (Eds.), *Clinical psychology and behavioral medicine: Overlapping areas.* Hillsdale, N.J.: Erlbaum, 1982.

Graham, D. T. Psychosomatic medicine. In N. S. Greenfield and R. A. Sternbach (Eds.), *Handbook of psychophysiology.* New York: Holt, Rinehart & Winston, 1972.

Weiner, H. *Psychobiology and human disease.* New York: Elsevier, 1977.

8 MEDICAL SETTINGS AND PATIENT BEHAVIOR

||||||||||||||||||||||||||||||||||||||||||||||||||||||||||||||||||||||||||||||||||||||||||||||||||||||||||||||||

The study of patient behavior and the effects of various medical settings has been a mainstay of psychological study of health. Although many of the principles governing this behavior resemble those already associated with behavior in other settings, there are special twists and concerns in dealing with medical settings.

HOSPITALIZATION

The hospitalization of patients is often necessary when intensive or formal care procedures are required for treatment, expensive or scarce resources are needed, or tests are required. In many cases, the treatment people receive in the hospital is superior to what is available anywhere else. However, there are some negative aspects of hospitalization—affective and behavioral effects—that can interfere with proper treatment.

Hospitalization is often considered to be a negative experience. Some people associate hospitals with fearful things such as pain or death; others dislike the disruptiveness of a hospital stay, the extreme dependency and loss of control that accompany hospitalization, or the dehumanizing aspects of "processing" and treatment in the hospital. Some people dislike or fear the image of the hospital as a complex, chaotic, and confusing environment where more harm than good occurs. Consider the following accounts:

> *The pervasive hospital idiom reinforces this sense of lost identity and returns to helpless infancy: "Nurse, would you just pop off her things for me? I want to examine her." In hospital everything is "popped" on or off, "slipped" in or out. I don't think I met a single doctor who in dealing with patients didn't resort to this sort of nursery talk. I once heard one saying to a patient, an elderly man, "We're just going to pop you into the operating theatre to have a little peep into your tummy." Nurses too had people "popping" all over the place—in and out of lavatories, dressing-gowns, beds, scales, wheelchairs, bandages. (Toynbee, 1977, p. 10)*

161

Recently when I was being given emergency treatment for an eye laceration, the resident surgeon abruptly terminated his conversation with me as soon as I lay down on the operating table. Although I had had no sedative, or anesthesia, he acted as if I were no longer conscious, directing all his questions to a friend of mine—questions such as What's his name?, What occupation is he in?, Is he a real doctor?, etc. As I lay there, these two men were speaking about me as if I were not there at all. (Zimbardo, 1969, p. 298)

We are not suggesting that these kinds of experiences are typical. But errors are sometimes made with lethal results, and these are usually publicized (fictionalized in books or movies or reported by the media), instilling fear in incoming patients. These "incoming" concerns are met with indifference in many cases, and hardly assuaged by the intake and treatment procedures frequently utilized by hospitals. Such fears are then compounded by the real problems hospitals must deal with—treating people as if they were objects, withholding desired information, and so on.

One of the more dramatic and stubborn problems creating patient distress is the depersonalization of hospital patients by the staff. **Depersonalization** refers to treating a patient as if he or she were not a person. Too often patients are treated as an insurance number, a body to be operated on, a mouth to be fed medication, or an object to be watched, moved, or treated. Of course, some concern for the patient is demonstrated, but, as Goffman (1963) has noted, the patient is expected to remain passive, cooperative, and uninvolved in treatment. Staff members tend to develop this one-dimensional view of patients because it facilitates staff operations and increases the number of people who can be treated.

Consider a "visit" to the hospital. When you arrive, you are feeling a little anxious and would rather not be there. But you report to the admissions desk. There, anger and impatience supplement your fears as you are required to complete several different forms and answer questions about how you will pay for your hospitalization. Following admission you are given hospital clothes to wear—just like everyone else's—and are left in a sterile and uninviting room, shared with at least one other patient. Your freedom to see friends and family is restricted to certain hours, and you are subjected to numerous tests, some performed with little or no explanation. Through all of this, you are shunted from room to room.

Not everyone experiences this kind of routinization. Some hospitals have attempted to personalize their systems and some physicians provide more information, but most must rely on depersonalizing procedures in order to cope with shortages of beds and to process the many patients that arrive each day.

Compounding this depersonalization and placing the patient in a more vulnerable state are the status demands of hospitalization. Frequently doctors and staff treat patients as if they were children, and sometimes they make patients feel guilty if they ask for information about or help with routine matters (Taylor, 1979). Some patients are made to feel that such requests are an imposition on a busy physician or nurse. As Taylor (1979) has noted, the patient must *yield control* of his or her body to people who are relative strangers and who are not treating him or her with normal respect. In many hospital settings, patients are extremely dependent on the staff. Additionally, patients must temporarily *submerge their identities*—job activities cease, social relationships are disrupted, and the patient is literally pulled from his or her normal surroundings and plunked down in an alien setting. The patient, shorn of most vestiges of his or her identity, becomes a minute element in a large organizational structure (the hospital) that cannot be controlled at the patient level. Adjustment to *loss of privacy* that accompanies living in a hospital is also necessary; plus the patient must learn and follow a new schedule of rules and regulations.

Finally, as we have noted, patients are often given very little information about the things of greatest concern—the outcome of tests, the progress of illness, and so on.

Fear, depersonalization, dependency, disruptiveness, loss of privacy, frustration, and other such problems reported as being stressful by hospital patients (see Volicer, 1973) may combine to have adverse effects on patient health and well-being. Research is needed to better understand how these conditions affect patient treatment and health. An interesting example of the kind of work that can be done is provided by an analysis of patient response to hospitalization by Taylor (1979). Her account of hospitalization deals with problems associated with depersonalization and loss of control, using the concept of learned helplessness that we discussed in Chapter 4.

GOOD AND BAD PATIENTS

Taylor's analysis assumes that depersonalization, loss of control, and lack of information are often characteristic of a patient's hospital experience. Patients realize that the staff would like them to be as invisible as possible and to behave "properly." In other words, they are supposed to remain cooperative, unquestioning, and passive. Most patients adopt this *good patient* role, suppressing their desires for more active involvement in their treatment. The good patient is usually well liked by the staff. Patients who are compliant, ask for little, and make few complaints facilitate staff functioning. Of course, nurses and technicians understand that every patient is ill and requires care, but the good patient does not add any demands or make the staff jobs any more difficult. However, some patients cannot or do not suppress these needs, and they may become angry and hostile. These patients assume a *bad patient* role. Taylor describes bad patient behavior in the following way: "In hospital patients, reactance is manifested behaviorally as petty acts of mutiny such as making passes at nurses, drinking in one's room, smoking against medical advice, and wandering up and down the halls." Acts of defiance, frequent requests, and apparent demands for more time and attention are all characteristic of the bad patient role.

Taylor (1979) argues that these roles may involve more than superficial compliance. While good patient behavior may be good for the staff, for instance, it may not be good for the patient. Conversely, bad patient behavior is disruptive to the staff, but it may have aspects that will facilitate the patient's recovery. Taylor's basic concern is the reasons for good patient behavior. Is good patient behavior deliberate? Are these patients trying to be cooperative, or is their behavior a result of having learned that they are helpless in hospital settings? It is not difficult to find sources of helplessness training, given the depersonalization and loss of control cues present in the hospital.

Tagliacozza and Mauksch (1972) have considered the fact that hospital patients

who conform to the good patient role are *not* generally as calm, accepting, cooperative, and happy as one might expect. Instead, they are in conflict, usually as a result
of wanting the attention from the staff that is typically reserved for good patients
but also wanting more information than they are routinely given. Asking for more
information is demanding, which is inconsistent with being a good patient. The
result of this kind of conflict may be a feeling of helplessness, compounding the
feelings of helplessness inherent in hospitalization.

If good patients appear to be passive and well behaved but are, in fact, experiencing helplessness because they cannot meaningfully reduce dependency, gain control,
or ask for information, what are the consequences for the patient? Taylor (1979) lists
several. First, the helpless patient will be less likely to try actively to improve his
or her condition. New pains or sensations may not be reported and other information
may be withheld, since the helpless patient believes that he or she is unable to
influence recovery. Second, helplessness may inhibit decision making. Patients asked
to make decisions about their care may be unable or unwilling to do so. Third, since
they are not active information seekers, helpless patients are probably ill informed,
and they run the risk of making decisions based on inadequate information. Helplessness involves the belief that one cannot meaningfully affect what happens. As a
result, helpless patients may expend little energy or attention in making decisions
when they must be made. Fourth, the helpless patient may have problems accomplishing the transition back to normal nonhospitalized life. This will depend on
many factors characterizing the patient's home life and on how long the patient was
hospitalized. Since helplessness does generalize, however, it is likely that difficulties
will emerge when the patient is suddenly placed back into a situation where he or
she must fend for him- or herself. Consistent with this, Coser (1962) has noted that
many patients, especially those who have been good patients, are unhappy about
leaving the hospital after a fairly long stay.

Good patients may also suffer unsuspected physiological problems. Research
has found limited evidence of norepinephrine depletion associated with helplessness,
depression, or loss of control (Schildkraut, 1965; Seligman, 1975; Weiss, Stone, and
Harrell, 1970). Adaptive reserves that could facilitate recovery may be depleted if
hospitalization is prolonged. And as we noted in Chapter 4, helplessness has been
associated with deteriorating health resulting sometimes in sudden death (Engel,
1968; Schmale, 1972). As a result, the good patient may experience a wide range of
problems. He or she may withhold valuable information that might help the treatment process, may have difficulty arriving at informed decisions, and may be in a
physical state of exhaustion or decline.

The next question is whether the bad patient is any better off. Taylor (1979)
describes this patient as reactant, refusing to become helpless and responding to
hospitalization with anger and attempts to gain control. Patients who try to regain
their lost control in hospitals seek to obtain information and demand that they be
treated as people. The staff, of course, may see these demands as annoying and as
interfering with their routine—hence the appellation bad patient. As we would
expect, this kind of behavior can have negative consequences for patient health. If
the patient begins to feel ignored or disliked (which may be an accurate perception,
since the staff may become irritated at the patient's behavior), arousal and suspicion

of the quality of care may result. A negative emotional and physical state may also result. Also the bad patient's important complaints may not be taken seriously by the staff, and health may suffer.

The bad patient, however, may have some advantages over his or her good counterpart. Since control has not been yielded, decision making may be more effective. And because this patient maintains at least the illusion of control over hospital routine, readjustment to normal life after release from the hospital may be easier.

The processes involved in good and bad patient behavior are summarized in Table 8.1 (Taylor, 1979). At this point they remain descriptive of the kinds of roles adopted in hospital settings and researchers are currently studying these issues. A recent study has reported evidence suggesting that "good" patients may indeed be a result of learned helplessness conditioned in the institutions (Raps et al., 1982). Attempts to provide control and responsibility in hospitals to counteract helplessness training have met with some success in countering this (see Hoge, 1964; Langer and Rodin, 1976). Clearly, the hospital setting can make contributions to patient health in numerous ways.

STRESS AND SURGERY

Many aspects of hospitalization are frightening: impending surgery, unknown examination procedures, and the like can all be stressful. Fortunately, the stressful nature of some of these procedures has been recognized, and stress-reducing interventions have been studied.

Stress generated by the need to undergo surgery has been implicated as a factor in healing and recovery. The apprehension and fear associated with the anticipation of surgery, as well as the alarm and distress commonly associated with recovery, may affect the ways in which a patient reacts to the situation and, consequently, the course of his or her recovery.

Janis (1958) was among the first to systematically study response to surgery. In one study he interviewed patients before and after major surgery. On the basis of the first interview, Janis classified patients as to the degree to which they exhibited anticipatory fear. Some were extremely fearful, expressing constant concern, anxiety, and feelings of vulnerability. Others expressed more moderate fear—their worries were real but less prominent, and they sought out information about their surgery from physicians and staff. A third group of patients exhibited little if any fear while awaiting surgery. Their reports suggested that they were denying fear rather than dealing with it, and these patients were more angry than worried.

Janis found that the moderate fear group—those patients who were fearful but who did not exhibit extreme fear—showed less postoperative emotional disturbance. A subsequent study with college students who had recently undergone surgery suggested the same thing. Adjustment following surgery was better among moderately fearful patients than among those showing extremely high or low levels of distress.

Janis explained this relationship by considering the ways in which different levels of fear could affect preparation for surgery. On an abstract level, he reasoned

TABLE 8.1   The Possible Consequences of Loss of Control, Good Patient Behavior, and Bad Patient Behavior in Hospital Patients

STATE	BEHAVIORS	COGNITIONS	AFFECT	PHYSICAL STATE	RESPONSE FROM STAFF
Loss of control (Depersonalization)	Nondiscriminant information seeking and use; complaints to staff.	Inadequate expectations; confusion.	Anxiety	Heightened physical reactions to symptoms and noxious medical procedures; possible increased need for medication, lenghtened hospital stay.	Nonperson treatment
Good patient behavior (Helplessness)	Compliance Passivity Learned helplessness Inability to take in information Failure to provide condition-relevant information	Feelings of helplessness, powerlessness, possible denial or fatalism.	Anxiety and depression	Possible norepinephrine depletion; helplessness also related to sudden death and gradual erosion of health.	Responsiveness to emergencies but routine failure to solicit information from patient.
Bad patient behavior (Reactance)	Complaints to staff Demands for attention, mutinous behavior Possible self-sabotage	Commitment to a right to know; suspicion (or paranoia) regarding condition, treatment and staff behavior.	Anger	Heightened catecholamine secretion and hydrocortisone production; possible aggravation of blood pressure, hypertension, tachycardia, angina. Eventual depletion.	Condescension; ignoring patients' complaints; "medicate to placate"; psychiatric referrals; possible premature discharge.

Reprinted, by permission of the publisher, from S. E. Taylor. Hospital patient behavior: Reactance, helplessness, or control? *Journal of Social Issues*, 1979, 35, 156–184.

that moderate levels of fear are optimal for developing defenses and coping strategies. Moderately fearful patients seemed to be realistic in approach, seeking information about what would happen to them and how to cope with these events. This information was rehearsed (learned) and provided a basis for confidence about the outcome of the surgery.

The excessive fear exhibited by some others appeared to be related to a history of psychological disorders, so their problems after surgery were regarded as a continuation of hyperemotionality. The poorer recovery of low-fear patients, however, was not as easily explained. Apparently, their fear was suppressed by their denial of it, which broke down once the undeniable pains and discomforts of the postoperative period were upon them. Since they had no reason to seek out and rehearse information, they had not developed the defenses necessary for adequate coping.

These explanations were supported by findings indicating that patients who had been given information about the unpleasant sensations that would follow surgery showed better recovery than did patients who had not received this information. Those who had been given information were less angry before surgery, showed greater confidence in their surgeon, and displayed less emotional disturbance after surgery.

Janis's (1958) research demonstrates a relationship between fear and surgical outcomes and provides a rehearsal mechanism—which Janis called the "work of worrying"—to account for these effects. If fear is excessive or absent, seeking and rehearsal of information will be inhibited, and feelings of helplessness and vulnerability will be more likely when the surgery is complete. The role of information in this relationship is perhaps the most important finding of the research and has itself generated a great deal of research. Studies done prior to or immediately after Janis's work suggested that provision of accurate information about likely sensations of pain reduces the aversiveness of these experiences when they occur (see Cobb et al., 1954; Grinker et al., 1946; Janis and Leventhal, 1965). Subsequent research has more directly addressed these issues.

Information

Three basic types of information may be given to patients awaiting surgery (or any frightening medical examination or procedure). The first concerns what people will *feel* (e.g., pains, discomforts). This kind of information is *sensory* in focus and corresponds fairly well with the kind of information Janis studied. The second deals not with sensations but rather with objective characteristics of what will be done during the surgery or examination. This procedural information is focused *externally* rather than on the patient. A third type of information deals with *coping* skills, providing ways of dealing with pain and discomfort when it arises. Research has indicated that these different kinds of information are not equally useful and that their effects vary across different situations (see Baum, Fisher, and Solomon, 1981; Johnson and Leventhal, 1974).

Imagine that you are in the hospital for surgery. You know that surgery can be dangerous and unpleasant and that recovery can be painful. Why would you want to know what you will feel after surgery? According to Janis, this information allows you to become acquainted with the problems you could encounter so that you are not surprised by them later. If you are told that, among other things, you might feel a sharp pain in your stomach, you will be less likely to experience surprise when such a pain materializes. If you do not have accurate expectations of what you might feel, such a pain might frighten you—you might think that something had gone wrong or that you were in danger. Armed with accurate expectations, however, you view pain as a normal result of the surgery and the recovery process rather than as a danger signal. As a result, the pain experience will be less threatening and hence less stressful.

One of Janis's (1969) subjects reported, "I knew there might be some bad pains, so when my side started to ache, I told myself that this didn't mean anything had gone wrong" (p. 98). A great deal of evidence of the effectiveness of having accurate sensory expectations in reducing distress has been reported.

Procedural information, which does not address interpretation of sensations, appears to reduce distress by providing patients with a sense of control over what is happening to them. By making the surgery or examination more predictable, this type of information gives patients some sense of control and confidence. Coping information, on the other hand, provides patients with real control, since it teaches them ways of relieving pain and discomfort when they wish to do so.

Research comparing these types of information has indicated that sensory information is more effective in reducing distress in medical settings than is procedural information. Coping information is effective when paired with sensory information—knowing how to cope with a pain is only useful when the pain is accurately anticipated.

Egbert et al. (1964) conducted one study demonstrating that sensory and coping information, when given together to patients prior to their abdominal surgery, reduced the need for analgesia and cut the average hospital stay for recovery by almost three days (see Figure 8.1). Subsequently, studies have demonstrated the effectiveness of sensory information alone and in combination with coping information (see Johnson, 1975; Johnson and Leventhal, 1974; Johnson, Morrissey, and Leventhal, 1973). A particularly vivid instance of the value of sensory information was reported by Johnson and Leventhal (1974), who studied responses to an extremely unpleasant medical examination. Their subjects underwent endoscopic examinations in which they were required to swallow a tube with a device on the end for examination of the gastrointestinal tract. Once the tube had been swallowed, it had to be retained for up to half an hour. Coughing, gagging, and breathing difficulties are common, and most patients find an endoscopic examination to be an aversive experience. By varying the type of information given to these patients, Johnson and Leventhal were able to show that sensory information was most effective in reducing distress. When combined with sensory information, instruction about coping skills was also effective.

Other studies found benefits of each kind of information separately. Patients given coping instructions, such as how to breathe to reduce pain, showed more rapid recovery from surgery (Lindeman and Van Aernam, 1971) and required fewer pain-killing analgesics (Healey, 1968). Patients given information about what they would feel showed improved recovery in a series of studies conducted by Johnson

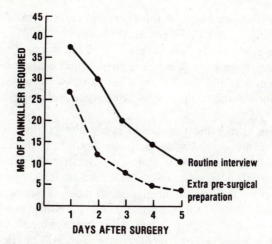

Figure 8.1   Graph depicting the different medication requirements of surgery patients given standard or experimental interviews before surgery. Those given extra information received less pain killer (morphine) after surgery.

Reprinted by permission from L. D. Egbert, G. E. Battit, C. E. Welch, and M. K. Bartlett. Reduction of post-operative pain by encouragement and instruction of patients. *New England Journal of Medicine,* 1964, *270,* 825–827.

(1973). In her studies, patients awaiting surgery were given information about sensations they would experience during aversive medical procedures *or* about the procedures themselves. A group receiving no information was also studied. Both information groups experienced less distress than the no-information group.

The relationship between information and distress to surgical outcome also applies to children (see Burstein and Meichenbaum, 1979; Knight et al., 1979). Several studies have found that information can reduce the distress children experience following an operation (see Cassell, 1965; Melamed and Siegel, 1975; Wolfer and Vistainer, 1975). In one study Wolfer and Vistainer provided some children with a combination of sensory and procedural information and some with regular care. Mothers were also given either additional information or regular information, and postoperative recovery of these groups was compared. Those children receiving information were rated as being less upset than those not receiving information, and they showed better recovery following surgery. In another study Melamed (1982) found that presurgical arousal was associated with lower levels of anxiety and retention of information. Arousal was interpreted as openness to the information provided.

Recalling Janis's (1958) description of low-fear subjects who consequently experienced heightened distress, it is clear that patients' *coping style* will affect the value of information in medical settings. Janis believed that the low-fear patients (who were also low-information patients) were using denial to cope with the stress of impending surgery. Lazarus and Cohen (1973) compared patients who used denial defenses with those who were extremely vigilant. Surgical patients were classified as deniers if they showed hesitation or reluctance in learning about their surgery or its consequences. Vigilant subjects, on the other hand, sought out such information in a compulsive, worrisome manner. A third group of patients was also studied—those who did not clearly exhibit either denial or vigilance.

Results indicated that vigilant patients fared the worst—they showed poorer recovery after surgery, spent more time in the hospital, and showed more negative reactions and complications than did any other patients. Surprisingly, patients using denial defenses showed the best recovery. Contrary to Janis's findings, denial seemed to aid in recovery from surgery.

Other studies have found that denial is not always a good strategy. Among children, moderate arousal and some vigilance appear to be more effective means of coping than denial, extreme arousal, and so on (Burstein and Meichenbaum, 1979). In addition, information seeking among children awaiting surgery has been shown to reduce some stress due to this threatening situation (Peterson and Toler, 1986). Similarly, Andrew (1970) studied surgical patients classified as vigilant, denial, or vigilant-denial subjects. Subjects who used both strategies benefited from presurgical information and showed the fastest recovery after surgery. The vigilant subjects were not affected by the information provided, and denial subjects showed poorer recovery when provided with information than when not given information.

Although different coping strategies will be more or less effective in different situations, it appears that some degree of involvement and information is beneficial in preparing for surgery. Information and active consideration of possible dangers before surgery seems to facilitate recovery from such experiences.

Other Surgical Interventions

Other cognitive and behavioral interventions designed to reduce distress have also been considered. Field (1974) used hypnosis to reduce surgical distress, but did not find any strong evidence of differential recovery or outcome. However, relaxation training among preoperative patients has been shown to reduce distress and facilitate recovery (see Egbert et al., 1964; Miller, 1977). Providing patients with support and reassurance has also shown benefits for surgical patients, though these effects are not consistently strong (e.g., Lindeman and Stetzer, 1973; Schmitt and Wooldridge, 1973).

One of the more promising of the noninformation-based interventions is the cognitive-behavioral approach taken by Langer, Janis, and Wolfer (1975). They gave patients one of four treatments. One group was given instruction on cognitive reappraisal-restructuring and reinterpreting situations in less threatening ways (recall that Lazarus and his colleagues demonstrated the effectiveness of reappraisal in determining stress generated by gruesome films). A second group was given information about surgery. The third group received information and reappraisal instruction, and the last group received neither. Before and after surgery, those patients given reappraisal instructions, whether alone or with information, fared better than the others.

HEALTH BEHAVIOR

Not surprisingly, behavior in medical settings is very complex—many factors determine response to hospitalization and help to determine recovery from surgery.

However, not all patient behaviors occur in the hospital. In fact, most of the behaviors of interest from a health standpoint occur outside the hospital. Although they are often called illness behaviors (see Mechanic, 1966), since these behaviors are related to health maintenance as well as to the etiology of illness, we will refer to them as health behaviors.

As you will recall from Chapter 3, there are three basic mechanisms linking behavior to illness or poor health. Two of these are of great relevance here—lifestyle and reaction to the sick role. Personal habits and patterns of behavior have been shown to influence the onset of a number of illnesses. In addition to behavior patterns, isolated or individual behaviors, such as drug taking, smoking, drinking, eating, and lack of exercise, can all impair health. One of the reasons this problem is difficult to address is that these behaviors occur while a person is healthy. The negative effects of excessive eating or of smoking are gradual and not always noticeable. The individual engaging in them receives little or no indication that health is being affected and may use the association between them and immediate health as "proof" that they are not dangerous.

Responses to the fact that one is or could be ill are more easily identified and have received a great deal of attention. Such responses involve attitudes toward seeking medical attention, methods of interpreting symptoms, and preferred styles of health care. (Compliance, perhaps the most thoroughly researched aspect of health behavior, will be treated separately in the next section.)

THE SICK ROLE

A number of researchers have focused their work on aspects of behavior associated with being sick—what people do when they are sick. To a certain extent, this research was generated by the repeated observation that certain types of behaviors or events were associated with illness. Hinkle and Wolff (1957), for example, found that over relatively long periods of time and with a relatively large number of subjects (nearly three thousand), the frequency of illness episodes was closely associated with social frustration, conflict, or both. However, the role of such events in causing illness could not be separated from the role of illness in causing or increasing frustration and conflict (Mechanic and Volkhart, 1961). As a result, interest also turned toward the effect on one's behavior of being ill.

Goffman (1961) discussed the drawbacks as well as the advantages of the sick role. On the one hand, sick people are excused from their normal responsibilities and obligations. On the other hand, they are stigmatized with all of the attendant social awkwardness and decreased attractiveness that being sick entails. Parsons (1951) also noted the mixed nature of the sick role, combining release from societal or group norms with the negativity of being sick. Parsons, however, pointed out the desirability of being excused or exempted from social obligations. Some people may be motivated to seek the protection that being sick entails, as a way of evading responsibilities.

These points have been modified somewhat, usually in the interest of pointing out that being sick is not necessarily a positive role to occupy. For example, Janis and Rodin (1979) have noted that people tend to make negative attributions toward sick people, and Coates and Wortman (1980) have discussed the social awkwardness typically involved in interaction with people who are ill. Yet research suggests that under trying times of stress many people opt for the sick role and the protection it affords (see Mechanic and Volkhart, 1961).

Illness behavior has a number of phases. Suchman (1965) has listed five states: *initial* (recognition and interpretation of symptoms), *assumption of the sick role, seeking assistance* (visiting a physician or clinic), *being a patient* (assuming a dependent role), and *recovery.* Mechanic (1978) has broadened these stages to include the types of information or inputs upon which people base decisions about their health. According to Mechanic, people attend to the *number and persistence of symptoms* that they experience, decide whether these symptoms are *recognizable* (if not, they may be cause for alarm), consider possible *disability* from symptoms, and look at *cultural and social definitions* of illness itself. Also considered at some point in the decision-making process is *prior knowledge* of general health as well as whether *treatment* can be obtained quickly and cheaply.

DETERMINANTS OF HELP-SEEKING

The degree to which people will seek medical attention depends on a number of factors, including perception and interpretation of symptoms, cultural or learned patterns of response to symptoms, and previous experiences in medical settings.

Symptom Perception
Although extensive literature on the perception of sensations extends back more than a hundred years, the ways in which sensations are interpreted as medically relevant or benign have not been satisfactorily determined. Many factors affect what sensations will be noticed and how they will be interpreted.

Symptoms are generally considered to be discrete sensations that are experienced at certain times. Nausea, headaches, cramps, and the like are episodic—they occur and recur for specific periods of time. Yet evidence suggests that many sensations called symptoms occur more or less continuously—most people experience these somatic sensations much of the time (see Krantz et al., 1980; Mechanic, 1972b; Zola, 1966). It is the degree to which people are *aware* of symptoms or are willing to report them and seek information about them that seems to vary. And this creates difficulty for research on symptom perception. Symptom reporting among Three Mile Island residents after the accident there, for example, has consistently and chronically increased (see Baum et al., 1980; Flynn, 1979). This increase may be interpreted as evidence of chronic stress among residents. Or it could reflect the fact that people are not experiencing more symptoms so much as they are more aware of them because they are afraid that the accident may have harmed them. It is also possible that these residents are simply more likely to report symptoms, just in case there might really be something wrong. As a local physician in practice near Three Mile Island indicated in a magazine interview, a sore throat, a routine symptom that would never have been reported in the past, is now seen as a call for alarm because it might be something dangerous caused by radiation. Fear of the possible long-term health consequences may have affected awareness and reporting of symptoms rather than actual experience of them.

The factors that influence the awareness and reporting elements just described are numerous. Situational constraints or excesses may increase or decrease awareness. Research has indicated that people become more aware of bodily sensations when they are bored, and less aware of sensations when they are fully occupied with a task (Fillingham and Fine, 1986; Pennebaker and Brittingham, 1982). Withdrawal appears to be associated with heightened awareness of symptoms (Baum, Aiello, and Davis, 1979; Pennebaker, 1979). How one views the world or how optimistic one is also affects symptom reporting (Scheier and Carver, 1985). The ways in which sensations are labeled and reported are determined by situational, cultural, and psychological influences (see Kasl and Cobb, 1966; Zola, 1963, 1966).

Interpretations of symptoms and subsequent action are affected by the actual sensations experienced. Discomfort in different intensities and/or locations is interpreted differently. However, a number of social psychological factors are also important. For example, women are more likely to report symptoms and to seek medical attention for them than are men (Mechanic, 1972). Partly due to this, women more accurately report the presence of symptoms when they are there, but also mention them more often when they are not present (Gonder-Frederick, Cox, Bobbitt, and Pennebaker, 1986). Lower social status is also associated with greater symptom reporting and help-seeking (see Koos, 1954). Help-seeking is not necessarily related to stress or to the extent of reported symptoms. Intervening factors such as social support and prior medical or psychological history appear to be reasonable predictors of help-seeking (see Baum et al., 1979; Bieliauskas, 1980; Bieliauskas and Webb, 1974; Rabkin and Struening, 1976).

Response to Symptoms

It is fairly clear that psychological distress and other psychosocial variables affect symptom perception, but it is less clear how these factors are related to help-seeking. The same variables that affect symptoms also appear to affect decisions regarding whether medical attention will be sought as well as general definitions of health (Mechanic, 1968). Psychological distress is a determinant of perceptions of health, and stress is important in determining whether people will use health care services (see Mechanic and Jackson, 1968). Another study identified only two influential variables: distress was associated with greater use of health care, and women were found to use health care services more often than men (Tessler, Mechanic, and Dimond, 1976).

Distress is not the only variable affecting utilization of health services. Mechanic (1978) has reported a study in which the patterns of health care use by a large sample of college students were monitored. Distress was important, but so were the student's sex and relationship to social networks. Higher status, less religious students were most likely to seek psychiatric help, younger students were most likely to seek counseling assistance, and women were most likely to use health services in general.

Other research has placed a great deal of emphasis on the effects of one's social environment on help-seeking. One's friends and family have clear impacts on the decision to use health care, either because they suggest it or because they confirm that a symptom may be serious. Thus friends and family can encourage or discourage help-seeking. Research has suggested that people with strong family ties may have less need for health consultations because their kin provide advice instead (McKinlay, 1972). Other studies, however, suggest that people with a moderate or high level of social support are *more* likely to seek health care (see Baum, Davis, and Aiello, 1979; Salloway and Dillon, 1973). The fact that psychosocial variables such as friendship networks can affect people's decisions regarding whether or not to go to a physician for care is not surprising.

PREFERENCES FOR TYPE OF CARE

Different people have different preferences for the type of care they receive. Some like to get a lot of information—what the physician is doing and finding and what it means—while others do not. Some want to take care of themselves; others want professionals to do it. Some want friendly physicians; others want businesslike interactions. Recent research has looked at whether these kinds of preferences represent any systematic bias in patterns of using health care facilities.

For example, how much should a doctor tell his or her patients? Regardless of whether a patient is dying or in the best of health, should he or she be told everything, or should the doctor use discretion in deciding what to divulge? On the one hand there is the patient's right to know. On the other side is the potentially negative impact of complete information on health and recovery. If the doctor believes that divulging everything will endanger the health of a patient, what should he or she do?

Questions relating to patient preferences and health care have been studied by Krantz, Baum, and Wideman (1980). Research on providing information to surgery patients has indicated that choice or control enhances recovery from surgery. But other studies suggest that there are not always *direct* benefits of increased patient control. By the same token, some individuals may benefit more than others from an active and informed role in their health care. Research has, for example, shown that personality differences and coping styles make individuals more or less suited to particular styles of health care (see Cromwell et al., 1977; Shipley et al., 1978). An example of this research has been modification of the locus of control concept and development of a health-specific index of locus of control (see Wallston and Wallston, 1984). This scale, which discerns the degree to which an individual feels able to control his or her health, has had success in identifying people who benefit from differently focused programs.

Personality variables are only one of a number of variables that may affect preference for, or receptivity to, different treatment approaches. Krantz and his associates developed research that attempted to include a number of such variables into a broad-based, two-factor preference measure. The scale they used, the Health Opinion Survey, measured patients' preferences for more or less *active participation* in health care and for a more or less *informed role* in this process.

The items in this scale (see Table 8.2) assess the degree of involvement patients desire in making decisions about their health, preferences for self-care (as opposed to letting health professionals take care of them), and preferences about what they are told about their health.

The Health Opinion Survey (HOS) was validated in several settings. Residents

TABLE 8.2   Health Opinion Survey

The following questions ask for your opinions about different kinds of health care. For each statement below, decide whether you *agree* or *disagree* and circle the answer which *best* fits your opinion. Each person is different, so there are no "right" or "wrong" answers. Please try to circle an answer for each question, and don't leave any blank. Even if you find you don't completely agree or disagree with a statement, choose the *one* answer that comes *closest* to what you believe.

	For each question, circle only one answer that comes CLOSEST to what you believe:
1. I usually don't ask the doctor or nurse many questions about what they're doing during a medical exam.	AGREE DISAGREE
2. Except for serious illness, it's generally better to take care of your *own* health than to seek professional help.	AGREE DISAGREE
3. I'd rather have doctors and nurses make the decisions about what's best than for them to give me a whole lot of choices.	AGREE DISAGREE
4. Instead of waiting for them to tell me, I usually ask the doctor or nurse immediately after an exam about my health.	AGREE DISAGREE
5. It is better to rely on the judgments of doctors (who are experts) than to rely on "common sense" in taking care of your own body.	AGREE DISAGREE
6. Clinics and hospitals are good places to go for help since *it's best for medical experts to take responsibility* for health-care.	AGREE DISAGREE
7. Learning how to cure some of your illness without contacting a physician is a good idea.	AGREE DISAGREE
8. I usually ask the doctor or nurse lots of questions about the procedures during a medical exam.	AGREE DISAGREE
9. It's almost always better to seek professional help than to try to treat yourself.	AGREE DISAGREE
10. It is better to trust the doctor or nurse in charge of a medical procedure than to question what they are doing.	AGREE DISAGREE
11. Learning how to cure some of your illness without contacting a physician may create more harm than good.	AGREE DISAGREE
12. Recovery is usually quicker under the care of a doctor or nurse than when patients take care of *themselves.*	AGREE DISAGREE
13. If it costs the same, I'd rather have a doctor or nurse give me treatments than to do the same treatments myself.	AGREE DISAGREE
14. It is better to rely less on physicians and more on your own common sense when it comes to caring for your body.	AGREE DISAGREE
15. I usually wait for the doctor or nurse to tell me about the results of a medical exam rather than asking them immediately.	AGREE DISAGREE
16. I'd rather be given many choices about what's best for my health than to have the doctor make the decisions for me.	AGREE DISAGREE

of a college dormitory, students reporting to the college infirmary for routine treatment for minor illnesses, and students enrolled in a medical self-help course at the same school were administered the scale. As expected, students in the self-help course scored higher on the behavioral-involvement subscale of the HOS than did the dormitory residents. They also scored higher on the information scale. People in a self-help course were more interested in involvement in their health care as well as more inquisitive about it. Users of the infirmary, by contrast, scored *lower* than the dormitory sample on the behavioral involvement scale. Individuals who made use of clinic services for minor illnesses were less oriented toward self-care than the unselected population and more likely to seek help.

Findings also indicated that among students using the infirmary, the higher the degree of desire for involvement, the lower the reported use of clinic facilities. College students who desired a good deal of involvement in their health care were less likely to use infirmary services for minor illness complaints. Presumably this was because they were more likely to try to treat themselves.

In another study, a clinic nurse rated a variety of patient behaviors during a medical exam. These behaviors related to information seeking (e.g., asking questions) and active involvement in treatment (e.g., attempts to self-diagnose). The number of questions asked by the student-patients during their exams was affected by preferences—information scores were associated with greater inquisitiveness. Further, those who indicated a stronger desire for active involvement were more likely to attempt to diagnose what was wrong themselves.

In stressful health care situations, there is evidence that the HOS can be a useful way of matching patients to treatment interventions in a way that minimizes stress and maximizes favorable health care outcomes. One study of patients undergoing oral surgery (Auerbach et al., 1983) varied the type of information given prior to the procedures. It was shown that when patients were given specific preparatory information about procedures, patients with high information preferences showed better adjustment during surgery. However, when patients were given only general information, patients with low information preferences fared better. In a second study (Martelli et al., 1987), patients were given preparatory interventions that were either emotion-focused (designed to reduce negative emotion and distress), problem-focused (offering objective information about surgical procedures and sensations), or mixed (involving interventions that combine both features). Again, results indicated that adjustment and satisfaction were better when high HOS information-preference subjects were given problem-focused information and low HOS information-preference subjects were given emotion-focused information.

These data indicate that attitudes toward treatment approaches can be measured reliably and that these preferences influence a variety of health and illness behaviors. However, since these studies dealt with minor illnesses, we do not yet know whether differences based on these preferences extend to serious or chronic illness. Probably these beliefs are shaped by a complex of processes, including cultural and demographic factors and past experience with illness and with medical professionals. Strong associations between preferences and demographic characteristics may have implications for developing modes of treatment for different population groups. Whatever the outcome of future research, it is important to appreciate that the attitudes people bring to the health care setting are important determinants of their receptivity to different kinds of care.

COPING WITH CHRONIC ILLNESS

One of the most challenging aspects of the management of patient behavior and of the relationship between health and behavior involves chronic illness. Most of us have been ill for more than a day or two, but few of us have been ill for weeks, months, or years. Many diseases, such as diabetes, hypertension, heart disease, and cancer, are not illnesses that one gets over and forgets. Diabetes and hypertension, for example, are not cured by medical treatment but are instead controlled: use of dietary restrictions, insulin, diuretics, beta-blocking drugs, and vasodilating drugs may allow people with these diseases to live normal lives, but the underlying conditions remain. These diseases are for life and require special coping skills and health care. Physical problems, related to the illness as well as the nature of treatment, must be dealt with. Thus patients must cope with pain, other symptoms that produce discomfort, physical impairment, and/or changes in cognitive abilities associated with their disease and with their treatment. Some forms of treatment, such as chemotherapy for cancer or various antihypertension medications, have side effects that may be more uncomfortable and disruptive than symptoms of the disease.

Some of the resources that people need and use in coping with chronic illnesses come from family and friends. While the social strains that are likely following diagnosis of chronic illness vary by disease and are affected by a number of variables, support from social sources is often crucial to patients. Thus friends and family may draw away from victims of AIDS or cancer, even though their support may be extremely important to the patient. The effects of chronic illness on one's family, for example, are complex, but there is some evidence of families drawing together in the face of such a crisis (Masters, Cerreto, and Mendlowitz, 1983).

Studies also suggest that treatments for major chronic illnesses can create difficulties for patients and care providers. Research on cancer patients, for example, has focused on variables that affect how well-adjusted patients are, particularly in the face of one or more of the very unpleasant treatments currently in use. The side effects of chemotherapy, many of which can be experienced in advance of treatment, include nausea and vomiting, and radiation therapy can cause a number of fears and side effects as well (Adersen, Karlson, Anderson, and Tewfick, 1984). Management of anxiety before, during, and after these procedures is an important issue that requires research attention.

Conditioning also appears to be important in how one copes with cancer, and hence, how the disease progresses and may interact with personality variables. Anticipatory nausea has been identified as an important conditioned response to chemotherapy cancer treatment. Normal side effects of such treatments include severe nausea and vomiting, and research has indicated that various stimuli associated with chemotherapy—the hospital, clinic, the nurse, and so on—may come to elicit these symptoms before administration of the drugs that cause these responses (see Lyles, Burish, Krozely, and Oldham, 1982). This can cause several problems, including reluctance to go for treatment, but little is known about why some people are more likely to develop anticipatory nausea than are others, since estimates show that 25 to 50 percent of patients develop this reaction (Van Komen and Redd, 1985). Studies have found that the severity of the chemotherapy, high levels of anxiety and arousal, attitudes toward illness, and other variables are associated with this response (see Morrow, 1982; Schulz, 1980).

More recently, a study by Van Komen and Redd (1985) examined one hundred cancer patients undergoing chemotherapy, one-third of whom experienced anticipatory nausea and, consequently, greater distress during therapy. Those who developed anticipatory nausea were also found to be higher in trait anxiety (i.e., chronic anxiety) than were those not getting sick in advance. They also scored higher on the Millon Behavioral Health Inventory (see Chapter 9), indicating that people with bleaker, more pessimistic outlooks, who feel more isolated, anxious, and inhibited, were most likely to develop anticipatory nausea.

We shall not discuss the details of coping with the great variety of chronic illnesses common in modern life. Many of the issues span diseases, and several psychological concepts, such as denial and control, are important. Instead, we shall consider rehabilitation and coping in patients who have experienced a heart attack as an exemplar of the issues underlying management of chronic illness. Clearly, the problems of active participation, as in the case of insulin self-administration in diabetes or the severe side effects of treatment and fears associated with cancer or terminal illnesses, make them somewhat different from heart disease (see Davis, Hess, Van Harrison, and Hiss, 1987; Van Komen and Redd, 1985). For our purposes here, however, discussion of post-heart attack demands will be illustrative of many major variables and processes.

RECOVERING FROM HEART ATTACK

One of the most important aspects of coping with chronic or serious illness is the process of rehabilitation and management of illness. Once someone has a disease, what can be done about it, particularly when it is a chronic illness such as heart disease? **Secondary prevention** refers to the problem of preventing or reducing further deterioration caused by a disease that has already taken hold. Modification of risk factors is an important part of cardiac rehabilitation. Getting patients to quit smoking is very important, as is modification of diet to lower cholesterol and fat intake, weight control, and medication adherence to control blood pressure (Krantz and Blumenthal, 1987). For example, if people who have had a heart attack or myocardial infarction (MI) continue to smoke, their risk of dying from heart disease will be nearly double that of post-MI attack patients who quit smoking (Sparrow, Dawber, and Colson, 1978; Wilhelmsen et al., 1975).

Recovery from an MI, however, is more than a medical problem; many of the nonmedical problems resulting from the onset of coronary disease are almost as severe as the primary illness itself. Complex and demanding social, vocational, and psychological adjustments are required of patients and their families. Recovery from heart attack requires the interaction of medical and psychological processes at many levels, and important recovery outcomes may depend on the patient's interpretation of illness and the success and failure of psychological coping mechanisms.

WHY WORRY ABOUT BLAME?

Who is blamed for misfortune has important implications for behavior and health. The "just world hypothesis" (Lerner, 1980) is a commonly held belief that the world is just, that victimization and negative events do not happen randomly. Bad things do not come to good people (Wortman, 1983). Thus people try to convince themselves that victims deserve their plight, that they have done something to warrant it. When confronted with a person who has cancer or who has been raped or injured in an accident, people may decide that the person caused the disease or accident or that he or she is a bad person who deserves to suffer (e.g., if so, then the victimization is consistent—caused by something—and the world is not random). Walster (1966) argued people want to view the world as orderly, not unpredictible. People may blame patients for their misfortune to retain a sense of control and preserve the consistency and orderliness of the world.

The flip side of blaming others for their problems is the tendency people have to blame themselves. Again, blaming oneself for negative outcomes maintains belief in control by holding that one caused his or her misfortune, but it also carries with it negative connotations about responsibility and deservingness. Janoff-Bulman (1979) has distinguished between two types of self-blame. The first, behavioral, involves blaming misfortune on aspects of one's behavior that are easily changed, such as effort or interest. Such an attribution would have an individual blame a health problem on his or her not trying hard enough to prevent it. Someone who fails to get a flu shot and then gets sick may say it was because he or she couldn't find time to get vaccinated. By doing so, the event is still controllable, and one's sense of control may be maintained by altering this behavior in the future in order to prevent a recurrence of the illness or similar illnesses (Janoff-Bulman 1979).

Timko and Janoff-Bulman (1985) found that among breast cancer patients, attributing cancer to one's personality (stable factor) was negatively associated with adjustment while attributing it to less stable behaviors was positive. Those women who believed they could have avoided becoming ill by changing behavior, such as not having taken birth control pills or eating different foods, were more likely to believe that they could avoid a recurrence. Behavioral self-blame was also shown to have positive effects on adjustment in a study of diabetic children (Tennen et al., 1984). Those children who viewed their disease as having been caused by behavioral factors such as diet were rated as coping better and having the disease under better control than were children who attributed the disease to uncontrollable factors such as heredity.

Related to the difficulties in coping with chronic illness is the tendency of care providers to withhold or oversimplify information. Twenty-five years ago a survey of physicians on whether they would inform patients about cancer diagnoses and prognoses found that 90 percent preferred not to do so (Oken, 1961). The primary reason for this was the fear that patients would become depressed or suicidal (Mount et al., 1974). Another study also found that physicians were reluctant to fully disclose information to patients (Mount et al., 1974). The tendency of physicians to withhold information has diminished somewhat since the 1960s and 1970s; most physicians now tell some or all patients about their cancer diagnoses (Novak, Greenwald, and Nevitt, 1982). However, some information is still frequently withheld, which poses problems for patients (Bedell and Delbanco, 1984).

Many cancer patients are often faced with many different alternative choices regarding treatment, ranging from surgery to chemotherapy and radiotherapy. Within each, further choices may be made. In such cases, it is possible that patients' involvement may backfire; faced with the task of choosing from among several noxious treatments whose complexities defy fully informed choices, they may become distressed and indecisive. For some, having medical personnel make some decisions and deferring to the expertise of the physician can ease this stress, and it has been assumed that greater patient control and input into such decisions is good (see Fiske and Taylor, 1984). Our discussion of blame raises the issue of who should assume responsibility for choices or treatments that fail—should the physician assume responsibility, as many have suggested? (see Clements and Sider, 1983). A study by Wagener and Taylor (1986) that compared kidney transplant patients for whom procedures had been successful or unsuccessful provided some support for this. Compared with successful transplant patients, those whose surgery had failed tended to assume little responsibility for the decision to have the surgery. The tendency to reduce distress by blaming others for negative events appeared to be stronger than the need to maintain a sense of control by assuming responsibility oneself.

The Impact of Illness on Work and Family

The process of recovery from heart disease is usually divided into an acute (in-hospital) phase and a convalescent (posthospital) phase. Three of the major concerns of the recovering heart patient after release from the hospital involve survival (fears of death and recurrence of disease), the effects of illness on the ability to resume work activities, and the effects of illness on sexual functioning (Croog, 1983; Dillard, 1982). It appears that most post-MI patients are reemployed after one year, with delays or failures to resume work occurring more often among blue-collar workers, relatively less educated people, and patients with long-lasting depression or emotional distress (Doehrman, 1977; Krantz and Deckel, 1983).

Evidence from several studies suggests that many, if not most, patients do not return to their previous levels of sexual activity after an MI. This is probably caused more by psychological and interpersonal concerns than by physiological factors such as decreased desire, depression, anxiety, wife's decision, and fear of death (Hellerstein and Friedman, 1970). The family can play an important role in influencing the course of patients' recovery and rehabilitation. As most coronary patients are middle-aged males, particular emphasis has been placed on how the wife can affect the way the husband copes with his disease (Croog, 1975, 1983). Conflicts between husband and wife or overprotectiveness on the part of the spouse can interfere with the recovery process (Garrity, 1975; Wishnie, Hackett, and Cassem, 1971).

PSYCHOLOGICAL PERSPECTIVES ON RECOVERY FROM HEART ATTACK

Defense Mechanisms and Coping Dispositions

Different investigators have conceptualized the patient's psychological reactions to heart attack in several ways. One view focuses on psychodynamic **defense mech-**

anisms and coping dispositions (particularly denial and depression) used in response to the acute stress of illness. Cassem and Hackett (1971) have developed a model for the time course of emotional reactions of the person who suffers an MI in which denial is considered the focal mechanism for the coronary patient. It is proposed that a patient feels heightened anxiety when first admitted to a coronary care unit (CCU). Denial is soon mobilized, and the patient finds it difficult to believe that he or she has really had a heart attack. (See Figure 8.2.) Subsequently, anxiety declines for a period and the patient often protests his or her detention in the CCU, insists on returning to normal activities, and becomes difficult to manage. However, after several days, the patient becomes more cognizant of the limitations of his or her true condition and experiences depression.

This model implies that patients who use denial will experience less anxiety in the CCU than those who do not and, because of the stress-reducing effects of denial, those who use this defense mechanism will show facilitated recovery. In support of this view, several studies have found that patients who use denial tend to be less anxious in the early phases of illness than those who do not (Froese, Hackett, Cassem, and Silverberg, 1974; Garrity et al., 1976). However, long-term follow-up studies examining the relationship between denial and longevity have not been able to test this hypothesis conclusively. In summary, it appears that patients' use of denial may make for better coping with the early stress of illness. In the long term,

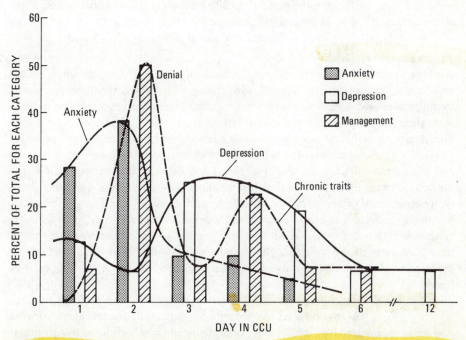

Figure 8.2 Curves representing emotional responses and requests for psychiatric management in a coronary care unit (CCU).
Reprinted with permission from T. P. Hackett and N. H. Cassem. Psychological adaptation to convalescence in myocardial infarction patients. In J. P. Naughton and H. K. Hellerstein (Eds.), *Exercise Testing and Exercise Training in Coronary Heart Disease.* New York: Academic Press, 1973.

however, patients who use denial excessively may endanger their chances of recovery by ignoring medical recommendations that are important for satisfactory rehabilitation. Conflicting results relating denial to long-term outcomes suggest the need for further research on this question.

Depression is considered to be one of the major problems in cardiac convalescence and rehabilitation (Hackett and Cassem, 1973). During recovery, patients must confront the realities of disability and deal with changes in lifestyle that are forced upon them. Moreover, after the period of hospitalization, some patients are reluctant to resume their normal activities or to return to work—often to an extent not justified by their medical disability. One common reaction of this group of patients, termed **cardiac invalidism,** is characterized by excessive dependency, helplessness, and restriction of activity.

There is some evidence that depression may be associated with worsened recovery (Pancheri et al., 1978) and that the negative effects of depression can be countered in coronary patients by brief cognitively oriented psychotherapy. Gruen (1975) exposed a random sample of cardiac patients to brief cognitive psychotherapy designed to facilitate coping with illness. Results of this study indicated that treated patients, compared to a matched control group, had shorter stays in the hospital, were less likely to develop medical complications, showed fewer manifestations of depression or anxiety, and were more able to return to normal activities at four-month follow-up. The cognitive treatments consisted of reassurance and encouragement and of strengthening the patient's positive beliefs and coping resources. These interventions, directed at several psychological processes, demonstrate the efficacy of brief psychotherapy during the acute phase of illness.

Perceptions of Health

Another approach to understanding psychosocial aspects of cardiac rehabilitation emphasizes the patient's perceived health status. This view is based on the notion that illness-related behaviors result from a series of decisions based on how patients view their current health situations (Garrity et al., 1976). Therefore, a patient's understanding of his or her clinical status is seen as equally important as actual physical status in determining behavioral health outcomes such as return to work and resumption of activities. Patients' mood and behavior concerning their illness are seen as resulting from what they believe about how severe their disorder is, and, within the limits of the patient's actual physical disability, recovery is bound to health perceptions. The health perception model is conceptually similar to the more general **health-belief model** used to study preventive and other health behavior (discussed later in this chapter) (Kasl and Cobb, 1966; Rosenstock, 1966). Both models emphasize decisions made by patients in order to reduce threats posed by illness.

This **health perception approach** has received major stimulus from research (Garrity 1973a; 1973b) designed to explain why some MI patients return to work and recreational activities and achieve acceptable levels of morale although others do not. In this research, patients who perceived their health to be poor in the hospital had lower morale and were less likely to have returned to work or to other involvements six months later compared to those patients who rated their health as relatively good in the hospital. The patients' perceptions of health was only weakly related to medical measures of physical health status. Therefore, perceptions of health had an independent relationship to measures of recovery and adjustment; after controlling for the influence of physical health, perceptions of health were still related to recovery outcomes.

The health perceptions model suggests several interventions to improve the patient's self-assessed health status. Individuals involved in acute coronary care may be able to affect a patient's behavioral rehabilitation several months later by modifying his or her perceptions and encouraging as much as is realistic a belief in the optimistic aspects of physical recovery (Garrity, 1973a, 1973b). Patient perceptions can be altered through education, instruction, various nursing care procedures, or brief psychotherapy interventions such as those used by Gruen (1975).

The "Control and Predictability" Model

A third psychological approach toward understanding recovery from heart attack is based on the fact that the onset of acute MI is a stressful and potentially uncontrollable crisis for most cardiac patients (Krantz, 1980; Krantz and Deckel, 1983). In addition to physical pain and fear of death, patients are confronted with uncertainties about employment and family activities. Restrictions of lifestyle and some fear and uncertainty may persist for months or even years beyond the acute phase of illness. The control-and-predictability model of heart attack recovery (Krantz, 1980) suggests that adverse consequences occurring after acute MI are mediated in part by feelings of helplessness induced by illness and potentially threatening hospital procedures. According to this view, individuals, who feel relatively more competent, less depressed, and less threatened (all reflections of perceived helplessness) during the acute phase of illness will fare better emotionally, behaviorally, and physiologically at later points in the recovery process. In addition, procedures that enhance the patient's behavioral control (providing choices, encouraging participation) or cognitive control (providing information, increasing environmental predictability) should facilitate recovery from acute MI. Evidence bearing on the control-and-predictability model derives from two studies that were originally not conducted for the specific purpose of testing this model.

Transfer from a CCU: Effects of Increasing Predictability

When patients are ready to transfer from a coronary intensive care unit to the general medical ward, adverse reactions are frequently observed as the nurse-patient and physician-patient relationships in the CCU may be suddenly disrupted. Klein et al. (1968) undertook a study of seven patients to observe their reactions to an abrupt transfer, without choice or warning. These researchers found that five of the seven patients showed adverse emotional reactions to the transfer, including increased excretion of catecholamines, along with some form of cardiovascular complication. Apparently, despite the fact that transfer was intended as a sign of recovery, the patients showing adverse reactions interpreted being moved as a sign of rejection by the staff. In addition, the patients felt considerable uncertainty about who their physician would be and about other aspects of their treatment because changes in treatment programs between the two locations were often abrupt.

Therefore, for a second group of seven patients, Klein et al. (1968) introduced a number of alterations in the CCU and ward procedures that acted to decrease uncertainty and increase the predictability of the environmental change. These changes included having the patients prepared in advance for the transfer, having the same physician-nurse team follow each of the patients, and having the patients visited daily by the same nurse who provided information and helped with adjustment. This second group of patients, who experienced an intervention designed to heighten predictability, experienced no new cardiovascular complications or untoward emotional reactions to transfer. Thus this study provides support for the notion that unpredictable facets of treatment can heighten stress and jeopardize recovery in the acute phase of coronary disease.

Nursing Factors and Recovery: Effects of Increased Patient Control

Practitioners treating coronary patients often assume that proper nursing and psychological care can reduce patient distress. A question that often arises in this regard is how much control is optimal for patients to exercise over their own treatment. Cromwell, Butterfield, Brayfield, and Curry (1977) studied patient care procedures that appear to represent, in part, mixtures of various types of personal control. Acute MI patients were randomly assigned to a combination of one of three nursing care procedures. The first intervention, called *information,* involved systematically providing patients with different amounts of information concerning the physiology, causes, and treatment of heart attack. A second intervention, *participation,* was accomplished by varying the extent to which patients were allowed to initiate and engage in activities relating to their own treatment. (Patients in high-participation conditions were allowed to turn on an electrocardiogram machine when they wished to test themselves and show the results to their physician and they were allowed to perform mild foot-pedaling exercises under nursing supervision.) A third intervention, called *diversion,* consisted of giving patients different degrees of access to television, visitors, and reading materials.

The major findings of this study concerned length of hospital stay. There was a complicated interaction among the three interventions, such that if patients had been given high information but low levels of diversion or participation, hospital stay tended to be long. In contrast, high information together with high participation or high diversion led to short hospital stays. Thus the results indicate that if an acutely ill MI patient is told about the severity of his or her condition, the patient also should be allowed to actively participate in treatment or at least be given some opportunity for diversion. No negative effects were associated with a short hospital stay, and there were obvious economic and psychosocial benefits of the favorable treatment combinations.

In terms of the control-and-predictability model, several issues and questions are raised by Cromwell et al. (1977). First, it appears that the effects of various treatments in an acute coronary care setting depend on the meaning to the patient, which in turn depends on the particular way in which the treatments are presented. This study also raises questions as to how much participation and responsibility are optimal to facilitate recovery from MI. In some cases, patients may neither prefer nor expect responsibility for medical decisions, and their perceptions of excessive responsibility, choice, or information may not be beneficial either psychologically or medically. As noted earlier in this chapter, recent research suggests that in health care situations, patients may differ in their receptiveness to self-care and information. The most favorable outcomes therefore may result from matching particular patients with particular treatment interventions (Auerbach et al., 1983; Martelli et al., 1987).

In health care settings, the patient's role in treatment is a major factor distinguishing traditional medical model approaches and newer behavioral approaches. Unlike the former, the behavioral approaches encourage the patient to become an active participant in treatment. Common sense suggests that the most efficacious approach to patient participation and control in treatment would maximize patients' abilities to cope with stressful aspects of illness without leading them to develop unrealistic expectations or to make medical decisions beyond their realm of competence (Johnson and Leventhal, 1974; Mills and Krantz, 1979).

COMPLIANCE WITH MEDICAL REGIMENS

Perhaps the most thoroughly researched aspect of health behavior is compliance—following a physician's advice or prescribed medical regimen. Yet progress in improving patient attendance and maintenance of doctor's orders has been very slow. Apparently, reasons for not following these orders are deeply ingrained and resistant to modification. This is problematic, since failure to follow a prescribed regimen may cause a serious breakdown in the treatment process. By not following doctors' orders, people risk more serious illness or prolongation of current problems, and failure to take prescribed preventive measures (such as getting a vaccine) can also have serious consequences. Not all failures to follow doctors' orders are potentially dangerous. Doctors do make errors and prescribe unnecessary procedures. However, most of the time, following doctors' orders is important.

Before going any further, we should define compliance. **Compliance** is the term generally used to refer to adherence or cooperation—doing as the doctor suggests or following advice to adopt certain attitudes concerning health or health-related behaviors. Taking medication when one is supposed to and not discontinuing it until told to do so, going on a prescribed diet, quitting smoking—these are all instances of complying with a physician's advice. **Noncompliance** refers to failure to follow advice—the degree to which a patient does not adhere to what he or she was told (Sackett and Haynes, 1976).

At a minimal level, failure to comply is not necessarily harmful, although prescribed regimens are less effective if not followed completely. A higher level of noncompliance may cause more serious problems. Let us say you have gone to see your doctor and have been given a prescription. The prescription should help you if the doctor's diagnosis is correct. If you fail to follow this prescription (and your condition does not improve), the doctor must question either your compliance with the regimen, the diagnosis, or the prescription. If you add to the problem by falsely insisting that you have taken your medicine, the doctor may be forced to assume (incorrectly) that your failure to improve was due to incorrect diagnosis and so prescribe an irrelevant treatment. Compliance is basic to an effective doctor-patient relationship and increases the effectiveness of the physician's treatment.

EXTENT OF NONCOMPLIANCE

How much of a problem is noncompliance? Unfortunately, this question is not easily answered. There are many different kinds of compliance—prevention, medication-taking, and lifestyle alteration—and our ability to measure them is often very limited. Estimates that have been made are alarming. Studies of treatment of a wide variety of illnesses, including hypertension, glaucoma, coronary heart disease, and diabetes, have indicated that only 40 to 70 percent of patients comply with physicians' prescriptions or advice (Becker and Maiman, 1975; Haynes, Taylor, and Sackett, 1979). Other estimates are even more dismal (see Davis, 1966), and rates of compliance with preventive procedures advised by the physician are still lower (see Gordis, Markowitz, and Lillienfield, 1969). However, compliance with some forms of treatment appears to be better. Compliance with chemotherapy for cancer patients, for example, appears to be very high among adults, with estimates of better than 90 percent of patients complying with treatment (see Taylor, Lichtman, and Wood, 1984).

Noncompliance is manifest at many points in the medical process. Some patients do not show up for appointments; others do not follow advice. It has been found that many patients fail to fill prescriptions for medication, discontinue medication early, fail to make recommended changes in daily routine, and miss follow-up appointments (Sackett and Haynes, 1976).

Unfortunately, inability to measure noncompliance precisely hinders interpretation of these data. The various ways in which compliance and noncompliance are assessed are not always accurate, and each one provides a separate set of problems. Should patients simply be asked what they have done? Can patient reports be assumed to be reliable? There is some evidence suggesting that these reports are accurate (see Francis, Korsch, and Morris, 1969), but most studies suggest that this is not a good way to measure noncompliance (see Park and Lipman, 1964; Sheiner et al., 1974). Since most patients wish to be thought of positively, they can not be expected willingly to portray themselves negatively by admitting to failures.

Research also indicates that asking physicians for estimates of their patients' rates of compliance is not reliable either (Davis, 1966; Kasl, 1975). More objective measurements appear to be somewhat better, but they remain problematic as well. Counting pills remaining in a patient's prescription is one possibility, as are pharmacy checks to determine when prescriptions are refilled. This quantitative approach tells us if the proper amount of medication was removed from its container in a given interval. It really does not tell us much more. Patients can and do dispose of remaining medication to make doctors think they took all of it, and these counts do not allow any inferences about whether the medication was taken properly or all at once.

Using clincial outcomes—whether or not the patient improves—as an index of compliance also has obvious limitations. Such an approach assumes that proper adherence to regimen will always effect a cure and that cures will not be achieved if a patient does not comply. There are many factors governing a patient's progress, of which compliance is only one.

Perhaps the most basic way to measure compliance is to assay a patient's blood or urine for traces of a prescribed medication. Examination of urine can yield concentrations of a prescribed drug, and studies using this kind of measure have yielded somewhat more reliable estimates of compliance than have other methods (see Fox, 1958; Gordis, 1976; Marston, 1970). However, there are a number of problems with this approach as well. Unless repeated measurements are taken, these assays provide estimates of drug usage at a given point in time only. It cannot be determined, for example, whether a patient with the appropriate drug concentration has been taking the medication regularly or did so just before his or her appointment. Similarly, differences in metabolism or biochemical response to drugs across individuals can cloud the meaning of these assays.

Measurements of compliance and noncompliance are imperfect estimates of patient behavior. When used together they are somewhat better, but should never be assumed to be 100 percent accurate. Obviously, a patient who reports that he or she has failed to comply with a regimen, who does not show improvement, and who does not show traces of medication in blood samples may be confidently labeled as a noncomplier. When multiple measures are not used, or when these measures do not correspond (e.g., patient says he or she did not comply but urine assay suggests he or she did), interpretations are more difficult.

DETERMINANTS OF COMPLIANCE

As complex and difficult as the study of compliance is, a large number of studies have been addressed to understanding causes of noncompliance and identifying factors that affect compliance. A number of approaches have been taken, including searches for personality variables or demographic characteristics that could be related to compliance, examination of the role of the interaction between doctor and patient, and consideration of health beliefs as a factor. Before turning to each of these approaches, we should consider general factors that may affect compliance. For example, aspects of the prescription itself are likely to affect compliance: if there are unpleasant side effects of the prescription or if it is too complex ("take two blue pills every three hours, a white pill after meals and at bedtime, and two green pills two hours after each white pill"), compliance will probably be low. Compliance decreases as the length of treatment increases. If medication is prescribed over a long time, for example, it is more likely to be discontinued early (Haynes, 1976). Further, if the financial cost of complying is great, compliance will be less likely. The greater the effort required for compliance or the greater the lifestyle change necessitated, the lower compliance is likely to be. In other words, a number of social or environmental factors are likely to exert fairly general influences on adherence to regimens (see Kasl, 1975). For example, having social support from family and friends appears to be associated with better compliance (Doherty et al., 1983; Sherwood, 1983).

Personality and Background

Some researchers have focused on personal attributes that may affect compliance. Ley (1977) has noted that some patients are complainers and that others accept advice more readily. Those who complain regardless of what is done or said will be less satisfied with the physician and, as a result, less compliant. Some patients are generally predisposed not to follow advice. Evidence for such personality effects, however, has not been found (see Lutz et al., 1983). It is also possible that certain personal attributes predispose an individual to be more or less compliant. A psychodynamic approach to compliance issues might suggest that patient behavior is actually symptomatic of underlying psychological problems (see Balint, 1964; Blum, 1972; Strain and Hamerman, 1978). Although there is no experimental evidence yet for this hypothesis either, clearly phobias, depressive episodes, obsessions, and the like play some role in compliance behavior and must be considered by doctors when diagnosing and prescribing for patients.

Another approach emphasizing personal attributes has been to examine the relationships between various background demographic variables such as education and adherence to prescribed regimens. There has been some evidence suggesting that factors relating to cultural, social, or educational status or income level are correlated with compliance (Strain, 1978). If a person cannot read, cannot afford to fill a prescription, or has social or cultural objections to certain prescriptions, compliance may be affected. Yet very few studies have shown any relationships between such variables and compliance. Backeland and Lundwall (1975) have noted the role of a sense of well-being in compliance behavior, but very few studies have found evidence of demographic variables affecting compliance (Haynes, 1976).

Before we consider alternatives, we should note that although evidence indicates little support for the notion that background determines degree of compliance, some attributes will certainly affect adherence to regimen. Economic factors cannot be excluded; physicians must be sensitive to costs, in terms of both money and time off work (see Hieb and Wang, 1974). Social factors and responsibilities may, at times, be in conflict with compliance.

Research has suggested that when these factors are used in combination—more than one or two are used to predict noncompliance—or when specific factors are related to specific illnesses or situations, better prediction can be attained. Korsch, Fine, and Negrete (1978) were able to identify almost 90 percent of noncompliant patients using multiple background variables, and other studies have enjoyed similar success when using more than one predictor (see Gordis, Markowitz, and Lillienfeld, 1969). There is, therefore, some reason to believe that a constellation of variables that describe a patient's background can be useful in understanding causes of noncompliance. However, the search for determinants of compliance has taken other courses as well.

Satisfaction and Compliance

One approach focuses on patient satisfaction with the physician as a primary determinant of compliance. If patients are satisfied, they will be compliant; if they are dissatisfied, they will be less compliant. People appear to be more resistant to persuasive appeals made by physicians with whom they are dissatisfied. A number of variables inherent in the doctor-patient relationship will determine satisfaction.

Evidence for these hypotheses comes from a number of sources. Studies of satisfaction with medical consultation, for example, indicate that a number of variables are important in determining a patient's attitudes toward a physician. Davis (1968) found that formal and businesslike interactions between doctor and patient were associated with dissatisfaction, as were passive interactions. The ways in which physicians obtained and provided information were also important. Antagonistic or authoritarian styles were not satisfying, but physicians' ability to reduce tension in the consultation was associated with satisfaction.

Korsch and her colleagues (Korsch, Freeman, and Negrete, 1971; Korsch, Gozzi, and Francis, 1968; Korsch and Negrete, 1972) examined the satisfaction with medical consultation of children. Mothers' satisfaction with consultation and treatment of their children was assessed, and communicator variables were again implicated as determinants of satisfaction. If doctors were seen as businesslike, satisfaction was lower than if doctors were thought to be warm and caring. Further, more than 80 percent of those who thought the physician had been understanding were satisfied, as compared to only a third of those who did not feel that the doctor tried to understand their concern. Mothers who rated their children's doctors as good communicators were more satisfied than were mothers who saw the doctors as poor communicators (Korsch, Gozzi, and Francis, 1968). Finally, mothers whose expectations were thwarted—information that they expected to receive was not provided—were less satisfied than were mothers who were provided with what they expected to receive. If they expected a diagnosis, a discussion of causes of an illness, or some other piece of information and it was not provided by the physician, satisfaction with the physician was reduced.

The relationship between satisfaction and compliance with medical advice was investigated by Francis, Korsch, and Morris (1969). If dissatisfied with the communicator (doctor) or the content of the consultation, mothers were less likely to comply with the advice. Table 8.3 (Francis et al.) illustrates this relationship. Further supporting this are recent findings indicating that physicians' nonverbal skills are associated with patient satisfaction and compliance (DiMatteo, Harp, and Prince, 1986).

Comprehension and Compliance
Ley and Spelman (1967) have argued that cognitive and informational factors are largely responsible for failures to comply with prescribed regimens. The failure of many people to follow doctor's orders is due not to dissatisfaction, personality, or

TABLE 8.3   Patient Satisfaction and Compliance with Medical Advice

PATIENTS' REPORT	PERCENT HIGHLY COMPLIANT
Doctor businesslike	31
Doctor friendly and not businesslike	46
High satisfaction with consultation	53
Moderate satisfaction with consultation	43
Moderate dissatisfaction with consultation	32
High dissatisfaction with consultation	17

Reprinted by permission from V. Francis et al. Gaps in doctor–patient communication. *New England Journal of Medicine,* 1969, *280;* 535–540.

the like, but to genuine problems in understanding and remembering what they are told. In one study more than half of the patients studied misunderstood doctors' instructions; in another, almost half of what was told to patients was quickly forgotten (see Boyd et al., 1974; Ley and Spelman, 1967). Patients generally know that the doctor is trying to help them, and noncompliance for reasons such as "I don't like the doctor" should be less common than noncompliance because "I don't understand what I am supposed to do." In support of this, Ley and Spelman list three determinants of failure in the doctor-patient interaction:

1. Often the material presented by the doctor is too difficult for patients to understand.

2. Patients sometimes do not understand basic physiology or anatomy and do not possess elementary medical knowledge.

3. Sometimes patients are under misconceptions that are so incorrect as to interfere with proper comprehension.

There is evidence indicating that people often lack basic technical information. Boyle (1970) found that half of those people studied did not know where the kidneys, stomach, lungs, or heart were located, and that a quarter of these people did not know where the intestine was. Riley (1966) asked people about their understanding of doctors' orders, and found that erroneous information about even common aspects of diet and medication was frequent. For example, almost three-fourths of those tested did not know that Alka-Seltzer contained aspirin.

Problems associated with misconceptions about basic physiology are also important. Roth et al. (1962), for example, found serious misconceptions about peptic ulcers that inhibited compliance with prescribed regimen. Many subjects knew that acid was involved in the development of ulcers, but only one in ten understood that this acid was secreted by the stomach, and some thought that the acid was secreted in the mouth. Others thought that the brain was involved; whenever food was chewed or swallowed, acid was secreted. The importance of this kind of misbelief is illustrated in an example provided by Ley (1977): ". . . consider the case of the patient with a peptic ulcer, who thinks that (a) acid causes ulcers, and (b) acid is secreted by the brain when he swallows. If he is told to eat small, frequent meals this is, in his view, telling him to put into his mouth small, frequent doses of what is causing his ulcer" (p. 21).

The Health Belief Model

Yet another way of predicting compliance is by identifying factors associated with the doctor who communicates the medical advice, the advice itself, and characteristics of the patient that make acceptance of advice more or less likely. This involves application of the health belief model (Rosenstock, 1966) to the area of compliance. We already know that behaviors of the physician that increase satisfaction or trustworthiness affect compliance and that discrepancy of prescribed and preferred behaviors is also influential. What other factors will affect acceptance of doctor's orders?

The health belief model considers three levels in predicting people's behavior. First, one must take into account the patient's *readiness to act,* or perceived necessity of action. This is determined by the perceived *severity* of the disease state that exists or that could occur and the perceived *susceptibility* to the illness or its consequences (how likely he or she feels disease onset really is). If a patient does not believe an illness is severe or does not believe that he or she has a good chance of becoming ill, readiness to act will be low. There will be no reason for such readiness. If, on the other hand, the illness is seen as severe and the patient believes that there is a good chance of coming down with it, readiness to act will be higher. We are far more likely, for example, to get flu shots if the strain of flu expected is believed to be severe, unusual, and highly contagious than if it is thought to be mild and relatively rare. Risk perceptions, then, are important determinants of health behavior and tend to be more optimistic than is warranted (Kulik and Mahler, 1987).

The second act of considerations in this model involves estimation of *costs and benefits* of compliance. In order to comply, the patient must believe that the advocated regimen will be effective and that the benefits of following it will outweigh the costs. Side effects, disruptiveness, unpleasantness, and other negative aspects of a regimen must be countered by the benefits of treatment—reduction of severity or susceptibility to an illness—if patients are to be expected to comply.

The health belief model also posits the need for a *cue to action,* something that makes the subject aware of potential consequences. Internal signals that something is wrong (e.g., pain, discomfort) or external stimuli such as health campaigns or screening programs are necessary to initiate health behaviors and motivate the analysis of readiness, costs, benefits, and so on.

This model has been useful in predicting compliance. Although the doctor's perceptions of the severity of the patient's condition do not affect compliance, perceptions of severity and susceptibility *by the patient* are related to compliance (Becker, 1976; Becker and Maiman, 1975). Particularly when preventive health behaviors are considered, patients who believe they are likely to become ill and that this eventuality would have negative consequences are more likely to take some action. This has been demonstrated in many areas, including treatments prescribed during preventive dental instruction, cancer screening, and heart disease testing (see Fink, Shapiro, and Roester, 1972; Haefner and Kirscht, 1970; Kegeles, 1963).

Research has also considered perceptions of efficacy of treatment and cost-benefit analyses in decisions on whether or not to comply with prescribed regimens. When medication is involved, simple beliefs regarding the likelihood that it will improve the patient's condition are very potent determinants of compliance (see Becker, 1976, Elling, Whittemore, and Green, 1960). Any questions of safety of treatment, side effects, or distress associated with treatment become very powerful suppressors and reduce the likelihood that patients will do as they were told (see Becker, 1974).

These kinds of findings are neither surprising nor difficult to explain. What the health belief model attempts to do is consider patients' subjective states regarding their health rather than objective characteristics of it. *Actual severity* of an illness is not related to compliance, but *patient perception* of severity is. Revisions in the model have expanded its range to include intentions as well as beliefs (Becker, 1974). Whether or not patients intended to comply prior to learning about vulnerability or severity can thus be considered. Yet the fact that various beliefs or intentions are correlated with compliance does not mean that they *cause* an individual to comply. The health belief model provides a useful way of predicting compliance but does not tell us how it is determined.

Naive Health Theories

Another consideration of determinants of compliance, related to the health belief model in its social psychological approach, has been proposed by Leventhal, Nerenz, and Leventhal (1984). Like the health belief model, this approach considers patient beliefs in determining compliance, but it does so with greater emphasis on the processes involved. Also called common-sense models of illness (Meyer, Leventhal, and Gutmann, 1985), these notions about health, symptoms, and illness can lead patients to drop out of treatment. Thus one major determinant of compliance is the naive theory that a patient constructs in order to explain or predict an illness, as in the case of a patient with high blood pressure who complies periodically with medication-taking. The patient believes that whenever her blood pressure is high, she gets headaches. This naive causal connection is reinforced by the fact that whenever she gets a headache, she takes her blood pressure and finds that it is elevated. Thus she takes her medicine only when she gets a headache. If she were to take her blood pressure at times when she did not have a headache, she would see that it was elevated then as well and the basic fallacy of her theory would be exposed. Yet this selective monitoring effectively reinforces her belief and makes it a central aspect of self-treatment. In addition, once these naive theories are developed, they affect the way in which new information is interpreted and remembered (Bishop and Converse, 1986).

This description is particularly powerful because it can explain noncompliance by someone who intends to comply, believes that severity and vulnerability are sufficient to warrant action, and so on. The headaches serve as a cue to action, and this account is therefore consistent with the health belief model. Despite the fact that research indicates that people cannot reliably predict changes in blood pressure by focusing on symptoms such as headaches (Bauman and Leventhal, 1985), people connect events together in naive theories that reduce compliance. These theories also provide readily testable interventions aimed at exposing the fallacious aspects of patients' common-sense theories about their health.

INCREASING COMPLIANCE

All of the theories or explanations of compliance and noncompliance have been used in attempts to improve patients' adherence to advice or prescription. Attempts to increase compliance have focused on a number of aspects of patients' relationship to treatment. Correcting erroneous beliefs about either health or illness and bodily function in general has been attempted in a number of educational campaigns. These have not been particularly successful (Haynes, 1976). Information about drugs has been provided by pharmacists as patient package inserts, and physicians and their assistants have attempted to provide patients with information about their treatment (see Neufeld, 1976; Schneider and Cable, 1978; Vidt, 1978). These attempts have been somewhat successful but do not provide an adequate solution to the problem.

Other attempts have considered personalization of treatment to reduce the costs of compliance. Here the treatment regimen is designed to fit with a given individual's lifestyle. Disruptiveness—the degree of change required to comply—can thereby be minimized, and health behaviors can be attached to well-learned aspects of an individual's daily routine. On an individual level such tailored regimens are easier to comply with, and some attempts on a larger scale have reported encouraging results (Haynes, Taylor, and Sackett, 1979; Schneider and Cable, 1978). Again, there is reason to believe that such an approach helps, but this solution does not address the whole range of noncompliers.

Some approaches attempt to modify doctor behaviors so as to make physicians more informative, better communicators, or just warm and sensitive. If doctor behaviors can be made more satisfying for patients, compliance should increase. Korsch et al. (1971) have outlined such a program. Although it has not been tested experimentally, it is consistent with research findings and makes good sense. The program suggests that doctors address patients' worries and concerns, provide clear, jargon-free information, and adopt a friendly, caring attitude. By doing so, doctors should be able to be more informative and increase patient satisfaction with them. Maguire and Rutter (1976) have discussed a training program that addresses these issues.

Other programs have been directed toward making communication between doctor and patient more effective and comprehensible. Thus increasing the number of questions that patients ask increases their involvement in health care, may give them more information, and appears to increase satisfaction with the physician visit (Roter, 1984). Ley et al. (1976) examined these issues in a study of the effects of increasing patients' understanding of medicine-taking. Many of these patients were unclear about some of what they had been told when medication was prescribed. They did not know, for example, what they should do if they forgot to take a pill, or whether or not the effects of the medication would be immediately apparent. These aspects of the regimen about which little was known were associated with decreasing compliance. In order to reverse this problem, leaflets were prepared that provided information about medications. These leaflets were of three kinds; some were easy to understand, some were moderately difficult, and the others were difficult. Some patients received no leaflet, and others received a leaflet of one of the three levels of difficulty. Results indicated that the leaflets improved the accuracy of pill-taking, but *only* when the leaflets were of easy or moderate difficulty. Very difficult leaflets did not significantly improve compliance.

A second study (Ley et al., 1976) was concerned with hospitalized patients. One-third of those studied received an extra five-minute visit from their physicians every ten days that was devoted to physician attempts to increase patient understanding of information that had already been provided. A second group of patients also received extra visits, but these visits were restricted to noninformation topics. Remaining patients did not receive any extra visits. Predictably, subjects in the first group were more satisfied and informed than the other patients when they were all followed up after discharge from the hospital.

Not all efforts at improving compliance by increasing knowledge about illness and treatment have been successful. Taylor et al. (1978) reported a study of hypertension patients that was less than successful. They presented a slide show and booklet about hypertension and its treatment, emphasizing the benefits of treatment and regular medication. After six months most of the patients receiving the information had mastered it, showing more knowledge of the disease and treatment than did patients not seeing the slide show and booklet. Despite this greater understanding, however, there were no differences in compliance or effectiveness of blood pressure control between patients who had and had not been given the educational program. However, programs that provide information about the problems people will face in trying to adhere to a regimen and focus on changing peoples' interpretation of their relapses have been more successful in promoting compliance (Belisle, Roskies, and Levesque, 1987).

Supervision has also been considered an effective way to increase compliance, because the act of reporting regularly to someone that you are following your regimen and your health is improving is a reinforcing situation. Consider the elementary school student who works hard so that she can get good grades. When she takes these grades home and shows her parents, she is made to feel good about herself; she is proud, is reinforced by parents, and comes to associate good feelings with good grades. On the other hand, presenting one's parents with poor grades is aversive and humiliating. One can apply this to the hypertensive patient. The patient who complies with prescribed medication and diet and who achieves some degree of blood pressure control is made to feel good when visiting the doctor. On the other hand, the noncompliant patient may be scolded and generally made to feel uncomfortable whenever visiting the doctor. Thus increased supervision or more frequent visits to the doctor should improve compliance, as the patient seeks to avoid the aversive consequences of having failed to do what was supposed to be done.

A number of studies have addressed this point, and they have found increases of up to 60 percent in compliance as a result of increased contact with medical personnel (see McKenney et al., 1973; Taylor et al., 1978; Wilber and Barrow, 1969). The impact of increasing supervision is further highlighted by the fact that when supervision is subsequently reduced to normal levels, compliance returns to its initial levels. The effects of increasing supervision do not generalize beyond the program of treatment; once supervision is decreased and the aversiveness of reporting to the doctor after having been noncompliant is reduced, compliance is no longer increased.

Related to this strategy is the use of self-monitoring or self-supervision to increase compliance. Haynes et al. (1976), for example, asked noncompliant hypertensive patients to keep a record of their blood pressure and found increased compliance during self-monitoring. However, this program was successful only when the records were reviewed by medical personnel. When patients were left on their own, compliance decreased. Without the threat of confrontation with a disapproving authority, self-monitoring did not have a lasting effect on compliance.

Generally attempts to increase compliance have been only moderately successful. Rodin and Kristeller (1981) argue that the general view of compliance is not specific enough to account for patient behavior over the entire course of treatment. Their three-stage model distinguishes among temporal phases in treatment and notes that patients have different concerns that must be addressed at different points in the process. This important distinction should allow for better success in improving compliance if different phases are handled in different ways.

The influences of medical environments, personal preferences and beliefs, information, and such are undeniable. The patient is a behaving organism, processing information and responding to different settings in ways that can influence health. The study of health behavior and response to medical settings is one of the most important aspects of health that psychologists can study. Since the psychological perspectives are focused more on these issues than on other biomedical fields, unique and lasting contributions can be made.

SUMMARY

In this chapter we reviewed the effects that various medical settings have on patient behavior.

Although hospitalization is necessary for some treatment, the hospital stay is often considered a negative experience. The patient is *depersonalized* through the structuring of activity, dress, visiting hours, and food and through lack of understanding of the procedures being applied; the patient is forced to *yield control* of his or her body to people who are strangers; and the patient must *submerge identity* and *adjust to loss of privacy*.

Patients who assume a cooperative role have been termed *good patients*, while those who are less cooperative are considered *bad patients*. While good patient behavior may help the staff, there is evidence that the noncompliant patient may retain more control and have an easier time readjusting to life outside the hospital.

Janis (1958) showed that patients who behaved moderately fearfully had less postoperative emotional disturbance. Janis reasoned that moderate levels of fear are optimal for defense and coping strategy development. Researchers have also conducted studies demonstrating that sensory and coping information given to patients before surgery reduces the need for analgesia and cuts the average period of recovery in hospital by several days. The same effect has been demonstrated during unpleasant medical examination and with children undergoing surgery. Other researchers have studied the effect of information given to patients before surgery. Depending on the patient's coping strategy, the information generally facilitated recovery.

Other studies indicate that reassurance, especially when given with information, helps in recovery. Other interventions, including hypnosis, relaxation training, and cognitive reappraisal-restructuring have also been applied with varying degrees of success.

Much interesting health behavior occurs outside the hospital. Response to illness has received a lot of attention and the *sick role* has been the subject of much study. Zbrowski (1952) studied cultural influences and the ways people react to symptoms of illness. Studies among residents of Three Mile Island show that symptom reporting of routine symptoms increased because of the fear of long-term health effects.

Interpretations of symptoms are affected by the actual sensations experienced.

Social factors are also important. Prior history of medical or psychological factors appear to be predictors of help-seeking.

Other research shows that social environment has an effect on help-seeking. Not only are friends and family likely to influence the decision to seek help, but those with a high level of social support are more likely to seek health care.

Some people seem to prefer different care styles. The *Health Opinion Survey* measures patients' preferences for more or less *active participation* in health care. Attitudes toward treatment approaches can be measured reliably, and these attitudes influence a variety of illness behaviors.

We discussed the topic of coping with chronic illness, including the consequences of cancer chemotherapy and recovery from heart attack. Three psychological perspectives on heart attack recovery were discussed, including a defense mechanism model linking denial to recovery, a health perceptions model emphasizing perceived health, and a model stressing predictability and personal control.

Compliance is the most researched area of health behavior. Compliance is a measure of adherence or cooperation with doctor's advice. Various things influence compliance, including patient satisfaction with the doctor, the information supplied, and the personality background of the patient. The *health belief model* (Rosenstock, 1966) predicts compliance by identifying aspects of doctor-patient communication that will affect compliance.

Some patients construct a *naive health theory,* connecting an unrelated symptom with a disorder and complying only when the symptom arises. This often explains noncompliance in those that intend to comply.

Attempts at increasing compliance have included making physicians better communicators, increasing patients' satisfaction by other means, and increasing contact with medical personnel. They have met with varying degrees of success.

RECOMMENDED READINGS

Baum, A., Taylor, S., and Singer, J. E. (Eds.). *Handbook of psychology and health, vol. 4: Social psychological aspects of health.* Hillsdale, N.J.: Erlbaum, 1984.

Burish, T. and Bradley, L. A. *Coping with chronic disease.* New York: Wiley, 1983.

Krantz, D. S., and Blumenthal, J. A. (Eds.) *Behavioral assessment and management of cardiovascular disorders.* Sarasota, Fla.: Professional Resource Exchange, 1987.

9 PSYCHOLOGICAL ASSESSMENT IN MEDICAL SETTINGS

|||||||||||||||||||||||||||||||||||||||||||||||||||||||||||||||||||||||||||||||||||||||||||||||||||||||||||||||||||||

Until relatively recently, the major form of psychological assessment conducted in medical settings involved the use of evaluation methods developed for psychiatric populations. A significant problem with this practice is that patients in a medical population are not necessarily similar to patients in a psychiatric population. Of course, such standard psychological tests may provide some general information about overall level of emotional health and the presence of such potentially debilitating symptoms as anxiety and depression. However, the interpretation of results obtained with a medical population on a diagnostic test with statistical norms and clinical signs developed for a psychiatric population may not be valid. As a result, assessments such as tests, questionnaires, and interviews that address "normal" medical issues and/or that have been standardized with nonclinical populations are needed.

Fortunately, a number of diagnostic tests have recently been developed with medical populations in mind. Before discussing these tests, we shall briefly review traditional psychiatric classification and assessment methods that are still commonly employed in many medical settings.

CLASSIFICATION OF PSYCHOLOGICAL DISORDERS

Classification involves the arrangement of various forms of abnormal behavior into specific categories. The descriptive categories help organize our thinking concerning the causes, symptoms, and treatment of abnormal behavior. They also aid in communicating the various types of psychological problems that individuals may experience.

German psychiatrist Emil Kraepelin is credited with developing the first systematic and widely accepted classification system of mental disorders. The first edition of this classic textbook in psychiatry, entitled *Lehrbuch der Psychiatrie,* was published in 1883. Through the years, he constantly continued to work out new details and revise old ones, so that the ninth edition of the text, published in 1927, one year after Kraepelin's death, was a two-volume work consisting of 2,425 pages. In his textbooks, he painstakingly integrated a great deal of clinical data in order to delineate the symptoms associated with specific mental disorders. He noted that certain symptom patterns occurred with sufficient regularity to allow one to identify and classify mental disorders on the basis of these symptoms. The classification schema he developed is the basis for the present-day diagnostic system.

A guiding philosophy behind Kraepelin's works was the belief that once various forms of mental illness had been successfully distinguished and classified, one would be able to predict the outcome of a specific type of disorder. The classification system would also provide a framework through which medical research could begin looking for agents responsible for the disease and treatment methods for curing it. The **nosological** or classification system he developed greatly influenced the field of psychiatry for many years, during which time the description and classification of disorders was heavily emphasized. Adhering primarily to an organic viewpoint or **medical model,** Kraepelin viewed mental disorders as diseases. This viewpoint, which did not emphasize the importance of psychological (psychogenic) factors in many disorders, seriously limited the subsequent usefulness of the Kraepelinean system. Although serving as a broad framework, it was significantly modified when the DSM, the classification system currently employed in the United States, was developed.

The *Diagnostic and Statistical Manual of Mental Disorders* (DSM) was adopted by the American Psychiatric Association in 1952 as its official classification schema of mental disorders. In 1968 a modified version (the DSM-II), developed in collaboration with the World Health Organization, was adopted. Some serious problems of validity and reliability were associated with these first two versions of the DSM (see Mears and Gatchel, 1979), and newer versions (DSM-III and DSM-IIIR) were published. The intent of this classification system is to allow mental health professionals throughout the world to compare types of disorders, incidence of occurrence, and other relevant data concerning mental disorders. It categorizes the wide variety of psychological disorders seen in hospital and clinical settings. These disorders differ greatly in terms of severity, degree of impairment produced, and the factors that determine them.

The manual provides a very comprehensive list of diagnostic categories. Moreover, the manual illustrates each disorder in terms of various dimensions. The first dimension spells out the *essential features of* each disorder or syndrome, giving an overview of the salient behaviors of the disorder. In addition, *associated factors,* or accompanying symptoms, are listed along with *age of onset, progression* or *course,* and social *impairment* characteristic of the disorder. The sixth dimension deals with the *complications* of each disorder, including disorders or events (such as suicide) that may result from the initial problem. Depression, for example, is a disorder that may have complications such as drug abuse.

The seventh dimension for each disorder lists *predisposing factors.* For instance, for the diagnostic category "Attention Deficit Disorder with Hyperactivity," retardation, epilepsy, forms of cerebral palsy, and neurologic problems would be listed as predisposing factors. *Prevalence,* the proportion of adults who may develop this problem is stated, as is the *sex ratio,* or relative frequency of the diagnosis for women and men. Finally, *familial pattern* (whether a disorder is more common among family members) and *differential diagnoses* are listed. Here disorders with features similar to those of the problem in question are noted. For example, opioid withdrawal is a problem that is remarkably similar to influenza. Thus influenza would be considered a differential diagnosis—a problem that would need to be distinguished for opioid withdrawal.

MULTIAXIAL CLASSIFICATION

One of the hallmarks of the DSM-III is what is called multiaxial classification. The DSM-II, like other classification systems, is basically a unicategory system. This means that the person normally receives only one diagnostic label and is placed into one category. The unicategorical approach assumes, for example, that schizophrenics do not ordinarily have sexual deviations or any other major problem. In a sense, the unicategorical approach is based on the assumption that the subject being assessed is a member of either *one* psychiatric category or *no* psychiatric category. Thus a neurotic might be coded as a hysterical, conversion type, but could not receive any other superimposed diagnosis. The DSM-III sees this unicategorical approach as being highly unrealistic and impractical.

The newer classification system attempts to avoid the possibility that a person with several disorders could be falsely placed in a single category. In order to capture unique individual factors, each individual is scored according to the following broad categories or axes.

Axis I: **Clinical Psychiatric Syndromes and Other Conditions.** This axis includes the major psychiatric disorders, with the exception of personality and specific developmental disorders.

Axis II: **Personality Disorders (Adults) and Specific Developmental Disorders (Children and Adolescents).** This axis includes personality and developmental disorders and may be used to further code prominent personality styles of the person being assessed.

Axis III: **Physical Disorders.** On axis III, physical disorders are to be recorded. The DSM-III considers knowledge of the general physical health of the person to be a major part of the total diagnostic picture.

Axis IV: **Severity of Psychosocial Stressors.** Axis IV enables the clinician to record specific psychosocial events "that are judged to be significant contributors to the development or exacerbation of the current disorder" (DSM-III, p. 2). For example, death of a spouse, financial condition, occupation status, and parenting status may have etiological significance and therefore be considered psychosocial stressors.

Axis V: **Highest Level of Adaptive Functioning During the Past Year.** Axis V permits the clinician to indicate his or her subject's highest level of adaptive functioning over the past year. There are provisions for the subject's adaptive success to be assessed in three areas: social relations (family and friends), occupational functioning, and use of leisure time. The clinician can rate his or her client with levels of scores ranging from superior through grossly impaired.

One primary purpose of the revisions of the DSM is to allow multiaxial diagnoses. By ensuring that a diagnosis is based on all five axes, the DSM-III reduces the probability that a single diagnostic category will be used to represent a unique individual. The fact that patients with a similar psychiatric diagnosis differ markedly on a host of dimensions was often lost in traditional diagnostic systems. While all diagnostic systems will probably continue to be inexact as a means for representing a functioning human, the DSM-III is certainly a far better system than the two earlier versions of DSM.

In Chapter 7 we discussed the general topic of psychophysiological disorders. Traditionally these disorders have been the disturbances with which psychiatrists and psychologists have had major involvement in medical settings. The DSM-III includes not only traditional psychophysiological disorders under the section "Psychological Factors Affecting Physical Condition," but also any physical condition in which psychological factors are found to be significant in the initiation or exacerbation of the disorder. (See box.)

TRADITIONAL PSYCHOLOGICAL ASSESSMENT PROCEDURES

The attempts to develop an effective classification system stimulated simultaneous efforts to construct effective and reliable techniques for the assessment of psychological disorders. The techniques developed have been quite diverse. In general, the different assessment tests can be classified into two major categories: projective techniques and nonprojective techniques. Before reviewing these two categories, we shall discuss a clinical method of assessment that cuts across all the theoretical orientations and clinical settings—the clinical interview.

THE CLINICAL INTERVIEW

The clinical interview, a basic and widely employed method of assessment, is effective for exploring and delineating specific concerns, feelings, and problems that an individual may be experiencing. The type of information collected in the interview tends to differ depending on the interviewer's theoretical orientation. For instance, a behaviorally oriented assessor might be concerned with determining the specific stimulus/environmental conditions associated with an abnormal piece of behavior. In contrast, a psychodynamically oriented assessor would be interested in reconstructing the person's early developmental history as a means of determining underlying psychological characteristics that may be causing certain behaviors of clinical concern.

The degree to which an interview is structured may vary greatly. The vast majority of interviews are conducted in a very loose, unstructured format in which the interviewer determines the types of questions asked and the manner in which

DSM-IIIR: PSYCHOLOGICAL FACTORS AFFECTING PHYSICAL CONDITION

A clinician may want to note that psychological factors contribute to the initiation or exacerbation of a physical condition. The physical condition, which should be recorded on Axis III, will usually be a physical disorder, but in some instances may be only a single symptom, such as vomiting.

This manual accepts the tradition of referring to certain factors as "psychological," although it is by no means easy to define what this term means. A limited but useful definition in this context is the meaning the person ascribes to environmental stimuli. Common examples of such stimuli are the sights and sounds arising in interpersonal transactions, such as arguments, or the news that a loved one has died. The person may not be aware of the personal significance of such environmental stimuli or of the relationship between them and the initiation or exacerbation of the physical condition.

The judgment that psychological factors are affecting the physical condition requires evidence of a temporal relationship between the environmental stimuli and the meaning ascribed to them and the initiation or exacerbation of the physical condition. Obviously, this judgment is more certain when there are repeated instances of a temporal relationship.

This category can apply to any physical condition to which psychological factors are judged to be contributory. It can be used to describe disorders that in the past have been referred to as either "psychosomatic" or "psychophysiological."

Common examples of physical conditions for which this category may be appropriate include, but are not limited to: obesity, tension headache, migraine headache, angina pectoris, painful menstruation, sacroiliac pain, neurodermatitis, acne, rheumatoid arthritis, asthma, tachycardia, arrhythmia, gastric ulcer, duodenal ulcer, cardiospasm, pylorospasm, nausea and vomiting, regional enteritis, ulcerative colitis, and frequency of micturition.

This category should not be used in cases of Conversion Disorder or other Somatoform Disorders, which are regarded as disturbances in which the specific pathophysiologic process involved in the disorder is not demonstrable by existing standard laboratory procedures and which are conceptualized by psychological constructs only.

Diagnostic criteria for 316.00 Psychological Factors Affecting Physical Condition

A. Psychologically meaningful environmental stimuli are temporally related to the initiation or exacerbation of a specific physical condition or disorder (recorded on Axis III).

B. The physical condition involves either demonstrable organic pathology (e.g., rheumatoid arthritis) or a known pathophysiologic process (e.g., migraine headache).

C. The condition does not meet the criteria for a Somatoform Disorder.

From American Psychiatric Association. *Diagnostic and Statistical Manual of Mental Disorders,* IIIR. Washington, D.C.: APA, 1987.

they are asked. This unstructured format, of course, can present a problem if one is interested in comparing the content and material gathered for certain patients by different interviewers. The differing experiences and clinical skills of the interviewers will make comparisons across interview data difficult, if not impossible.

An alternative is to impose more structure on the interview situation. One such structured interview system is the Current and Past Psychopathology Scales (Spitzer and Endicott, 1969). It consists of an interview guide gauged to gather specific information. The clinician focuses attention on a uniform set of typical patient characteristics. Responses to a set of specific questions are scored on six-point scales that measure the degree to which certain behaviors and feelings are present. Questions are always phrased in an identical manner so the responses elicited can be scored and compared across patients. Assessment of the Type A behavior pattern with the Structured Interview procedure, which we reviewed in Chapter 5 and which we will further discuss later in this chapter, is another example of a structured interview method.

Spitzer (1966) also developed the Mental Status Examination Record, an automated, computer-scored form for describing a patient's clinical characteristics. It is a standardized and quantitative method that allows a clinician to compare individuals over time and also to compare different patient groups, because they are assessed on the same items and rated in the same categories. This automated procedure permits the collection of objective and quantifiable interview data and produces a diagnostic statement about an individual.

PROJECTIVE TECHNIQUES

Projective techniques were developed by psychoanalytically oriented theorists interested in the hidden or covert aspects of an individual's personality. These methods, which are referred to as unstructured tests, present the individual with a stimulus for which there is little or no well-defined cultural pattern of responding, so that the individual must "project" upon that ambiguous situation his or her feelings, attitudes, motives, and manner of viewing life. According to psychoanalytic theory, these factors, which are assumed to be largely at the level of the unconscious, make up the person's "core" personality structure and determine the way in which an individual will behave. The two most frequently used projective tests in psychiatric settings have been the Thematic Apperception Test and the Rorschach Inkblot Test.

The Thematic Apperception Test (TAT)

The TAT was developed in 1938 by the Harvard psychologist Henry Murray. It consists of a series of thirty pictures with personal connotations and one blank card. The cards are presented one at a time, and the respondent is requested to make up a story (as complete and detailed as possible) suggested by each picture shown. Murray's main goal was to have respondents interpret the cards according to their tendencies to perceive in a certain way (i.e., **apperception**). Recurrent themes presented by the respondent are then interpreted in terms of **needs** or internal motivators (such as achievement or aggression) and **presses** or environmental determinants (such as rejection by others or danger).

Unfortunately the TAT has no generally accepted system of scoring and interpretation. Rather, the clinician uses a great deal of subjective interpretation of the possible meaning and significance of various aspects of the stories. This seriously limits the reliability and validity of it. As a result, the test as a whole is currently not widely used in psychiatric or medical settings. However, there have been some special scoring procedures developed to measure specific themes on the TAT, such as the need for achievement (McClelland, Atlanson, Clark, and Lowell, 1953) and the need for power (McClelland, David, Kahn, and Wanner, 1972).

The Rorschach Inkblot Test

The Rorschach was developed by Swiss psychiatrist Hermann Rorschach, who published his major work on the test in 1942. The test is administered by an examiner who presents a series of ten bilaterally symmetrical inkblots. The respondent is asked to describe what he or she sees or what the inkblot suggests. After responding to all ten inkblots, the respondent is shown the inkblots again, and the examiner asks what characteristics of the inkblot determined the responses and interpretations. The respondent's answers then are usually scored for location (the part of the card used in the response), quality, content, and other determining factors, including color, shape, movement, and human or animal characteristics. The responses and scores are interpreted as "signs" reflecting the respondent's personality characteristics.

Unlike the TAT, there have been a number of major scoring systems developed for the Rorschach test (see Beck, 1961; Exner, 1974; Klopfer, Ainsworth, Klopfer, and Holt, 1954). Exner is especially noteworthy for his efforts toward standardizing and developing objective criteria and norms for both children and adults. However, it should be noted that the Rorschach was not developed with a medical population in mind. Thus, although it may provide some general information about overall level of emotional health, it has not been demonstrated to be a useful diagnostic tool with a medical population.

NONPROJECTIVE TECHNIQUES

Many clinicians became dissatisfied with projective tests because of problems of reliability and validity produced by the need for subjective interpretation of the test responses. As a result, more psychometrically sound tests were developed that could be objectively scored and quantified. Out of this tradition, a variety of **structured tests** were devised to measure personality characteristics. Statistical norms for these tests are usually developed by administering the test to large groups of individuals at different times, so that the way one individual responds to test items can be compared with the way certain kinds of other people tend to respond.

MMPI

One of the most popular and widely used personality tests is the Minnesota Multiphasic Personality Inventory, which was originally developed by Hathaway and McKinley (1943). It was developed in order to provide mental health professionals with a comprehensive method to use in the description and diagnosis of abnormal behavior. The test consists of 550 items covering a wide range of subjects, including statements concerning current and past behaviors, beliefs, attitudes, symptoms, and traits.

The test is scored for ten psychiatric-personality scales as well as three "validity" scales used to check for the subjects' faking, misunderstanding, or sloppiness in taking the test. The ten "clinical" or psychiatric-personality scales are as follows:

1. *Hs: Hypochondriasis scale.* Assesses whether subjects have an exaggerated concern about their physical health, often with somatic complaints that have a psychological basis.

2. *D: Depression scale.* Assesses intense unhappiness and depression.

3. *Hy: Hysteria scale.* Assesses psychologically caused physical symptoms in persons with an apparent unconcern or indifference about their condition.

4. *Pd: Psychopathic deviate scale.* Assesses the degree of difficulty in social adjustment, the presence of delinquency and other antisocial behaviors, and the tendency to "act out."

5. *Mf: Masculinity-femininity scale.* Assesses the degree to which individuals engage in typical sex-role type behaviors and have feelings and attitudes traditionally ascribed to one or the other sex.

6. *Pa: Paranoia scale.* Assesses paranoid symptoms such as feelings of persecution, suspiciousness, worriedness, and interpersonal sensitivity.

7. *Pt: Psychasthenia scale.* Assesses whether individuals experience unreasonable fears, high anxiety levels, excessive doubts, and feelings of guilt.

8. *Sc: Schizophrenia scale.* Assesses whether individuals have characteristics indicative of the various subtypes of schizophrenia, such as hallucinations and social withdrawal/isolation. A high score on this scale may also indicate a somewhat artistic individual who engages in abstract thinking, or simply a socially withdrawn person.

9. *Ma: Hypomania scale.* Assesses impulsivity, excessive activity, and degree of manic excitement.

10. *Si: Social introversion-extroversion scale.* Assesses the degree of sociability.

The three "validity" scales are as follows:

1. *L: Lie scale.* Assesses the subject's frankness or deception in answering the questions. It contains items that describe socially desirable but improbable behaviors; answering "false" to such statements as "I sometimes put off till tomorrow what I might do today" and "I get angry sometimes" would indicate deception.

2. *F: Infrequency scale.* Assesses the degree of carelessness, confusion, or effort to deceive by subjects in answering the questions. Containing items that are answered in the same direction by at least 90 percent of normal subjects, it is a

measure of how similar the subject's responses are to those of the general population.

3. *K: Defensiveness scale.* Another method, although more subtle, for assessing test-taking attitudes. It was designed to detect defensiveness or subtle faking.

After the MMPI was developed, it soon became evident that the test could not be used successfully because individuals obtaining high scores on a particular scale often did not fit precisely into that diagnostic category. Moreover, it was found that many apparently normal individuals scored high on the clinical scales. Subsequently, though, it was discovered that useful diagnostic discriminations could be made by assessing combinations or patterns of scale scores. This is the manner in which the MMPI is currently used. For example, individuals with a high score on both the Pd and Ma scales (not just the Pd scale) were found to be associated with psychopathy and other antisocial forms of behavior. Empirically based manuals, containing profile patterns along with case descriptions of patients with these profile patterns, have been developed for clinical and personality assessment (e.g., Dahlstrom, Welsh, and Dahlstrom, 1972). These manuals are "cookbook" interpretations of the MMPI that provide clinicians with standards against which to match their cases. These cookbook manuals have added to the popularity and widespread use of this personality inventory. There are even computer services that score MMPI profiles and provide a detailed printout of the cookbook interpretation.

The MMPI generally produces characteristic patterns for an individual suffering from a psychophysiological disorder that can be used to differentiate the person's behavior from symptoms of other clinical disorders and from nonpsychiatric patterns of behavior. The MMPI pattern shown in Figure 9.1 is typical for an individual suffering from a psychophysiological disorder. This 1-2-3 profile pattern (elevations in hysteria, depression, and hypochondriasis scales) is associated with symptoms that occur in various psychophysiological disorders.

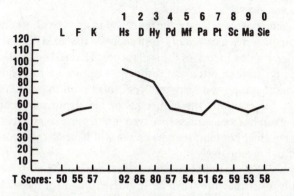

Figure 9.1 A 1-2-3 MMPI profile pattern (elevations in hysteria, depression, and hypochondriasis scales) which is typical for an individual suffering from a psychophysiological disorder.
From H. Gilberstadt and J. Duker. *A Handbook for Clinical and Actuarial MMPI Interpretation.* Philadelphia: Saunders, 1965. Copyright © 1965 by W. B. Saunders Company. Reprinted by permission of Holt, Rinehart and Winston, CBS College Publishing.

Psychophysiological disorders are not limited to this one profile pattern. Other pattern types have been found to diagnose specific forms of psychophysiological disorders. For example, specific profile patterns have been found to be associated with ulcer patients (Sullivan and Welsh, 1952), headache patients (Dahlstrom and Welsh, 1960), neurodermatitis patients (Gilberstadt, 1962), as well as those patients complaining of pain (Meehl, 1951).

A word of caution is necessary about interpreting scores on the MMPI or any other single psychological assessment test. The fact that a person shows a profile pattern similar to that of a psychosomatic patient group does not necessarily mean that he or she is actually suffering from a psychophysiological disorder. It indicates only that the person is answering a series of questions on the inventory in a manner similar to the way in which a diagnosed psychophysiological patient might answer. Other factors can also cause this type of responding. Results of the test are only suggestive and should not be employed as the sole basis for making a diagnosis. Before one can expect to make an accurate assessment, data generally must be gathered from multiple sources (such as self-report, observation by others, and physiological testing).

Structured Psychological Tests and the Problem of Response Bias

One potentially significant and well-demonstrated difficulty associated with structured personality tests is the presence of response sets or biases (Mears and Gatchel, 1979). A **response set** or **bias** is a particular test-taking attitude that causes a person not to answer items on a test in terms of their manifest content. That is to say, he or she has a characteristic and consistent way of responding to items on the test regardless of what the items actually say. Three major forms of response sets have been shown to affect structured psychological tests: response deviation or dissimulation, response acquiescence, and social desirability.

Response dissimulation or **deviation** is the tendency to answer items in an uncommon direction in order to present an overly favorable or unfavorable picture of oneself. The MMPI validity scales were developed in an attempt to control for this factor to some degree.

Response acquiescence refers to the tendency to agree with test items no matter what their content. On a personality test such as the MMPI, the questions are worded so that agreement increases the scale score. That is, the total score on a scale is a direct function of how often the respondent agrees or responds "yes" to the items. The more often a person answers "yes" to an item that is part of the MMPI depression scale, for example, the higher his or her depression score will be. If a nondepressed person has an acquiescence response set and so answers "yes" to these items regardless of their content, then he or she will have a scale score that suggests the presence of depression.

Social desirability is the tendency to answer items in the most socially desirable manner, regardless of what the truth is. In order to control for social desirability, certain inventories use a forced-choice question format. In this format, pairs of self-reference statements are presented simultaneously to the respondent, who is to choose the statement that is the most self-descriptive. The alternatives in each pair of statements are made equivalent in terms of social desirability. An example of a forced-choice format inventory, developed as an alternative to the MMPI, is the

Edwards Personal Preference Schedule (Edwards, 1959). The inventory contains 225 pairs of items, with the items in each pair being comparable in social desirability ratings. For example, a respondent would be asked to choose which of these two statements is more descriptive of him or her:

(A) I feel like blaming others when things go wrong for me.
(B) I feel that I am inferior to others in most respects.

Obviously a clinician has to be sensitive to the possibility of individuals falsifying their responses on a test. Many tests have validity scales to help isolate those cases in which falsification of responses occurs. Moreover, in most medical settings it can be assumed that a patient seeking professional help would not want to falsify his or her responses.

PSYCHOLOGICAL ASSESSMENT METHODS DEVELOPED FOR MEDICAL SETTINGS

We now turn our attention to assessment procedures specifically developed with a medical population in mind. In recent years the number of such procedures has been growing. We will review the most widely known and utilized of these methods. The first two to be discussed—the SCL-90 and the Millon Behavioral Health Inventory—are similar to the MMPI in their focus on the assessment of psychopathology. They are different, however, in that they were developed for use with a medical population rather than solely with a psychiatric population. We shall then review methods that were developed to assess psychological characteristics associated with physical illness. The first of these—the Life Experiences Survey—was constructed to evaluate life change events, the stress of which has been shown to be associated with physical illness. It was developed in response to problems associated with the first scale of this type, the Schedule of Recent Experiences. Procedures developed for the assessment of Type A-B behavior characteristics, specifically the Structured Interview and the Jenkins Activity Survey, will then be reviewed. Finally, the oldest form of psychological assessment in medical settings—neuropsychological assessment—will be discussed.

THE SCL-90 RATING SCALE

The SCL-90 and SCL-90R (Derogatis, 1977) are ninety-item self-report symptom inventories that were developed to measure psychopathology in both psychiatric and medical outpatients (Derogatis, Lipman, and Covi, 1973). It was one of the first such scales developed with a medical population in mind. Each item is rated on a five-point scale of distress (0 to 4) from "not at all" to "extremely." The inventory is scored on nine primary symptom dimensions plus three global indices of pathology. The nine primary dimensions are as follows:

Somatization, which measures subjective distress arising from the perception of bodily dysfunctions.
Obsessive-compulsive, which is analogous to the clinical syndrome.

Interpersonal sensitivity, which gauges hypersensitivity to perceived self-deficiencies and strong feelings of inferiority compared to others.

Depression, which reflects a broad range of concomitants of the clinical depressive syndrome.

Anxiety, which is viewed as a pervasive negative affective state present to some degree in almost all clinical syndromes and the predominant clinical feature in some.

Hostility, which gauges thoughts, feelings, or behaviors that may be characterized as manifestations of anger, resentment, hostility, or aggression.

Phobic anxiety, defined as a persistent fear response to a specific individual, place, object, or situation that is characterized as being irrational and disproportionate.

Paranoid ideation, which is a disordered mode of thinking characterized by factors such as suspiciousness, projective thought, concerns over loss of autonomy, and persecutory themes.

Alienation, which measures mild idiosyncratic thought and interpersonal distancing at one extreme and full-blown symptoms of psychosis at the other.

The three global indices of pathology are as follows:

Global severity index, which combines information on the number of symptoms and intensity of distress.

Positive symptom distress index, which measures intensity of distress only.

Positive symptom total, which communicates data on the number of symptoms only.

Derogatis, Rickels, and Rock (1976) have demonstrated a high degree of convergence between the nine primary symptom dimensions and the scales on MMPI considered to measure a corresponding symptom construct. Thus the SCL-90 may prove to be a useful clinical inventory that can provide an alternative to much more time-consuming inventories such as the MMPI. Moreover, as it was developed for use with outpatients, not just psychiatric patients, it may be useful in a variety of research situations as well as diagnostic ones.

THE MILLON BEHAVIORAL HEALTH INVENTORY

The Millon Behavioral Health Inventory (MBHI) was developed in response to the need for a psychological assessment device specifically for use with individuals undergoing evaluation or treatment in medical settings for physical disorders. It is a more carefully standardized and psychometrically sound inventory than the SCL-90. Its major intent is to provide information to clinical personnel (e.g., physicians, psychologists, nurses) who are required to make behavioral assessments and treatment decisions about individuals with physical problems. Information is provided concerning factors such as the patient's style of relating to health care personnel and major psychosocial stressors as well as probable response to illness and treatment interventions. As we noted at the beginning of this chapter, traditional assessment methods designed for psychiatric populations (such as the MMPI) may not be totally valid for a medical population because the statistical norms and clinical signs may differ significantly. The MBHI was developed and standardized on an actual medical population.

The MBHI, a 150-item self-report inventory, is the first comprehensive psychodiagnostic instrument developed specifically for the physically ill. It provides twenty clinical scales that measure dimensions found to be relevant for psychosocial assessment and decision making with medical populations. These twenty scales are organized into four broad areas including personality and coping styles based on Millon's (1969) theory of personality and health behavior, psychogenic attitudes related to stress, psychosomatic correlates such as allergic tendencies, and prognostic indices that predict complications or difficulties associated with illness.

An attractive feature of the MBHI is the availability of an automated computer interpretation system. Clinical profile interpretations can be provided through an actuarial-based computer-generated narrative. In the close-up at the end of this chapter, a sample profile and portions of the accompanying computer-generated narrative report are presented to give the reader the flavor of the automated interpretation system.

The MBHI should prove to be of value in medical settings, though we do not know as much about this instrument as we do about others. One of the reasons why the test has not been used as widely as it could is the fact that scoring keys for the test are not available, and scoring must be contracted for through National Computer Services, Inc. The cost involved in this has limited the use of the MBHI and has impeded the development of a larger data base. In addition, a critical review of its test construction procedures (Mitchell, 1985) may have also stimulated some caution regarding its use.

Nevertheless, some recent research has demonstrated the utility of the MBHI with certain medical problems. For example, Gatchel, Deckel, Weinberg, and Smith (1985) evaluated the use of the MBHI in predicting the response of chronic headache sufferers to a behavioral treatment program. Results demonstrated that a number of scales significantly predicted response to treatment, as measured by daily number of headaches, duration, intensity, and medication use. The Emotional Vulnerability scale was found to be the most general predictor of treatment outcome. High scorers for this scale (who are generally poor responders to treatment programs) demonstrated the least amount of improvement in the headache measures.

In another study Gatchel et al. (1986) evaluated the use of the MBHI in predicting improvement in physical functioning of chronic low back pain patients undergoing a comprehensive multidisciplinary treatment program. Results revealed that various MBHI scales, especially the Emotional Vulnerability scale, were predictive of improvement in the overall physical functioning of these patients.

LIFE CHANGE ASSESSMENT

In Chapter 3 we discussed research demonstrating a relationship between life stress (defined in terms of self-reported life changes) and physical illness. The instrument most widely used in life stress research has been the Schedule of Recent Experiences

(SRE), developed by Holmes and Rahe (1967). The SRE is a self-administered questionnaire containing a list of forty-three events to which subjects respond by checking those events that they have experienced during the recent past (previous six months or one year). Unfortunately there is a major problem associated with this instrument. The SRE was based on the assumption that life changes per se are stressful, regardless of the desirability of the events experienced. In this inventory both desirable and undesirable events are combined in determination of the overall life stress score. However, research has suggested that undesirable events (e.g., the death of a close family member) may have a significantly different, and perhaps a more detrimental, impact on individuals than desirable and positive events (e.g., outstanding personal achievement) (see Sarason, Johnson, and Siegel, 1978).

A related problem with the SRE involves the quantification of life changes. Individuals differ greatly in how they are affected by events. Therefore, the values derived from group ratings (which are used with SRE) may not necessarily reflect the impact that events have on particular individuals.

In response to these problems, Sarason et al. (1978) developed a new measure of life stress called the Life Experiences Survey (LES). It is a fifty-seven-item self-report measure that allows the respondent to indicate events that he or she experienced during the past year. There are two portions of the scale. Section 1, designed for all respondents, contains a list of forty-seven specific events plus three blank spaces in which respondents can indicate other events that they have experienced. The events listed in this section correspond to life changes that are common to people in a wide range of situations. Section 2 consists of ten events designed primarily for use with students, but they can be adapted for other populations. The events deal specifically with changes experienced in the academic environment.

Sarason and colleagues have shown that negative life change scores are significantly related to a number of stress-related dependent measures such as personal maladjustment, depression, and anxiety. These results suggest that the LES may be a useful research and clinical tool. A more detailed evaluation of its usefulness awaits further research.

STRUCTURED INTERVIEW

As we saw in Chapter 5, the Type A behavior pattern has been recognized as an independent risk factor for coronary heart disease. Much of the original work conducted in this area employed the Structured Interview (SI) procedure developed by Friedman and Rosenman (1974). The SI was conceived and developed to elicit characteristics of the Type A syndrome. In its most recent form (see Rosenman, 1978a), it takes about ten minutes to administer. The box presents the SI.

The effective administration and assessment of the SI requires a period of supervised training. This is because assessment involves not only the evaluation of the specific content of answers, but also the general stylistics and mannerisms of the individual as he or she answers the questions. The way something is said in the interview may be more important than what is actually said. Obviously there is a certain amount of subjective evaluation involved in the SI; because it is not totally

BEHAVIOR PATTERN INTERVIEW

Introduction: "I would appreciate it if you would answer the following questions to the best of your ability. Your answers will be kept in the strictest confidence. Most of the questions are concerned with your superficial habits, and none of them will embarrass you."

1. May I ask your age *please?*

2. What is your occupation or job?
    a. How long have you been in this type of work?

3. Are you *satisfied* with your job level? (Why not?)

4. Does your job carry *heavy* responsibility?
    a. Is there any time when you feel particularly *rushed* or under *pressure?*
    b. When you are under *pressure* does it bother you?

5. Would you describe yourself as a *hard-driving, ambitious* type of *man (woman)* in accomplishing the things you want, getting things done as *quickly* as possible, *or* would you describe yourself as a relatively *relaxed* and *easygoing* person?
    a. Are you married?
    b. How would your *wife (husband)* describe you—as *hard-driving* and *ambitious* or as relaxed and easygoing?
    c. Has she ever asked you to slow down in your work? *Never?* How would she put it—in *her (his) own* words?

6. When you get *angry* or *upset,* do people around you know about it? How do you show it?

7. Do you think you drive *harder* to *accomplish* things than most of your associates?

8. Do you take work home with you? How often?

9. Do you have any children? When they were around the ages of six and eight, did you *ever* play competitive games with them, like cards, checkers, Monopoly?
    a. Did you *always* allow them to *win* on *purpose?*
    b. *Why* (or *why not*)?

10. When you play games with people your own age, do you play for the fun of it, or are you really in there to *win?*

11. Is there any *competition* in your job? Do you enjoy this?
    a. Are you competitive off the job, sports for example?

12. When you are in your automobile, and there is a car in your lane going *far too slowly* for you, what do you do about it? Would you *mutter* and *complain* to yourself? Would anyone riding with you know that you were *annoyed?*

13. Most people who work have to get up fairly early in the morning—in your particular case, uh-what-time-uh-do-you-uh, ordinarily uh-have-uh-to-uh-uh-get-up?

14. If you make a *date* with someone for, oh, two o'clock in the afternoon, for example, would you *be there* on *time?*
    a. If you are kept waiting, do you *resent* it?
    b. Would you *say* anything about it?

15. If you see someone doing a job rather *slowly* and you *know* that you could do it faster and better yourself, does it make you *restless* to watch him?
    a. Would you be tempted to *step in and do it* yourself?

16. What *irritates* you most about your work or the people with whom you work?

17. Do you *eat rapidly?* Do you *walk* rapidly? After you've *finished* eating, do you like to sit around the table and chat, or do you like to *get up and get going?*

18. When you go out in the evening to a restaurant and you find eight or ten people *waiting ahead of you* for a table, will you wait? What will you do while you are waiting?

19. How do you feel about waiting in lines: *Bank* lines, or *supermarket* lines? *Post office* lines?

20. Do you *always* feel anxious to *get going* and *finish* whatever you have to do?

21. Do you have the feeling that *time* is passing too *rapidly* for you to *accomplish* all the things you'd like to *get done* in one day?
    a. Do you *often* feel a sense of *time urgency? Time pressure?*

22. Do you *hurry* in doing most things?

All right that completes the interview. Thank you very much.

From R. H. Rosenman. The interview method of assessment of the coronary-prone behavior pattern. In T. M. Dembroski et al. (Eds.), *Coronary-Prone Behavior.* New York: Springer, 1978, pp. 68–69.

objective, the SI cannot yield a truly numerical quantification. In spite of the subjectivity problem, however, it has produced a high degree of interrater agreement in the categorization of Type A and B behavior (from 75 to 90 percent in various studies reviewed by Rosenman, 1978).

Using the SI, one can classify people as Type A-1 or A-2, Type B or Type X (Rosenman, 1978a). Type A-1 characteristics include general expressions of vigor, energy, alertness, and confidence, and loud, rapid, tense, or clipped speech. This category also is indicated by acceleration of speech at the end of long sentences, frequent interrupting, explosive speech, hostility, impatience, and use of abrupt one-word responses such as "Never!" or "Absolutely!" Type A-2 people are not as extreme as A-1's. Thus a Type A-2 might be in a hurry but not extremely impatient, occasionally use explosive speech, interrupt, or accelerate his or her speech, or otherwise show less hostile or aggressive characteristics of Type A-1. Type B subjects show little or no evidence of any of these characteristics: they are relaxed, do not interrupt, give long responses, speak in quieter voices, and do not exhibit hostile responding.

A Type X person is one who exhibits in almost equal proportions characteristics attributed to Type A and Type B patterns. The Type X pattern occurs in only about 10 percent of the population.

QUESTIONNAIRE ASSESSMENT OF TYPE A BEHAVIOR

Because of the subjectivity involved in the SI assessment, a number of paper-and-pencil scales were developed in an attempt to provide a more objective and efficient means for assessing Type A behavior. As we pointed out in Chapter 5, the most notable of these has been the Jenkins Activity Survey (JAS) (Jenkins, Rosenman, and Friedman, 1967). The JAS includes many of the questions used in the SI. It was hoped that it would provide an objective and quantifiable continuous scale of Type A-B behavior, based on a weighted combination of responses to the various questions. Unfortunately, as was noted in Chapter 5, the JAS correlates only moderately with the SI ratings (from 50 to 75 percent) and even less well with actual incidence of coronary heart disease (Rosenman, 1978a). The basic weakness of scales such as this has been attributed to the fact that they assess only self-report, which can be significantly affected by self-appraisal and response-set effects, whereas the SI takes into account both the subject's verbal and nonverbal behaviors.

NEUROPSYCHOLOGICAL ASSESSMENT

As we mentioned at the beginning of this text, behavioral medicine or medical psychology is a relatively young discipline. However, the collaboration between psychology and one medical specialty—neurology—has a much longer history. Beginning as a part of clinical psychology and then taking on an identity of its own, neuropsychology extends at least as far back as World War I. It represents the first major category of psychological practice addressed to nonpsychiatric medical patients. It can be viewed as the principal forerunner of modern behavioral medicine/medical psychology.

Neuropsychological assessment involves the search for behavioral manifestations or patterns of performance aberrations that are associated with specific brain disorders. It is an important assessment method because many of the currently used medical-neurological tests—the angiogram X-ray technique to detect a brain tumor, the measurement of the electrical activity of the brain, the examination of the retina to detect blood vessel damage, and the evaluation of perception and motor coordination—can assess gross brain damage but usually cannot detect more subtle dysfunctions. Neuropsychological test results may provide clues about the nature of such subtle disturbances (Lezak, 1976).

The neuropsychological evaluation can serve several purposes:

1. It can aid the physician in arriving at the diagnosis of presence/absence of organic brain dysfunction.

2. It can help to confirm or support a tentative diagnostic decision based on other assessment methods.

3. It can provide more definitive evidence of the behavioral/cognitive effects associated with a brain dysfunction condition.

4. It can serve as a baseline measure of a patient's abilities, against which to compare later performance changes produced by surgery, medication, rehabilitation efforts, or just time.

5. In providing a thorough assessment of the patient's condition, it can yield some valuable information about the prognosis for improvement.

Halstead (1947) developed the first comprehensive neuropsychological test battery for the assessment of brain damage. It was subsequently revised by Reitan (1955), and further modified by Matthews and Klove at the University of Wisconsin. Reitan (1964) has empirically demonstrated that the neuropsychological test battery can reliably identify the etiology and location of certain brain lesions with a high degree of accuracy. The norms used in such identification were developed by comparing test performance patterns of patients with known organic disorders in specific parts of the brain to those of normal individuals with no known brain disorder.

The **Halstead-Reitan Battery (HRB)** consists of eight tests that yield ten scores. For each of these, an empirically derived cutoff is employed to give a dichotomous classification of impaired-neurologic or unimpaired-normal. The **impairment index** derived is simply the number of scores in the impaired range. The following tests make up the HRB:

Category Test, which measures abstracting ability. It is a nonverbal concept attainment test that requires the subject to abstract a general principle from a series of geometric stimuli. For example, figures varying in size, shape, color, and location, grouped by abstract principles, are projected on a screen. The subject's task is to figure out the principle involved. The principle might be that green is correct.

Tactual Performance Test, which measures tactile perception. Subjects are required to do the Sequin Form Board blindfolded, first using the preferred hand, then the nonpreferred, then both. The scorers measure time to completion. The subject is then asked to draw the board from memory, placing drawings of the block forms and locations where he or she remembers them to be.

Trail Making Test, which measures visual attention and visual-motor tracking coordination. In this test the subject is requested to connect circles in correct numeric or alphanumeric sequence.

Finger Tapping Test, which measures manual dexterity. Rapid finger movement in a counter device is measured for both hands.

Speech Perception Test, which measures auditory perception. The subject listens to a series of tape-recorded nonsense words such as "theeks" or "theez." On an answer sheet, he or she must select the correct word from among several alternatives.

Rhythm Test, which also measures auditory perception. This test, taken from the Seashore Scales of Musical Talents, requires the subject to make same-different judgments of rhythmic patterns.

Aphasia Screening Test, which tests for aphasia (the loss of the ability to read, write, or understand). This test, which assesses relatively gross sorts of aphasic symptoms, requires the subject to draw geometric figures. It is scored as normal, impaired in language, impaired in drawing, or impaired in both language and drawing.

Sensory Examination, which tests for touch, visual, and auditory functions derived from the classical neurologic examination.

In addition to these tests, the Wechsler-Bellevue Intelligence Scale I or the Wechsler Adult Intelligence Scale (WAIS), which measures a variety of cognitive-verbal and motor-performance tasks, and the MMPI are frequently administered in order to provide an even more comprehensive understanding of the cognitive-psychological functioning of the individual.

It should be noted that actuarial or cookbook interpretation methods, similar to those discussed earlier for the MMPI, are being developed for neuropsychological test interpretation (see Reitan and Davison, 1974). They provide clinicians with standards against with which to match their cases and make the interpretation of test-battery results much more objective.

Finally, if there is a problem with neuropsychological techniques, it is that these tests are still undergoing research validation. Moreover, there is not yet a full understanding of normal brain organization and functioning. Neuropsychological test interpretation methods will need to be revised continually as more information is accrued about brain functioning.

SUMMARY

In this chapter we have discussed the traditional forms of psychiatric classification and assessment methods and the more recent diagnostic tests developed with a medical population in mind. Early attempts to develop an effective psychiatric classification system stimulated simultaneous efforts to construct effective and reliable techniques for the assessment of psychological disorders. Although the techniques developed have been quite diverse, they can be classified into two major categories: projective techniques, such as the TAT and Rorschach Inkblot Test, and nonprojective techniques, such as MMPI. None of these tests, however, was developed with a medical population in mind. In recent years a number of assessment procedures have been developed specifically for a medical population. We reviewed the most widely known and utilized of these methods—the SCL-90, the Millon Behavioral Health Inventory, the Schedule of Recent Experiences, the Life Experiences Survey, the Structured Interview, and the Jenkins Activity Survey. Finally, we also discussed the oldest form of psychological assessment in medical settings—neuropsychological assessment.

RECOMMENDED READINGS

American Psychiatric Association. *Diagnostic and statistical manual of mental disorders, IIIR.* Washington, D.C.: American Psychiatric Association, 1987.

Derogatis, L. R., Rickels, K., and Rock, A. F. The SCL-90 and the MMPI: A step in the validation of a new self-report scale. *British Journal of Psychiatry,* 1976, *128,* 280–289.

Kleinmuntz, B. *Personality and psychological assessment.* New York: St. Martin's Press, 1982.

Lezak, M. D. *Neuropsychological assessment.* New York: Oxford University Press, 1982.

Rosenman, R. H. The interview method of assessment of the coronary-prone behavior pattern. In T. M. Dembroski et al. (Eds.), *Coronary-prone behavior.* New York: Springer-Verlag, 1978.

Sarason, I. G., Johnson, J. H., and Siegel, J. M. Assessing the impact of life changes: Development of the Life Experiences Survey. *Journal of Consulting and Clinical Psychology,* 1978, *46,* 932–946.

10

COGNITIVE–BEHAVIORAL TREATMENT TECHNIQUES IN MEDICAL SETTINGS

||||||||||||||||||||||||||||||||||||||||||||||||||||||||||||||||||||||||||||||||||||||||||||||||||||||||||||||||||||||||||||||

In this chapter we shall discuss a variety of cognitive-behavioral treatment procedures that have been effectively employed with problem behaviors often seen in medical settings. We will not consider traditional psychotherapy methods, since they have not been in the mainstream of the relatively new and growing field of behavioral medicine. The various cognitive-behavior therapy techniques we will review have been found to effectively treat a wide range of maladaptive behaviors that have been resistant to other types of traditional treatment. Such findings highlight the clinical potency of such methods as well as the learning principles upon which they are based.

MAJOR LEARNING PRINCIPLES

CLASSICAL CONDITIONING

Ivan Pavlov (1849–1936), the eminent Russian physiologist, first described the process of classical conditioning with his work on the conditioned reflex. Reflexes are specific, automatic, and unlearned reactions elicited by a specific stimulus. If you ever touched a surface you did not know was hot, such as a hot stove, you demonstrated a reflexive behavior—immediate withdrawal of your hand from the stove. Similarly, if a piece of dust suddenly enters your eye, your eye will automatically blink and begin to secrete tears. Such **unconditioned reflexes** are automatic and have a great deal of survival value for the organism. Pavlov demonstrated that such unconditioned reflexes could be **conditioned,** or learned. Pavlov, while studying dogs in order to more fully understand the digestive process, began to notice that many of the dogs secreted saliva even before food was delivered to them. He observed that this phenomenon occurred whenever the dogs either heard the approaching footsteps of the laboratory assistant who fed them or had a preliminary glimpse of the food. In order to more systematically investigate this phenomenon, Pavlov developed a procedure for producing a conditioned reflex. This procedure came to be called **classical conditioning.** It is one of the most basic forms of learning.

Pavlov conducted a series of well-known studies on the process of classical conditioning using dogs as experimental subjects. In these studies Pavlov demonstrated that if a neutral stimulus or event such as a bell was presented to a dog just prior to the presentation of food (an unconditioned stimulus that normally elicits an automatic unconditioned reflex of salivation), after a number of such presentations the bell (now a conditioned stimulus) would elicit a conditioned or learned salivation response when presented by itself in the absence of food. The conditioned reflex of salivation would occur to the bell alone. This represents the process of classical conditioning, and is based on the learned association or connection between two stimuli, such as the bell and food, that have occurred together at approximately the same point in time. An association is learned between a weak stimulus (such as the bell) and a strong stimulus (such as the sight of food) so that the weak stimulus comes to elicit the same response originally controlled only by the stronger one (i.e., salivation). Pavlov called this tendency to respond to the neutral conditioned stimulus (CS) as though it were the unconditioned stimulus (UCS) **stimulus substitution.** Such conditioned reflexes are automatic responses to an eliciting stimulus or event. Such behavior is termed **respondent** because it responds to some event in the environment. Classical conditioning is often referred to as **respondent conditioning.** In contrast to respondent behavior, the term **operant behavior** is used when the organism responds voluntarily and operates on the environment to produce some effect (we will discuss this in the next section).

There have been a number of behavioral treatment techniques developed on the basis of classical conditioning principles. One of the most widely used of these—systematic desensitization and its variants—will be discussed later in this chapter.

OPERANT CONDITIONING

Operant or instrumental conditioning is an approach that was originally formulated by the American psychologist Edward Thorndike, and then more comprehensively developed by B. F. Skinner in the United States and Jerzy Konorski and Stefan Miller in Poland. Unlike classical conditioning, **operant conditioning** develops new behaviors that bring about positive consequences or remove negative events. In classical conditioning a new stimulus (such as a bell) is conditioned to elicit the same responses that had previously occurred to the unconditioned stimulus, whereas in operant conditioning a new response is learned. Behavior that produces food, social approval, or other positive consequences, or that reduces damaging or aversive events, illustrates operant behavior. The behavior "operates" on the environment to bring about changes in it.

Animal training, such as that involved in the learned performance of circus animals, involves basic principles of operant conditioning. Although operant training has existed for centuries, Skinner, Konorski, and Miller were the first to carefully delineate the methods and procedures of operant conditioning under which such training could be accomplished most efficiently. The key stimulus is reinforcement. **Reinforcement** refers to any consequence that increases the likelihood that a particular behavior will be repeated, or that strengthens that behavior. **Extinction** involves the gradual decrease in the strength or tendency to perform a response due to elimination of reinforcement.

An important procedure used in operant conditioning is shaping. In work on operant conditioning, the bar-pressing response of rats has been one of the most frequently studied processes. It is an easy response for rats to perform, it is a well-defined act, and it is easy to record automatically; thus it is a reliable measure. However, when put in a new situation rats will not spontaneously find the correct sequence of behavior (approach the bar, rise up on hind legs, place front paws on the bar down toward the floor). Instead of waiting for the rat to accidentally stumble on the correct sequence, the experimenter will employ a method called shaping, which is based on the process of successive approximations. This training method was formally developed by Skinner. In the **shaping** procedure the animal is reinforced for demonstrating closer and closer approximations to the desired response (the reinforcement used is usually food or water, with the rats being food- or water-deprived in order to increase their motivation to work for the reinforcement). The process of successive approximations works as follows. The first response that shows that the rat is on the right track (e.g., approaching the bar) is reinforced. After a number of such reinforcements, the rat will begin interrupting its behavior in order to approach the bar. The reinforcement is now withheld until the rat not only approaches the bar but also rises off the floor somewhat in front of the bar. Initially the rat may be reinforced for merely lifting one paw off the floor. Gradually, however, the experimenter reinforces the rat only if both paws are lifted high enough to reach the bar. Finally the experimenter will not reward the rat until the bar is actually pressed. This concludes the **successive approximations shaping procedure.** At this point the experimenter can introduce different **reinforcement schedules** in order to produce different patterns of responding. Also, a **discriminative stimulus** can be introduced, so that the rat receives reinforcement for pressing the bar only when a certain light is on in the cage. The animal will soon learn not to respond when the light is off. In this manner the rat's bar-pressing behavior comes under **stimulus** (e.g., light) **control.**

This same shaping procedure is used in training circus and other performing animals to perform complicated acts. For example, dolphins can be shaped to leap out of the water, and lions can be taught to jump through flaming hoops. These techniques are used in virtually every zoo and marine animal show. Such shaping procedures are so powerful that Skinner and two of his early associates—Fred Keller and Marian Breland—worked on a project during World War II called "Project Pigeon," with the goal of training pigeons to guide a bomb toward a predetermined target. They were well on their way to completing the training of these "pigeon soldiers" when the development of the atomic bomb ended the war, thus removing the urgent need for this research.

Numerous behavioral treatment programs employing operant conditioning principles have been developed. A number of these—biofeedback, contingency management, and stimulus control procedures—will be discussed later in this chapter.

OBSERVATIONAL LEARNING

There have been many examples of various complex forms of behavior being learned without any apparent direct form of external reinforcement. Indeed, there has been a great deal of recent research indicating that learning can occur through simple observation without the presence of any form of tangible direct reinforcement. Such learning, besides being called observational learning, is sometimes called imitation learning, cognitive learning, vicarious learning, or modeling. **Observational learning** is defined simply as that learning which occurs without any apparent direct reinforcement (Bandura, 1969). Many behaviors can be acquired if an individual sees the particular behavior performed or modeled by another person.

Examples of behavior acquired by observational learning abound. Aggressive responses, fear of particular objects or situations, and other complex adaptive and unadaptive behaviors can be developed through modeling (see Bandura, 1969; Kazdin, 1974). Also, observation learning may be used to increase desired behaviors or lessen undesired behaviors through presentation of a model that performs the appropriate responses. One of the earliest laboratory studies on observational learning, (Bandura et al., 1963), involved nursery school children. One group of children observed an adult model perform a series of aggressive acts, both verbal and physical, toward a large toy Bobo doll. Another group watched a nonaggressive adult, who simply sat quietly and paid no attention to the doll. A third group of children was not exposed to a model. Later, after being mildly frustrated, all children were placed in a room alone with the Bobo doll and their behavior was observed. It was found that the behavior of the two model groups tended to be similar to that of their adult model. That is, children who had viewed the aggressive adult performed more aggressive acts toward the doll in the free-play situation than the other groups and also made more responses that were exact imitations of the model's aggressive behavior. Those children who had observed a nonaggressive adult model performed significantly fewer aggressive responses than the aggressive-model group.

These results, as well as similar findings from many other experiments (Bandura, 1969), clearly demonstrate that learning can occur without an individual's ever having made a particular response himself or herself, or ever having received any type of tangible external reinforcement for the behavior. The fact that an individual can perform such novel behavior points out the importance of a person's internalization and cognitive abilities, which allow him or her to transform what has been observed into a number of new patterns of behavior. This highlights the importance of cognitive factors and explains why such variables are considered in currently developing learning approaches. We will discuss a number of recently developed cognitive-behavior therapy techniques later in this chapter.

BEHAVIOR THERAPY APPROACHES

SYSTEMATIC DESENSITIZATION

Systematic desensitization is a technique developed by Joseph Wolpe (1958) as a means of alleviating anxiety. He based his procedure on the principle of **counterconditioning,** in which an attempt is made to substitute relaxation (an adaptive behavior) through learning for anxiety (the deviant or maladaptive behavior) in response to a particular object or situation. The procedure typically involves the pairing of deep muscle relaxation, which is taught by a progressive muscle relaxation technique developed by Jacobson in 1938, with imagined scenes depicting situations or objects associated with anxiety. Wolpe had his patients imagine the anxiety-related objects or situations, because many of the fears treated were abstract in nature (e.g., fear of rejection by a loved one) and therefore could not easily be presented *in vivo* (in real life). However, even when the objects or situations can be presented in real life (e.g., fear of a specific object such as a bug), *in vitro* systematic desensitization is often employed.

In this treatment procedure a graded hierarchy of scenes is constructed, consisting of items ranging from low-anxiety to high-anxiety provoking situations. The individual gradually "works up" this hierarchy, learning to tolerate more and more difficult scenes as he or she relaxes. The relaxation response tends to inhibit anxiety from occurring with the imagined scenes. It is found that this ability to tolerate anxiety-related imagery of objects or situations produces a significant decrease of anxiety in the related real-life situations. The therapeutic procedure has been demonstrated to be effective with a great many anxiety-related disorders such as phobias (including fear of medical and dental procedures), insomnia, and stress-related psychophysiological disorders such as ulcers, asthma, and hypertension (see Rimm and Masters, 1974).

As an example of the effective use of systematic desensitization, let us briefly review a study reported by one of the authors (Gatchel, 1980). This study evaluated the efficacy of group-administered systematic desensitization in the treatment of individuals with an extreme degree of fear of dental procedures. An interesting aspect of this study was the fact that dentists from the community were trained to administer the treatment. Indeed, an attractive feature of a procedure such as systematic desensitization is the fact that it is standard and easily administered so that individuals can be trained to effectively administer it. The standard and objective characteristics of the procedure are further evidenced by the fact that computer-administered systematic desensitization has been successfully employed in the treatment of severely phobic individuals (Lang, Melamed, and Hart, 1970).

In a treatment investigation by Gatchel (1980), dental-phobic individuals were administered six therapy sessions. (Another attractive feature of this treatment is its time and cost efficiency and the fact that it can often be administered on a group basis.) The following anxiety hierarchy was employed with these subjects:

1. Thinking about going to the dentist.

2. Calling for an appointment with the dentist.

3. Getting in the car to go to the dentist's office.

4. Sitting in the waiting room of the dentist's office.

5. Having the nurse tell you it's your turn.

6. Getting in the dentist's chair.

7. Seeing the dentist lay out the instruments, one of which is a probe.

8. Seeing the dentist lay out the instruments, one of which is pliers used to pull teeth.

9. Having a probe held in front of you while you look at it.

10. Having a probe placed on the side of a tooth.

11. Having a probe placed in a cavity.

12. Getting an injection in your gums on one side.

13. Having your teeth drilled and worrying if the anesthetic will wear off.

14. Getting two injections, one on each side.

15. Hearing the crunching sounds as your tooth is being pulled.

It was found in this study that, compared to individuals who received no treatment, persons who were administered systematic desensitization demonstrated a significant reduction in dental anxiety and evidenced an almost 100 percent improvement in dental visitation/appointment-making behavior. The fact that all these individuals were originally extremely dental-avoidant testifies to the therapeutic efficacy of the desensitization procedure. This procedure has also been found effective in the treatment of a variety of medical phobias such as injection phobia and hemodialysis phobia.

PROGRESSIVE MUSCLE RELAXATION

Progressive muscle relaxation, which is an important component of the systematic desensitization treatment process, often can serve as a powerful therapeutic technique in its own right. Clinicians often use it by itself to treat a wide variety of disorders including generalized anxiety, insomnia, headaches, neck tension, and mild forms of agitated depression. Its use is based on the premise that muscle tension is closely related to anxiety and that an individual will feel a significant reduction in experienced anxiety if tense muscles can be made to relax. Other techniques, such as autogenic training (Schultz and Luthe, 1959), biofeedback (which we will discuss later in this chapter), transcendental meditation, and yoga, are also commonly used to reduce physiological activation, which is assumed to be closely tied to anxiety.

The teaching of progressive muscle relaxation skills generally follows a fairly

ABBREVIATED PROGRESSIVE MUSCLE RELAXATION TRAINING

The following are general guidelines for an abbreviated muscle relaxation training procedure:

1. Instruct the subject to "make a fist with your dominant hand [usually right]. Make a fist and tense the muscles of your [right] hand and forearm; tense until it trembles. Feel the muscles pull across your fingers and the lower part of your forearm." Have the subject hold this position for five to seven seconds; then say "relax," instructing him/her to just let his/her hand go: "Pay attention to the muscles of your [right] hand and forearm as they relax. Note how those muscles feel as relaxation flows through them" (10–20 seconds).

   "Again, tense the muscles of your [right] hand and forearm. Pay attention to the muscles involved" (5–7 seconds). "Okay, relax; attend only to those muscles, and note how they feel as the relaxation takes place, becoming more and more relaxed, more relaxed than ever before. Each time we do this you'll relax even more until your arm and hand are completely relaxed with no tension at all, warm and relaxed."

   Continue until subject reports his/her (right) hand and forearm are completely relaxed with no tension (usually 2–4 times is sufficient).

2. Instruct the subject to tense his/her (right) biceps, leaving his/her hand and forearm on the chair. Proceed in the same manner as above, in a "hypnotic monotone," using the (right) hand as a reference point (that is, move on when the subject reports his/her biceps feels as completely relaxed as his/her hand and forearm).

   Proceed to other gross-muscle groups (listed below) in the same manner, with the same verbalization. For example: "Note how these muscles feel as they relax; feel the relaxation and warmth flow through these muscles; pay attention to these muscles so that later you can relax them again." Always use the preceding group as a reference for moving on.

3. Nondominant (left) hand and forearm—feel muscles over knuckles and on lower part of arm.

4. Nondominant (left) biceps.

5. Frown hard, tensing muscles of forehead and top of head (these muscles often "tingle" as they relax).

6. Wrinkle nose, feeling muscles across top of cheeks and upper lip.

7. Draw corners of mouth back, feeling jaw muscles and cheeks.

8. Tighten chin and throat muscles, feeling two muscles in front of throat.

9. Tighten chest muscles and muscles across back—feel muscles pull below shoulder blades.

10. Tighten abdominal muscles—make abdomen hard.

11. Tighten muscles of right upper leg—feel one muscle on top and two on the bottom of the upper leg.

12. Tighten right calf—feel muscles on bottom of right calf.

13. Push down with toes and arch right foot—feel pressure as if something were pushing up under the arch.

14. Tighten left upper leg.

15. Tighten left calf.

16. Tighten left foot.

For most muscle groups two presentations will suffice. Ask the subject if he/she feels any tension anywhere in his/her body. If he/she does, go back and repeat the tension-release cycle for that muscle group. It is often helpful to instruct the subject to take a deep breath and hold it while tensing muscles, and to let it go while releasing. Should any muscle group not respond after four trials, move on and return to it later.

Caution: Some subjects may develop muscle cramps or spasms from prolonged tension of muscles. If this occurs, shorten the tension interval a few seconds, and instruct the subject not to tense muscles quite so hard.

Although the word hypnosis is not to be used, progressive relaxation, properly executed, does seem to create a state resembling a light hypnotic-trance state, with the subject more susceptible to suggestion. Relaxation may be further deepened by repetition of suggestions of warmth, relaxation, etc. Some subjects may actually report sensations of disassociation from their bodies. This is complete relaxation and is to be expected. Subjects should be instructed to speak as little as possible while under relaxation.

In bringing subjects back to "normal," use the numerical method of trance termination: "I'm going to count from one to four. On the count of one, start moving your legs; two, your fingers and hands; three, your head; and four, open your eyes and sit up. One—move your legs; two—now your fingers and hands; three—move your head around; four—open your eyes and sit up." Always check to see that the subject feels well, alert, etc., before leaving.

The subject should be instructed to practice relaxation twice a day between sessions. He/she should not work at it more than fifteen minutes at a time, and should not practice twice within any three-hour period. He/she should practice alone. Relaxation may be used for getting to sleep if practiced while the subject is horizontal; if the subject does not wish to sleep, he/she should practice sitting up. Properly timed, relaxation can be used for a "second wind" during study.

By the third session, if the subject has been practicing well, relaxation may be induced merely by focusing attention on the muscle groups and instructing the subject to "concentrate on muscles becoming relaxed, warm," etc. However, if the subject has difficulty following straight suggestions, return to the use of tension release.

standardized procedure, in which individuals practice muscle relaxation directly by first discriminating tension and stress in various muscle groups and then relaxing these groups. For example, an individual would be requested to wrinkle his or her forehead and notice the pattern and feeling of strain in these muscles. After maintaining the tension for about ten seconds, the subject would be told to let the forehead muscles completely relax and to notice the difference in sensation at those places where tension and strain were previously felt. After a few minutes of relaxation, the sequence is repeated again. The main goal of the training program is to teach individuals what relaxation of each muscle group feels like and to provide practice in achieving more relaxation. Once the individual is able to discriminate the patterns of tension in a particular muscle group, he or she is no longer told to tense before relaxing. Instead, he or she must relax the muscles from their present level of tension.

The relaxation procedure originally developed by Jacobson required training over many months, with hundreds of muscle sites trained. In normal clinical practice, however, a much more abbreviated form of training is usually employed. The following muscle groups are routinely attended to: right and left hand; forearm and wrist of both hands; biceps of both arms; shoulders; neck; forehead and eyes; mouth, cheeks, and jaw; chest and back; stomach; thighs; calves; and feet.

MODELING

Bandura and colleagues have shown that fear can also be reduced by having fearful individuals repeatedly observe models effectively engaging in the feared activities (see Bandura, 1971). It is based on the principle that the repeated observation that the feared performance does not lead to unfavorable or negative consequences will lead to the extinction or elimination of both anxiety responses and fear-arousing thoughts. This modeling procedure is often called **vicarious extinction.**

Bandura has found that even when one is using models, it is usually beneficial to employ a graduated hierarchy: models perform a sequence of activities beginning with those that are least feared and progressing to those that are most feared. For example, in one modeling study conducted by Bandura, Grusec, and Menlove (1967), fear of dogs was treated by having fearful children observe another child interact with a dog in a graduated sequence. The fear-producing quality of the interactions was gradually increased by controlling the physical restraints on the dog as well as the duration and degree of physical contact of the interactions. Subsequent studies have found that this modeling procedure is effective even when filmed models, and not live models, are used (Bandura, 1971).

Modeling procedures have been effectively employed to reduce hospital- and surgery-related anxieties in children. Melamed and Siegel (1975) showed one of two films to children (aged four to twelve) about to undergo surgery for hernias, tonsillectomies, or urinary-genital tract problems. One group of children was shown a film entitled *Ethan Has an Operation.* The film depicted a seven-year-old child who was hospitalized for a hernia operation:

The film, which is 16 minutes in length, consists of 15 scenes showing various events that most children encounter when hospitalized for elective surgery from the time of admission to time of discharge including the child's orientation to the hospital ward and medical personnel such as the surgeon and anesthesiologist; having a blood test and exposure to standard hospital equipment; separation from the mother; and scenes in the operative and recovery rooms. In addition to explanations of the hospital procedures provided by the medical staff, various scenes are narrated by the child, who describes his feelings and concerns that he had at each stage of the hospital experience. Both the child's behavior and verbal remarks exemplify the behavior of a coping model so that while he exhibits some anxiety and apprehension, he is able to overcome his initial fears and complete each event in a successful and nonanxious manner . . . film models who are initially anxious and overcome their anxiety [coping models] result in greater reduction in anxiety than models who exhibit no fear [mastery models]. (Melamed and Siegel, 1975, p. 514)

The control group of children was shown a film of similar interest level but that was totally unrelated to the hospital situation. Children in both groups also received the standard hospital preoperative counseling procedures explanation by a nurse of what would happen on the day of surgery, with pictures and demonstrations, and visits by the surgeon and anesthesiologist.

Prior to surgery and again three to four weeks after the surgery, self-report, observational, and physiological measures of the children's situational anxiety were obtained. It was found that the children who had viewed the hospital-related film demonstrated less anxiety than the control group of children on all measures at both preoperative and postoperative assessment periods. Thus this peer-modeling film had a significant effect on reducing anxiety in children above and beyond that produced by standard hospital preoperative procedures. Such peer modeling is probably especially important for young children, because it is often easier for a child to understand another child than it is for the child to understand an adult.

One of the important factors probably underlying the effectiveness of these modeling procedures is the information given to subjects. As we discussed in Chapter 8, there is a growing body of research literature demonstrating the effectiveness of presurgery information in reducing the distress associated with surgery.

CONTACT DESENSITIZATION

An effective variation of *in vivo* systematic desensitization that combines modeling and guided participation procedures is called contact desensitization. Originally developed by Ritter (1968), it involves having the therapist first *model* the appropriate behavior for the fearful individual and then *guide* the person through each step of the graduated hierarchy. For example, if the individual was afraid of snakes, the therapist might first model a variety of behaviors, starting with approaching and touching the snake and then gradually progressing to allowing the snake to crawl loose around the therapist's shoulders. The fearful individual is then requested to perform the lowest behavioral task on the hierarchy, with the therapist's aid. The client repeats each item of the hierarchy until the anxiety associated with that item has been extinguished. Although a graded hierarchy is used, relaxation training is not. The procedure is based solely on extinction.

This procedure has been found to be very effective. In fact, in the treatment of at least one phobia—fear of snakes—it has been found to produce even greater therapeutic improvement than systematic desensitization and modeling (Bandura, Blanchard, and Ritter, 1969).

BEHAVIORAL REHEARSAL

Allowing individuals to "act out" or "role play" their interpersonal problems and usual manner of behaving is a method used in many different forms of psychotherapy. In behavior therapy, role playing or behavioral rehearsal methods that attempt to simulate real-life situations have been developed and formalized to train individuals how to perform new behavior patterns. The therapist often "models" or "coaches" the appropriate behavior that a client may be lacking. A client lacking appropriate dating behavior, for instance, would be taught appropriate skills through behavioral rehearsal. Such procedures are being used more and more in teaching social skills for a variety of interpersonal situations.

Related to these procedures are assertiveness training techniques, which are used with individuals who experience a great deal of anxiety because of problems in asserting themselves. Salter (1949) was the first to give a great deal of attention to the fact that unassertive behavior often causes anxiety. Many individuals cannot stand up for their rights and greatly regret their inability to do so. This may create a great deal of interpersonal anxiety. Salter developed a method to teach such socially inhibited persons how to express their feelings to others more effectively and assertively. More recently, McFall and colleagues (McFall and Lillesand, 1971; McFall and Marston, 1970; McFall and Twentyman, 1973) have reported the therapeutic effectiveness of assertiveness training in reducing anxiety in various interpersonal situations.

Assertiveness training may be an especially valuable adjunctive treatment in dealing with certain psychosomatic disorders. Often, because of a lack of appropriate interpersonal social skills such as assertiveness training, an individual cannot adequately cope with stressors that are causing and/or exacerbating the physical symptoms. For example, an overly demanding boss or spouse may be causing a great deal of stress. This seems to be especially true in the case of migraine headache (Price, 1979). By providing an individual with means to more effectively deal with these unfair demands—new behaviors developed through assertiveness training—one can help him or her deal more adaptively with such stress situations.

CONTINGENCY MANAGEMENT

Contingency management refers to the process of changing the frequency of a behavior by controlling the consequences of that behavior. In the process of shaping a rat to press a bar, food reinforcement is developed only after the rat has made a correct response. The experimenter controls or manages the contingency between reinforcement (delivery of food) and a certain behavior (bar-pressing responses) in order to increase the frequency of that behavior. Any attempt to change the frequency of a behavior by systematically controlling consequences such as reinforcement is called **contingency management.** Indeed, we all use contingency management procedures in everyday life, albeit sometimes inconsistently: the parent rewards or punishes the child for some behavior, or the employer gives a bonus to an employee for some outstanding work performance. These are attempts to encourage or discourage particular behaviors by associating with them some consequence that is either desirable or undesirable. Behavior therapists have developed some systematic contingency management programs to alter a wide range of behaviors.

One particularly effective type of contingency management technique is the **token economy** program. Token economy programs have been shown to be effective in modifying and controlling deviant behaviors, even the bizarre behavior patterns and problems of schizophrenics in hospitalized settings (Ayllon and Azrin, 1968; Krasner, 1968). They have been found to be among the most successful rehabilitation programs for hospitalized patients as well as individuals in other structured settings such as classrooms. In these programs a person's undesirable behaviors are identified, and more desirable behaviors incompatible with the problem responses are defined (e.g., psychotic talk in patients is eliminated and replaced with normal nonpsychotic talk). Individuals are systematically reinforced with tokens whenever they engage in the socially desirable behavior. These tokens can then be exchanged for special goods, such as candy, or special privileges, such as community outings.

Token economy programs have been shown to be very effective in increasing the frequency of socially adaptive behaviors even in severely regressed hospitalized patients. They are also found to be effective in improving the individual's sense of responsibility and self-reliance and in decreasing feelings of helplessness.

Contingency management techniques such as this can be used effectively in a wide variety of nonmedical settings, such as schools and homes. They are also being used more and more to increase compliance to medical regimens. We discussed the topic of compliance in Chapter 8; in Chapter 11 we shall discuss the use of contingency management techniques in the treatment of chronic pain.

STIMULUS CONTROL

An important element in operant conditioning is the concept of a discriminative stimulus or cue. When we are driving a car, we routinely stop at a traffic light when it turns red. We are aware of the necessity of performing such a behavior in order to avoid getting a ticket or, even worse, being involved in a traffic accident. The traffic light serves as a discriminative cue or stimulus for the behavior (stopping the car) to occur. It informs us that a particular response is likely to be rewarded. As another example, a school-crossing sign is a discriminative stimulus for slowing down the speed of your car. Thus a discriminative stimulus tells us when and where it is appropriate to emit a certain behavior in order to receive reinforcement or avoid aversive consequences (e.g., receiving a traffic ticket for exceeding the speed limit). Strictly defined, a **discriminative stimulus** is an environmental cue that informs us when it is likely that a response or behavior will be reinforced. Discriminative stimuli provide an occasion for the potential occurrence of an operant response. Behavior that is prompted by a discriminative cue or stimulus is termed to be under **stimulus control.** A wide variety of problem behaviors are under stimulus control. Many behaviors occur more frequently in some situations than in others. As a consequence, treatment programs have been developed to take into account this principle of stimulus control.

In a classic report by Stuart (1967), the principle of stimulus control was employed in an obesity treatment program. Stuart's treatment program consisted of gradually restricting and eliminating stimuli that had come to elicit the maladaptive eating behavior. For example, the program involved guidelines such as restricting eating to specific times and places; not eating while engaged in other enjoyable activities like watching television, listening to the radio, and so on; ridding the house of fattening foods; avoiding passing a restaurant or going grocery shopping when hungry. Thus stimulus control is dealt with by restricting eating to appropriate times and places and eliminating eating cues from the environment. Using this stimulus control approach, Stuart's program produced remarkable success. At a one-year follow-up, clients in the program had lost from twenty-six to forty-six pounds. Although weight losses of this magnitude have not been consistently found in studies conducted since Stuart's initial report, the behavioral treatment of obesity has been found, on the whole, to be effective (Stunkard, 1979). Later in this chapter we will review another effective behavioral weight reduction program developed by Mahoney, Moura, and Wade (1973). That program employed principles of contingent positive reinforcement. Such behavioral treatment programs continue to show success in significantly modifying maladaptive overeating. Stimulus control procedures have also been found to be effective with a variety of other problem behaviors such as insomnia (Bootzin, 1973) and poor study habits (Goldiamond, 1965).

COGNITIVE BEHAVIOR THERAPY TECHNIQUES

Albert Ellis (1962) originally developed **Rational-Emotional Therapy (RET)** on the assumption that cognitions can produce emotions. He assumed that psychological disorders such as neuroses are caused by faulty or irrational patterns of thinking. Accordingly, he indicated that the focus of therapy should be directed at changing the internal or covert sentences that people say to themselves and that produce negative emotional responses. Summarizing the results of 172 case histories of clients he treated with either RET or traditional psychoanalytic therapy, Ellis (1962) found RET to be the more effective treatment. Although this was far from a controlled outcome evaluation study, it did suggest the potential effectiveness of his therapy technique. More important, it prompted more behavior therapists to begin to use his basic technique as a "cognitive restructuring" method with a variety of behavioral disorders (Goldfried and Davison, 1976).

COGNITIVE RESTRUCTURING

Meichenbaum (1972) has reported success in using **cognitive restructuring** techniques to modify anxiety. In this procedure the therapist determines the specific thoughts or self-verbalizations that are presumed to give rise to the anxiety. The therapist then assists the client in modifying these negative self-verbalizations and replacing them with positive self-statements.

Like systematic desensitization, cognitive restructuring has been demonstrated in controlled therapy evaluation studies to be highly effective in reducing anxiety. In terms of the differential effectiveness of these two therapy techniques, Rimm and Masters (1974) have suggested that systematic desensitization may be more effective with clients who show a relatively small number of phobias or fears, whereas those persons who experience multiple fears in a great many interpersonal situations might profit more from cognitive restructuring techniques. Additional research is needed to test experimentally the validity of their suggestion.

Another cognitive restructuring method that has recently been developed is *thought stopping.* It is used with clients who experience distress because of obsessive thoughts they have difficulty controlling. The technique, which is relatively straightforward, has been summarized by Rimm and Masters (1974):

> *The client is asked to concentrate on the anxiety-inducing thoughts, and, after a short period of time, the therapist suddenly and emphatically says "stop" (any loud noise . . . may also suffice). After this procedure has been repeated several times (and the client reports that his thoughts were indeed interrupted or blocked), the locus of control is shifted from the therapist to the client. Specifically, the client is taught to emit a subvocal "stop" whenever he begins to engage in a self-defeating rumination. (p. 430)*

As Rimm and Masters (1974) note, empirical evidence is very promising and shows that thought-stopping procedures are effective in dealing with obsessional thinking.

These cognitive restructuring procedures not only are effective in treating anxiety experienced by neurotic individuals but also are beneficial in dealing with anxiety and stress in general. They may be effectively employed to allow patients to more successfully cope with psychological stressors that are intimately linked with the precipitation or exacerbation of physical symptoms. Also, as we noted in Chapter 8, these procedures are being found to be effective in reducing distress associated with surgery.

SELF-CONTROL TECHNIQUES

There has been a great deal of interest in recent years in developing self-control or self-management strategies for modifying problem behaviors. How can we best train an individual to control and alter his or her own behavior through internalization processes? There have been a number of self-control strategies developed, with the main goal being to train individuals to use psychological self-management methods for dealing with problem behaviors. For example, the obese person is taught to use self-control methods to lose weight, the heavy smoker to decrease smoking, the exceedingly tense person to manage stress.

An example of a study that assessed different self-control methods for treating obesity is that of Mahoney, Moura, and Wade (1973). Five different groups were employed in this study:

1. *A control group,* which merely received information about the program but no specific treatment.

2. *A self-monitoring group,* which was requested simply to monitor its daily weight during the program.

3. *A self-reward group,* in which money was used for rewards. (In such a procedure, a therapist may instruct the client to set aside a specified amount of money toward the purchase of a desired item each time a certain amount of weight-loss occurs.)

4. *A self-punishment group,* in which a fine of a specified amount was levied if weight was not lost.

5. *A combined self-reward/self-punishment group,* in which the procedures of groups 3 and 4 were combined.

In the self-control groups, subjects were given suggestions on the contingencies to be used (e.g., reward yourself for *x* amount of pounds lost), but they were free to self-reward or self-punish as they saw fit. Thus the goal was to have them personally use a self-control strategy (contingent reinforcement) to help modify their weight gain.

Results of this study are presented in Figure 10.1. As can be seen, subjects in the two self-reward groups (groups 3 and 5) lost significantly more weight than the subjects in the self-punishment-only group (group 4). The fact that this latter group did not lose any more weight than the control and self-monitoring groups indicates that self-punishment is not a very effective procedure. Rather, self-reward strategies appear to be the more powerful and promising techniques for self-regulated change of behavior. In such procedures:

> *Individuals can reinforce themselves in a number of ways. Tangible rewards—such as money and gift certificates—have been shown to be effective in many applications. More recently, persons have been trained to self-reward privately (i.e., via a thought) as a means of strengthening or maintaining behavior. Likewise, they may enlist social support for their actions such that their self-reward strategies are supplemented by the compliments and encouragement of family and friends. (Mahoney and Arnkoff, 1979, p. 91)*

Self-control procedures show great promise for dealing with a wide range of problem behaviors. A comprehensive review of the various strategies being developed can be found in Mahoney and Arnkoff (1979).

BIOFEEDBACK

Before Harry Houdini performed one of his famous escapes, a skeptical committee would search his clothes and body. When the members of the committee were satisfied that the Great Houdini was concealing no keys, they would put chains, padlocks and handcuffs on him. . . . Of course, not even Houdini could open a padlock without a key, and when he was safely behind the curtain he would cough one up. He could

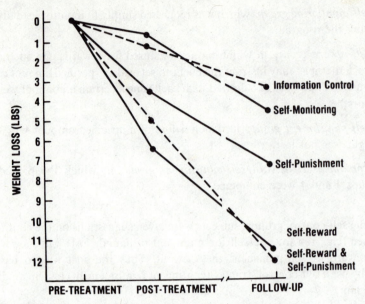

Figure 10.1   **Weight loss with different self-management procedures.**
From M. J. Mahoney, N. G. M. Moura, and T. C. Wade. The relative efficacy of self-reward, self-punishment, and self-monitoring techniques for weight loss. *Journal of Consulting and Clinical Psychology,* 1973, *40,* 404–407. Copyright © 1973 by the American Psychological Association. Reprinted by permission of the author.

hold a key suspended in his throat and regurgitate it when he was unobserved. . . .
The trick behind many of Houdini's escapes was in some ways just as amazing as the
escape itself. Ordinarily when an object is stuck in a person's throat he will start to
gag. He can't help it—it's an unlearned, automatic reflex. But Houdini had learned
to control his gag reflex by practicing for hours with a small piece of potato tied to a
string. (Lang, 1970, p. 23)

Through the years other unusual instances of voluntary control over physiological functions have been noted in the scientific literature. Lindsley and Sassamon (1938) reported the case of a middle-aged male who had the ability to control the erection of hairs over the entire surface of his body. McClure (1959) noted the case of an individual who could voluntarily produce complete cardiac arrest for periods of several seconds at a time. Numerous instances of voluntary acceleration of heart rate were reported by Ogden and Shock (1939). Russian psychologist Luria (1958) described a mnemonist who had attained remarkable control of his heart rate and skin temperature. This individual could abruptly alter his heart rate by forty beats per minute. He could also raise the skin temperature of one hand while simultaneously lowering the temperature of the other hand. It has also been documented that many yogis can control various physiological responses at will.

Such acts of bodily control have traditionally been viewed as rare feats that only certain extraordinarily gifted people could accomplish. However, in more recent years behavioral scientists have demonstrated that the average person can learn a degree of control over physiological responses. The principal training method developed and utilized in this learning process has been labeled **biofeedback.**

Starting in the 1960s, there has been a growing interest, among both the scientific community and the general public, in the area of biofeedback because of its many potentially important clinical applications. For example, it would be therapeutically valuable if we could teach patients with migraine headaches how to control the cranial artery dilation involved in the pain process, or teach patients with hypertension how to lower their blood pressure.

The biofeedback technique is based on the fundamental learning principle that we learn to perform a particular response when we receive feedback or information about the consequences of the response we have just made and then make appropriate adjustments. This is how we learn to perform the wide variety of skills and behaviors we use in everyday activities. For example, we learn how to drive a car by receiving continuous feedback about how much we need to turn the steering wheel in order to turn the car a certain distance, or how much pressure we must apply to the accelerator in order to make the car move at a certain speed. If we were denied this feedback—as, for instance, by being blindfolded—we would never receive useful information about the consequences of our driving responses. We would therefore never be able to learn the appropriate adjustments needed to perform a successful maneuver with the car. Information feedback is thus very important. Indeed, Annent (1969) has reviewed numerous experimental studies demonstrating the importance of feedback in the learning and performance of a wide variety of motor skills.

The availability of feedback is also important in learning how to control internal physiological responses. Since we do not receive feedback of these internal events in day-to-day life, we cannot control them. However, if a person is provided biofeedback of, say, blood pressure via a visual display monitor, he or she can become aware of the consequences of blood pressure changes and how adjustments can be made to modify and eventually control it. Receiving feedback removes one's "blindfold," thus enabling one to learn how to voluntarily control a response. The recent development of sensitive physiological recording devices and digital logic circuitry has made it possible to detect small changes in visceral events and provide subjects with immediate biofeedback of these events.

Since the initial pioneering experiments with animal subjects conducted in the late 1950s and early 1960s by Neal Miller (1969), there have been demonstrations of human subjects' learned control of a variety of what were once assumed to be "involuntary responses"—blood pressure, heart rate, sweat gland activity, skin temperature, neuromuscular activity, various brain wave rhythms, and even penile tumescence. Unfortunately, research evaluating the therapeutic effectiveness of biofeedback procedures has been plagued by a number of problems. There is still a lack of systematic, well-controlled studies that demonstrate conclusively the clinical effectiveness of these techniques. For the most part, claims of effectiveness have been based on uncontrolled group or single case studies. A great deal of research is needed to determine whether biofeedback techniques are active therapeutic procedures or merely powerful placebo conditions. Recent reports have suggested that placebo factors play a significant role in clinical applications of biofeedback (Gatchel, 1979;

Katkin and Goldband, 1979). Also, an important question that needs to be addressed in biofeedback evaluation research is whether biofeedback procedures are significantly superior to less expensive and more easily administered methods such as muscle relaxation training and other behavioral techniques. Nevertheless, biofeedback has become a very important and widely used behavioral treatment technique.

Gatchel and Price (1979) and Hatch, Gatchel, and Harrington (1982) have provided comprehensive surveys and evaluations of the clinical effectiveness of biofeedback with a variety of disorders/problem behaviors, taking the problems just discussed into account. A summary of the status of research on the clinical effectiveness of biofeedback follows.

ANXIETY

Gatchel and colleagues (see Gatchel, 1979) have found that heart rate biofeedback may be useful for inhibiting cardiac acceleration and self-reported anxiety during acute stress. There is no conclusive evidence that biofeedback on other physiological responses such as electromyogram (EMG) is any more effective than simple muscle relaxation training. The research by Gatchel and colleagues has also demonstrated the important role that placebo factors play in producing and maintaining fear reduction in a biofeedback treatment program. As Gatchel (1979) has noted, even if placebo factors are eventually found to be the major active ingredient in biofeedback treatment, such a finding would not detract from its therapeutic effectiveness *as long as clinicians realize this* so that they can best choose the appropriate treatment for their various patients. Indeed, there is a long-accepted maxim in medicine that states: "Treat many patients with new remedies while they still have the power to heal" (Shapiro, 1971).

ESSENTIAL HYPERTENSION

Research has shown a limited degree of success in reducing the symptoms of essential hypertension with biofeedback. The technique has not been shown, however, to reliably produce reductions in blood pressure of a clinically significant magnitude that transfer to the nonlaboratory environment. Thus it cannot be considered an alternative to pharmacologic treatment at this time. It should be noted, though, that a study reported by Luborsky et al. (1980) compared the relative efficacy of medication, relaxation training, and biofeedback during a six-week treatment program with mildly moderately hypertensive individuals. It was found that although patients given medication derived the most benefit even at moderate levels of medication, some patients experienced comparable benefits from the two behavioral treatments. These investigators suggest that hypertensive individuals who are strongly motivated to adhere to a behavioral treatment program should be encouraged to undergo such treatment first to assess whether it is beneficial, before being put on medication. This is an interesting suggestion that certainly merits additional investigation.

The usefulness of biofeedback as an adjunct to chemotherapy has not yet been evaluated, and such studies would be of much value. On the whole, research in this area has not advanced very far. Sample sizes are small, control groups are lacking, and follow-up data are unavailable far too often. These are serious shortcomings, and until additional research is performed to remedy these problems the usefulness of biofeedback in the management of essential hypertension cannot be determined.

POSTURAL HYPOTENSION

In some cases of high spinal cord injury, the reflex pathways that normally produce vasoconstriction when one assumes an upright posture are damaged, resulting in a lowering of the blood pressure to the point where some patients cannot stand or sit upright without fainting. There is no effective treatment for the disorder, and severely effected patients must remain in the supine position. Although controlled group outcome studies are not yet available, several good case studies have demonstrated that systolic blood pressure biofeedback training has enabled some patients to sit upright or to stand with crutches, which prior to training produced fainting (see Hatch, Gatchel, and Harrington, 1982).

CARDIAC ARRHYTHMIAS

The few case studies available indicate that heart rate biofeedback seems to be effective in the treatment of cardiac arrhythmias such as sinus tachycardia, atrial fibrillation, and premature ventricular contractions (see Hatch, Gatchel, and Harrington, 1982). However, judgment must be withheld with regard to therapeutic value of biofeedback for such disorders generally until more research is conducted.

RAYNAUD'S DISEASE

Raynaud's disease is a condition characterized by recurrent attacks of paroxysmal vasospasm in the hands or feet, commonly triggered by exposure to cold or emotional stress. Since specific vasomotor responding has repeatedly been shown to occur with skin temperature biofeedback in normal subjects (Taub, 1977), this would seem to be an appropriate technique for reducing vasospastic attacks of Raynaud's disease. However, several case studies and group outcome studies reported thus far have failed to produce conclusive evidence to this effect. Biofeedback-specific effects do not appear to be essential ingredients in producing therapeutic improvement. Simple muscle relaxation and autogenic training procedures seem to produce equal degrees of therapeutic improvement (see Hatch, Gatchel, and Harrington, 1982).

MIGRAINE HEADACHE

Although an abundance of published reports make positive claims for the clinical efficacy of biofeedback in treating **migraine headache,** a careful and critical review of this literature suggests that caution should be maintained. Many studies in the area are flawed by inadequate control groups, inappropriate statistical analysis, small sample size, brief pretreatment baseline and posttreatment follow-up periods, and the use of "treatment package" techniques that confound the effects of biofeedback with those of other components of therapy. Indeed, in a recent extensive review of the literature, Beatty (1980) concludes that there is currently no convincing evidence to indicate that biofeedback methods are any more efficacious in the treatment of migraine headache than are simple relaxation and placebo type interventions.

MUSCLE CONTRACTION HEADACHE

To summarize the results of experiments using EMG biofeedback as a treatment for muscle contraction headache, a number of controlled group outcome studies have shown that treatments involving biofeedback are more effective than inactive control procedures. A number of these studies have included follow-up evaluations conducted several months following the end of treatment, and the results indicate that clinical gains are often maintained. No definitive conclusions can be drawn at this time about the comparative value of biofeedback procedures and general relaxation procedures. It is not yet possible to determine whether a combined treatment involving EMG (electromyographic or muscle activity) biofeedback and verbal relaxation training is any more effective than either technique alone. A similar conclusion has been reached in a recent review of the biofeedback–tension headache literature by Cox and Hobbs (1980), who state that the only thing that can be concluded from the existing data is that EMG biofeedback is more effective than placebo in the treatment of tension headaches.

ASTHMA

Unfortunately there have been a number of methodological problems associated with EMG biofeedback–asthma reduction studies. Alexander and Smith (1979) have criticized these studies, noting that instructions to try to decrease the noncontingent biofeedback signal may lead to counterproductive frustration in no-treatment control group subjects. Alexander and Smith (1979) also note that measurement of peak expiratory flow rate (the common dependent measure) is highly dependent on patient motivation, cooperation, and physical effort; thus biofeedback treatment may affect that dependent outcome measure primarily through such nonspecific factors.

GASTROINTESTINAL DISORDERS

Although some of the research results on the biofeedback-assisted modification of gastrointestinal behaviors are encouraging, controlled studies with large samples have not yet been conducted. Thus there is little information concerning the specific contribution of biofeedback to the success of the techniques. The use of electric shock to eliminate rumination seems to work and may be the only available technique that will work with some patients; however, nonaversive techniques using the standard contingent feedback paradigm might find more widespread applicability among cooperative patients. Biofeedback treatments for peptic ulcer and irritable bowel syndrome require much additional testing and refinement of technique before they can be recommended for clinical use. Finally, the research suggesting the efficacy of biofeedback therapy for fecal incontinence should lead to controlled studies.

EPILEPTIC SEIZURES

At this time the amount of controlled group research concerning possible therapeutic effects of EEG biofeedback for the treatment of epileptic seizures is extremely small, and all but the most speculative conclusions would be premature. The positive results that have been reported, however, are encouraging and would seem to justify the more time-consuming and expensive research that must now occur to produce more conclusive answers. Many important issues remain to be resolved. One of the most basic concerns is how biofeedback affects brain electrophysiology and seizures. For example, do epileptic patients undergoing biofeedback therapy (1) learn to tonically modify their EEG rhythm, (2) learn to eliminate specific electrophysiological abnormalities, (3) learn to abort an impending seizure, or (4) simply learn to relax? Much research needs to be done before EEG biofeedback can be expected to have a clinically significant effect on the psychological control of epileptic seizures.

UPPER MOTOR NEURON DYSFUNCTIONS

A number of well-designed individual and multiple case studies have suggested the therapeutic effects of biofeedback in the treatment of **upper motor neuron disorders** such as paresis, cerebral palsy, and incomplete spinal cord lesions. However, controlled group experiments are lacking except in the biofeedback treatment of paresis, where results are negative or ambiguous. And the failure of therapeutic results to persist following removal of biofeedback remains problematic. Thus, although the intervention with biofeedback has been associated with therapeutic gains, it is not yet possible to distinguish between specific effects of biofeedback and associated nonspecific factors such as therapist attention, novelty, and placebo effects. At the present time, there is no compelling evidence for long-term clinically significant gains attributable to the specific effects of biofeedback for the treatment of upper motor neuron disorders.

LOWER MOTOR NEURON DYSFUNCTIONS

The case studies reporting the successful application of EMG biofeedback in the treatment of **lower motor neuron dysfunctions** (e.g., peripheral nerve injury, Bell's palsy) must currently be interpreted with some caution, given the lack of control procedures.

DYSKINESIAS

Biofeedback techniques have been used to treat a number of different **dyskinesias,** including spasmodic torticollis, Parkinson's disease, tardive dyskinesia, and Huntington's disease. Individual and multiple case reports suggest a possible use of EMG biofeedback in the treatment of these disorders. However, the role of the biofeedback is unclear since controls were not used, treatment procedures were not adequately described for each case, and the biofeedback was sometimes combined with some other behavior therapy technique such as aversive conditioning treatment.

MUSCULAR PAIN

Although tentative results are promising with regard to the biofeedback treatment of pain, the role of placebo factors is probably a potent one, as it is in many other pain syndromes, and needs to be more carefully evaluated. It should also be recognized that the etiology of many muscular pain disorders such as low back pain and

THE PLACEBO EFFECT

The *placebo effect* was originally shown to be an important factor in medical research when it was found that many times inert chemical drugs, which had no direct effect on physical events underlying various medical disorders, produced symptom reduction. Extensive literature on the placebo effect undeniably demonstrates that the *belief* by the patient that a prescribed medication is active, even if it is in fact chemically inert, often leads to significant symptom reduction (Shapiro, 1971). In a review of the placebo effect, Shapiro (1971) gives this definition:

> A placebo *is defined as any therapy, or that component of any therapy, that is deliberately used for its nonspecific, psychologic, or psychophysiologic effect, or that is used for its presumed specific effect on a patient, symptom, or illness, but which, unknown to patient and therapist, is without specific activity for the condition being treated.* . . . *A placebo, when used as a control in experimental studies, is defined as a substance or procedure that is without specific activity for the condition being evaluated.* . . . *The* placebo effect *is defined as the nonspecific, psychologic or psychophysiologic effect produced by placebos.* (p. 440)

In the area of drug therapy, Shapiro (1971) notes that for centuries the use of medication has been largely a placebo-effect process, with chemically inert or inactive drugs producing therapeutic improvement in people who believed that these drugs or "magic potions" would help them. Frank (1961) has presented evidence that improvement in various physical and psychological problems can occur after a patient ingests a pill that a physician has suggested will help alleviate the problem. Frank also notes that placebo effects are similar to many faith-healing procedures in which the individual believes he or she will be helped.

The placebo effect has also been found to be an active ingredient in psychotherapy/behavior therapy, especially when anxiety is being treated (Shapiro, 1971). As Shapiro (1971) indicates, the effect appears to be a "multidetermined phenomenon" that is not yet completely understood. It has also been shown to be an important factor in biofeedback treatment (Gatchel, 1979). One important psychological factor contributing to the placebo effect that has been shown to affect the outcome of psychotherapy is generalized expectancy of improvement (Wilkins, 1973). Research is continuing in this important field. In Chapter 11 we shall review some research suggesting the importance of endorphins (endogenous opiatelike substances emanating from the brain) in mediating the placebo effect. Regardless of the exact psychophysiological mechanism ultimately found to be involved in this effect, therapists and physicians need to be aware of the potentially powerful and positive impact that the placebo effect can have in the treatment of a wide range of medical and psychological disorders.

myofascial pain remains a mystery, and therefore it is difficult to determine the target physiological response to assess and modify.

SEXUAL DYSFUNCTIONS

As Geer (1979) recently concluded on the basis of a review of the literature, although genital responses have been shown to be responsive to both instructional control and biofeedback, there is currently no evidence that the direct conditioning of genital responses through biofeedback has therapeutic value. Geer does suggest, however, that biofeedback may have a role to play in guiding the development of erotic and nonerotic fantasy, which can, in turn, have significant therapeutic value. This is a relatively new area of biofeedback research that currently lacks well-controlled investigations. A great deal of additional research is needed.

CONCLUSIONS

It has been amply demonstrated that some degree of self-control is possible over behaviors long assumed to be completely involuntary. It has also been shown that, with biofeedback, it is possible to extend voluntary control to pathophysiological responding in order to modify this maladaptive behavior in the direction of health. These are highly significant achievements. However, many important questions still remain as to how medically effective biofeedback will be. To date, very few well-controlled clinical outcome studies have been conducted using large numbers of patients having well-confirmed medical diagnoses. Moreover, the few comparative group outcome studies that have been performed compared the relative effectiveness of biofeedback to that of various other behavioral techniques. It would be extremely helpful to also compare biofeedback techniques with more traditional medical treatments, some of which have fairly well established success rates. Combinations of medical and behavioral techniques should also be explored and evaluated. These studies will be most informative if they are designed so that the unique contribution of each individual technique, as well as the combined effect, can be isolated and reliably measured.

Unfortunately, claims for the therapeutic efficacy of biofeedback have been grossly exaggerated and sometimes even wrong. Overall, it is justified to conclude that relevant and encouraging data do exist, but at the present time the value of clinical training in biofeedback still has to be questioned in many areas. Moreover, terms such as biofeedback therapist and biofeedback clinic, which are now regularly encountered in many medical settings, are difficult to justify. They imply that a form of treatment exists that is more or less generally applicable to a variety of ills. Worse yet, they imply, at least in the minds of some, that biofeedback is a new alternative treatment modality. Currently, in the majority of areas in which it is applied, biofeedback should be viewed merely as an adjunctive treatment.

The potential of biofeedback in diagnosis, etiology, prevention, and rehabilitation should continue to be tested. Some of its most important contributions may prove to be conceptual rather than technological or directly therapeutic. Moreover, as one of the authors emphasized earlier, in order for the field of biofeedback to effectively develop and progress:

> *. . . the clinician or researcher employing biofeedback needs knowledge in a number of different areas; the pathophysiology of the disorder being treated and the physiology of the response systems to be voluntarily regulated, the relation of such response systems to the etiology and symptoms of the particular disorder, the electrical functioning of the feedback device itself, the nature of the self-regulation process involved in biofeedback "learning," and the knowledge and use of appropriate methodology. Without such expertise, it cannot be expected that useful and reliable biofeedback treatment procedures can be developed. (Price and Gatchel, 1979, p. 235)*

BROAD-SPECTRUM COGNITIVE BEHAVIOR THERAPY

Lazarus (1971) has coined the term broad-spectrum behavior therapy to emphasize the fact that most behavior therapists employ several different treatment procedures for a specific disorder in an attempt to deal effectively with all the important controlling or causal variables. Just as traditional psychoanalytic therapy attempts to determine the underlying unconscious or "root" cause of a behavior disorder, behavior therapy seeks to assess the major causes of such behavior. However, the search is not for underlying unconscious causes, which are difficult to reliably assess, but for the learned and environmental determinants or causes. As Bandura (1969) notes, if by "searching for the cause of a disorder" one means the search for the strongest and most significant causal and controlling variables, then the goal and task of all therapists, traditional psychotherapists as well as behavior therapists, is the same. The chief difference is that behavior therapists assume that the search for environmental determinants and the direct modification of behavior is heuristically the most feasible and effective approach, whereas traditional psychotherapists assume that it is more important to uncover and to attempt to treat unconscious motivations of behavior.

Most behavior therapists therefore use several different treatment procedures for a specific disorder in order to deal effectively with all the important controlling or causal variables. Fortunately, behavior therapists have a number of very effective procedures in their treatment arsenal—systematic desensitization and its variants, progressive relaxation training, behavioral rehearsal and assertiveness training, self-control techniques, cognitive restructuring and thought-stopping procedures, and biofeedback, to name a few that we have discussed in this chapter. For a more comprehensive review of these as well as other cognitive-behavioral techniques, there are a number of excellent books available (e.g., Bootzin, 1975; Goldfried and Davison, 1976; Mahoney, 1974; Meichenbaum, 1977; Rimm and Masters, 1974).

The availability of a variety of different treatment methods gives broad-spectrum behavior therapy a major advantage over traditional forms of psychotherapy, in which the same general form of therapy is applied to all disorders. The traditional "general" psychotherapy approach has not been very successful in dealing with the various forms of abnormal and maladaptive behavior (Mears and Gatchel, 1979). Cognitive-behavior therapy has taken the approach of developing specific treatment techniques to deal with particular disorders. In recent years there has also been more effort to individualize treatment so that the type of treatment employed is tailored to the specific disorder and characteristics of the patient. Goldstein and Stein (1976) published a text entitled *Prescriptive Psychotherapies* in which an attempt is made to outline the type of treatment that is most effective in dealing with spec ders. Such an approach helps ensure the appropriate matching of patient-treatment variables to produce the most successful therapeutic outcomes.

As an example of the broad-spectrum or multimodal approach to treatment, take the case of treating hypertension. In training an individual with hypertension to relax and voluntarily lower his or her blood pressure level, the therapist might initially use progressive muscle relaxation and then blood pressure biofeedback. The therapist might also teach the patient new methods for more effectively coping with stressful situations, as blood pressure can be temporarily elevated as the result of inability to cope with perceived aggression or frustration (see Hokanson and Burgess, 1962). The individual might need to learn interpersonal social skills, such as assertiveness training, or cognitive restructuring techniques in order to more successfully cope with such stressors.

SUMMARY

In this chapter we have discussed a variety of cognitive-behavioral treatment procedures that have been successfully employed with problem behaviors often seen in medical settings. These techniques were developed on the basis of some major learning principles demonstrated to modify behavior—classical conditioning, operant conditioning, and observational learning-modeling. Systematic desensitization, developed by Wolpe, has been found to be effective in the treatment of a variety of medical phobias. Progressive muscle relaxation, which is an important component of the systematic desensitization treatment process, can often serve as a powerful therapeutic technique in its own right for the treatment of stress-related disorders. Modeling procedures, originally developed by Bandura, have been found to reduce fear and anxiety. Contact desensitization is an effective fear-reduction therapy that combines elements of systematic desensitization and modeling. Behavioral rehearsal procedures, such as assertiveness training, are used in teaching social skills for a variety of interpersonal situations. Contingency management procedures can be used effectively in a wide variety of settings (schools, homes, hospitals) to change behavior. They are also being used more and more to increase compliance to medical regimens. Stimulus control procedures have been found to be effective with a variety of problem behaviors such as obesity and insomnia. We also reviewed a number of cognitive behavior therapy techniques, such as cognitive restructuring and self-control methods. In addition, we reviewed the use of biofeedback for medically related disorders and pointed out its clinical utility. Finally, we noted the current trend of multimodal or broad spectrum behavior therapy. This approach emphasizes the use of several different treatment procedures for a specific disorder in an attempt to deal effectively with all the important controlling or causal variables involved.

RECOMMENDED READINGS

Gatchel, R. J., and Price, K. P. (Eds.) *Clinical applications of biofeedback: Appraisal and status.* Elmsford, N.Y.: Pergamon, 1979.

Geer, J. H., and Messé, M. Sexual dysfunctions. In R. J. Gatchel, A. Baum, and J. E. Singer (Eds.), *Behavioral medicine and clinical psychology: Overlapping areas.* Hillsdale, N.J.: Erlbaum, 1982.

Hatch, J. P., Gatchel, R. J., and Harrington, R. Biofeedback: Clinical applications and medicine. In R. J. Gatchel, A. Baum, and J. E. Singer (Eds.), *Behavioral medicine and clinical psychology: Overlapping areas.* Hillsdale, N.J.: Erlbaum, 1982.

Mahoney, M. J., and Arnkoff, D. B. Self-management. In O. F. Pomerleau and J. P. Brady (Eds.), *Behavioral medicine: Therapy and practice.* Baltimore: Williams & Wilkins, 1979.

Meichenbaum, D. H. *Cognitive-behavior modification.* New York: Plenum, 1977.

Shapiro, A. K. Placebo effects in medicine, psychotherapy, and psychoanalysis. In A. E. Bergin and S. L. Garfield (Eds.), *Handbook of psychotherapy and behavior change: An empirical analysis.* New York: Wiley, 1971.

Turner, S. M., Calhoun, K. S., and Adams, H. E. *Handbook of clinical behavior therapy.* New York: Wiley, 1981.

11 PAIN AND PAIN MANAGEMENT TECHNIQUES

||||||||||||||||||||||||||||||||||||||||||||||||||||||||||||||||||||||||||||||||||||||||||||||||||||||||||||||||||||||||

Pain is an extremely common complaint in medical settings, with literally hundreds of thousands of individuals actively seeking relief from unbearable pain. It is a significant problem because of the frequent ineffectiveness of traditional medical approaches; success rates for certain chronic pain problems (e.g., low back pain) rarely exceed 60 percent, and long-term success rates are below 30 percent (Loeser, 1974). Traditionally, one of the contributing factors to this poor success rate has been the way medicine has dichotomized pain complaints as either "organic" or "psychogenic" in nature. Such an overly simplistic and naive conceptualization seriously hampered the physician's ability to understand the patient, and his or her pain, fully. As will be seen in this chapter, pain is a complex phenomenon that involves not only physiological sensations and mechanisms but also significant behavioral/psychological components. A model of pain that integrates both physiological and psychological components has the best chance of allowing a comprehensive understanding of the pain process—and has important implications and practical applications for the assessment and treatment of individuals with pain.

THE PHYSIOLOGY OF PAIN

Traditionally pain has been conceptualized as some specific type of activity in the sensory nervous system. As Melzack (1973) noted:

> The best classical description of the theory was provided by Descartes in 1644, who conceived of the pain system as a straight-through channel from the skin to the brain. He suggested that the system is like the bell-ringing mechanism in a church: a man pulls the rope at the bottom of the tower, and the bell rings in the belfry. So too, he proposed, a flame sets particles in the foot into activity and the motion is transmitted up the leg and back into the head, where, presumably, something like an alarm system is set off. The person feels pain and responds to it. (p. 126)

A more formal model of pain was proposed by Von Frey in 1894 (Melzack and Wall, 1965). This **specificity theory of pain** assumed that there were specific sensory receptors responsible for the transmission of sensations such as touch, warmth, and pain. The sensory receptors were thought to differ in their structure; these differences rendered them sensitive to specific kinds of stimulation. The receptors believed to be associated with the sensation of pain were assumed to be free nerve endings. Thus pain was viewed as having specific central and peripheral mechanisms similar to those of other bodily senses.

Approximately at the same time that Von Frey was proposing his specificity theory of pain, Goldschneider presented an alternative conceptualization that was labeled the **pattern theory of pain** (Melzack and Wall, 1965). Goldschneider argued that pain sensations were the result of the transmission of nerve impulse *patterns* originating from, and coded at, the peripheral stimulation site. Differences in the patterning and quantity of peripheral nerve-fiber discharge were viewed as producing differences in the quality of sensation. Thus a minimal tactile stimulus to an area might cause a feeling of touch, whereas stronger tactile stimuli would cause pain. If the same nerve fibers were being stimulated and discharged, it was argued, then the difference in sensation had to be due to an increased discharge and spatial summation. It was assumed that the pattern of stimulation produced by a specific stimulus had to be coded by the central nervous system. Therefore the experience of pain was deemed to be the result of central nervous system coding of nerve impulse patterns, and not simply the result of a specific connection between pain receptors and pain sites.

There has been some support for portions of both of these early theoretical formulations of pain. In support of the specificity theory, for example, Bonica (1953) reported that there is a unique and specific experience of pain originating in the skin when appropriate stimulation is administered. Moreover, he also identified two sets of sensory fibers that had stimulus-specific conducting properties that were clearly involved in the transmission of pain. In partial support of the pattern theory, Melzack and Wall (1965) demonstrated that skin receptors have some specialized properties by which they can transmit particular types and ranges of stimulation in the form of patterns of impulses.

In spite of such support for these two formulations, a number of reported findings cannot be accounted for by either of them. For example, research (to be discussed in the next section) has indicated that psychological factors such as an individual's anxiety level can significantly affect the pain experienced from a noxious stimulus. This intervening psychological mechanism is not taken into account by the specificity theory, which proposes a specific and direct stimulus-response chain. Another inadequacy of the specificity theory is its failure to explain why surgical intervention techniques directed at breaking the specific connection between the peripheral body damage site producing the noxious stimulation and the assumed central pain mechanism (e.g., through nerve severing) have not produced widespread therapeutic effects in alleviating chronic pain.

The pattern theory of pain, on the other hand, does not account for the physiological evidence of nerve-fiber specialization that Bonica (1953) originally reported. Thus, although both the specificity and pattern theories do account for certain physiological mechanisms of pain perception, neither of them can comprehensively deal with the complex mechanism of pain perception. Moreover, the ever-evolving field of neurotransmitter mechanisms and the enkephalin compounds have introduced additional complexities that these models cannot effectively incorporate. Pain is no longer viewed as the result of a straight-through transmission of impulse from the skin to the brain.

NOCICEPTION

Recent physiological research has demonstrated a number of structures within the nervous system that contribute to pain. The term **nociceptor** has replaced the older term **pain receptor** in order to highlight the fact that these sensory units contribute to the pain experience rather than create it. Peripheral nociceptors are specialized transducerlike units and bare nerve endings that have terminations in the skin, deep somatic tissues, and the viscera. Two major groups of these peripheral nerve fibers are involved in nociception: (1) **A-delta fibers**, which are small myelinated fibers that appear to mediate immediate or sharp pain. It is estimated that nearly 25 percent of these fibers are nociceptors; and (2) **C fibers**, which are even smaller fibers that are unmyelinated. These appear to mediate diffuse and dull or aching pain. It is estimated that approximately 50 percent of C fibers are nociceptors. There are also other fibers (**A-alpha-beta fibers**) that transmit other sensory modalities of a more innocuous nature.

There are two basic classes of these A-delta and C fibers. One class of these fibers are called **mechanical nociceptors** because they respond maximally to intense mechanical stimulation. Another class of fibers are called **polymodal nociceptors** because they respond maximally to mechanical and temperature stimulation. They may also be activated in tissue damage by various endogenous biochemicals such as serotonin, histamine, and prostaglandins.

These peripheral nerve fibers enter the spinal cord through the dorsal horn where they undergo considerable modulation from within the dorsal horn as well as from descending impulses from higher brain centers (this modulation is quite complex, and its scientific understanding is continually undergoing elucidation). The afferent pathway from the dorsal horn crosses to the opposite anterolateral segment of the spinal cord and then ascends in the spinothalamic tract. It ascends to the sensory cortex via the thalamus and also by alternative pathways to the reticular activating system, with widespread subsequent radiation to lower and higher brain centers (the role of many higher centers and their interaction with the lower brain stem system is understood quite poorly at this time). Moreover, the spinothalamic tract communicates with other levels in the spinal cord.

Thus nociceptive stimuli travel from the periphery to the cerebral cortex via specific afferent pathways to specific brain sites. However, these pathways are subject to modulation at various sites in the dorsal horn, the spinothalamic tract, and lower and higher brain centers. This helps to explain why an incoming peripheral pain signal can be modulated by downward afferent processes. As we shall see, recent conceptualizations of pain have taken into account the role of such higher central modulation effects.

THE GATE-CONTROL THEORY OF PAIN

In 1965 Melzack and Wall introduced the **gate-control theory of pain** in an attempt to more adequately take into account many of the diverse psychophysiological mechanisms that appear to be involved in the pain perception process. Although the theory has limitations, it did for the first time introduce to the scientific community the importance of central, psychological factors in the pain perception process. It gave credence to the potentially significant role that such psychological factors play.

This theory assumes that there are a number of structures within the central nervous system that contribute to pain. It is the interplay between these structures that is critical in determining if, and to what extent, a specific stimulus leads to pain. Thus pain is not viewed as the result of straight-through transmission of impulses from the skin to the brain. Rather, the pathway is far more complex, involving considerable opportunities for modulating the incoming pain signal by other afferent sensations and even by descending inhibiting impulses from higher centers.

In very basic terms, this gate-control theory proposes the presence of a neurophysiological mechanism in the dorsal horns of the spinal cord that serves a gatelike function, increasing or decreasing the flow and transmission of nerve impulses from peripheral fibers to the CNS. Thus sensory input is subjected to the possible modulating influence of the gate before it evokes any pain perception. It is further proposed that the degree to which this gate increases or decreases sensory transmission is determined by the relative activity in large-diameter fibers (A-beta fibers) and small-diameter fibers (A-delta and C fibers) as well as by descending efferent influences from the brain. Figure 11.1 presents a schematic of this gate-control theory.

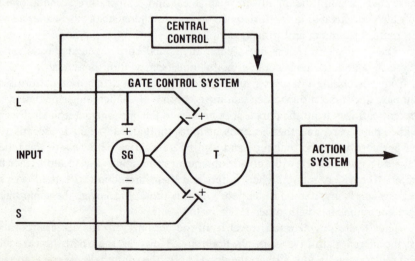

Figure 11.1   The gate-control theory of pain: (L) large-diameter fibers; (S) small-diameter fibers; (SG) spinal-gating mechanism; (T) spinal cord transmission cells.
From R. Melzack and P. D. Wall. Pain mechanisms: A new theory. *Science*, 1965, *150*, 971–979. Copyright © 1965 by the American Association for the Advancement of Science.

The following is a summary of the more specific propositions of this theory:

1. The substantia gelatinosa functions as a gate-control system that modulates the amount of input transmitted from the peripheral fibers to the dorsal horn transmission (T) cells.

2. The gate-control mechanism is influenced by the relative degree of activity in the large-diameter A-beta fibers and the small-diameter A-delta and C fibers. Activity in the large fibers closes the gate, tending to inhibit transmission; small-fiber activity opens the gate, tending to facilitate transmission.

3. This spinal-gating mechanism is influenced by efferent nerve impulses that descend from the brain. As a result, psychological processes such as anxiety, depression, attention, and past experience can exert their influence directly on the pain perception process. Melzack and Wall refer to this as the *central control mechanism*. This mechanism is assumed to play a major role in identifying sensory impulses from the periphery, assessing these signals in terms of past experience, and ultimately modulating properties of the gate-control system.

4. When the output of the spinal cord T-cells, determined by the interaction of the spinal-gating mechanism and the central control mechanism, exceeds a critical threshold level, it activates neuromechanisms that constitute the action system responsible for both pain perception and behavior.

This particular theory represented a significant advance in our conceptualization of pain. It is comprehensive enough to account for the evidence suggesting specific types of pain receptors, as well as allowing for the possibility that pain stimulation and transmission may occur in patterns of sensations. In addition, it allows for the significant role that downward CNS mediation can play in pain perception. It also partially accounts for different types of pain as well as the different effects of time variables on the pain process (Fordyce and Steger, 1979). Finally, it views pain as a complex set of phenomena rather than a simple specific or discrete entity. Of course, as our understanding of pain neurophysiology, neurotransmission, and endogenous opioids increases, a more refined model will evolve.

This theory has led to the development of a procedure for artificially stimulating the nervous system in order to relieve pain. Electrical stimulators have been developed that can be used on or beneath the surface of the skin, or implanted near the spinal cord. Electrical pulses can then be administered in the vicinity of areas where pain is reported or in the region of the major nerves serving these areas. This method is based on the assumption that electrical stimulation activates the large-diameter fibers and thereby "closes the gate." Stimulation of activity in these large fibers is believed to activate cells of the substantia gelatinosa and thus inhibit the activity of T cells that affect the action system responsible for pain response and perception. This electrical stimulation procedure often produces relief from pain both during the stimulation and for a period of time after the stimulation. It should be noted, however, that not all individuals benefit from this type of treatment; moreover, the relief from pain is usually only temporary (Long, 1976; Melzack, 1975).

NEUROCHEMICAL BASES OF PAIN

There has been an increasing amount of interest in recent years in *endorphins* and *enkephalins*—endogenous opiatelike substances that constitute a neurochemically based internal pain-regulation system. These **opioids** are produced in many parts of the brain and glands of the body, and have been implicated to play a significant role in pain reduction. The first major endogenous opioid to be clearly isolated was **enkephalin.** Since then numerous similar substances have been identified. Three basic families of these opioids are now usually considered (Akil et al., 1984): **beta-endorphin,** which produces peptides that appear to project primarily to the limbic system and brain stem; **proenkephalin,** which produces peptides that are widely distributed to the neuronal, endocrine, and central nervous systems; and **prodynor-phin,** which is distributed to the brain, gut, and the pituitary. This overall system of opioids is highly complex, with each family having a variety of forms, different potencies, and different active receptor sites.

Investigators still do not know all of the functions of the endogenous opioids and what factors are important in triggering their arousal. One possible interesting mechanism is beta-endorphin mediation of the **placebo effect** involved in the reduction of pain. In a number of painful conditions, it is commonly found that one-third of the patients experience significant relief from pain following the administration of a placebo (Beecher, 1956). The exact mechanism involved in this placebo analgesia effect is not entirely understood at this time. However, the analgesic placebo effect and the analgesia produced by active narcotics appear to have very similar effects. For example, with repeated use over a long period of time, placebo analgesia becomes less effective (i.e., tolerance develops), there is an urge to continue taking the placebo with a tendency to increase the "dosage" over time, and an abstinence-withdrawal syndrome appears when use is suddenly discontinued. Also, a placebo may partially decrease or reverse withdrawal symptoms in narcotics addicts, and individuals who react to placebos experienced significantly greater relief from postoperative pain after receiving narcotic analgesias (see Levine, Gordon, and Fields, 1978). Thus placebos appear to have a significant effect on reducing pain.

A study by Levine, Gordon, and Fields (1978) has demonstrated how beta-endorphins may be involved in this phenomenon. In this study, which was a double-blind investigation, the effects of a placebo medication and a drug called **naloxone** on postoperative dental pain (produced by a major tooth extraction) were evaluated. Naloxone is a pure opiate antagonist. It was assumed that if placebo-induced analgesia is mediated by the endogenous beta-endorphins, then naloxone, the opiate antagonist, would possibly block their effects. Three hours after surgery, half of the patients received the placebo medication; the other half of the patients received naloxone. Four hours after surgery, patients received the other medication. Patients were requested to report their degree of pain on two pain-rating scales after receiving their medications.

Results of this study indicated the following: (1) Patients given naloxone experienced, as expected, significantly greater pain than those who received the placebo. Since naloxone is an opiate antagonist, it would not be expected to reduce pain. (2) Patients administered the placebo were found to be either placebo responders whose pain was reduced or unchanged (39 percent) or placebo nonresponders whose pain increased (61 percent). It should be noted that this percentage of responders to nonresponders is similar to the one-third/two-thirds placebo responder-nonresponder percentage normally found in the research literature. (3) When naloxone was given as the second drug, it produced no additional increase in pain level in the nonresponders, but it did increase the pain levels of the placebo responders. Naloxone therefore appeared to block the beta-endorphins that were producing the pain reduction in the placebo responders. Thus the enhancement of reported pain produced by naloxone could be accounted for by its effects on placebo responders. The results from this study demonstrate that beta-endorphin release mediates placebo analgesia for dental postoperative pain. When beta-endorphins are blocked by naloxone, pain reduction no longer occurs.

Future research will hopefully delineate more clearly the variables actually involved in affecting beta-endorphin activity. Such research on these opioid substances also suggest additional mechanisms for the downward efferent pain-inhibiting mechanisms that currently are not adequately accounted for by the gate-control theory (Snyder, 1977). It also again indicates the importance of psychological processes in the pain perception process. In the next section, we shall discuss at greater length the influence of psychological processes on pain perception.

PSYCHOLOGICAL INFLUENCES ON PAIN PERCEPTION

As we have seen, the gate-control theory of pain allows for the significant role that downward CNS mediation can play in the pain perception process. There are a number of studies that demonstrate the important impact that psychological factors can exert on pain perception. Beecher (1956) was the first influential writer to emphasize the importance of the psychological status of an individual in determining his or her response to pain. His belief originally stemmed from his observation of wounded soldiers returning from battle during World War II. In a classic investigation Beecher (1956) compared the requests for pain-killing medication made by soldiers taken to combat hospitals following wounds received in combat at Anzio to those requests made by civilians with comparable surgical wounds. It was found that only 25 percent of the combat-wounded soldiers requested medication. Most of the soldiers either denied having pain from their extensive wounds or said they had so little that they did not think medication was necessary. In marked contrast, the civilians with similar wounds obtained during surgery experienced much more pain, with greater than 80 percent of these patients requesting pain medication. Beecher interpreted these results as suggesting that psychological factors such as an individual's emotional state and secondary pain/relief (most likely experienced by soldiers who were allowed to leave the aversive life-threatening combat zone because of their wounds and probably would eventually be sent home) can significantly affect the experience of pain.

There have been other studies demonstrating the importance of the psychological state of an individual on pain. For example, Sternbach (1966) has reported that pain tends to increase as the anxiety level of the individual increases. In an earlier study Hill, Kornetsky, Flanery, and Wilder (1952) demonstrated that induced-anxiety conditions were associated with higher intensities of pain than no-anxiety conditions. Another interesting finding of this study was that morphine was much more effective in decreasing pain when the patient's anxiety level was high; it had little or no effect if that individual's anxiety level was low.

Cultural and social factors have also been shown to greatly influence the perception of pain (see Weisenberg, 1977a,b). For example, Tursky and Sternbach (1967) and Sternbach and Tursky (1965) demonstrated significant differences in reactions to electric shock among ethnic groups: "Yankees" (Protestants of British descent) had a "matter of fact" orientation toward pain and assumed it was a common experience; Irish subjects tended to inhibit their pain expressions and suffering; Italians demonstrated an immediacy of pain experience and emotionally exaggerated their pain, demanding fast relief; Jews also emotionally exaggerated their pain and had great concerns about the meaning and any future implications of the pain. Christopherson (1966) also demonstrated that there are significant differences in the magnitude of pain responding to identical pain stimulation as a function of the cultural background of an individual.

These differences in attitudes and responses to pain appear to be learned. In Chapter 10 we discussed the fact that modeling or imitation learning is an important form of learning. For example, investigations of dental fears in children have demonstrated that the attitudes and feelings of a child's family toward dental treatment are important in determining that child's own anxiety toward dental treatment. In one such study it was found that children with anxious mothers showed significantly more emotionally negative behavior during a tooth extraction than did children of mothers with low anxiety (Weisenberg, 1977b).

In a rather dramatic demonstration of how pain perception and response can be modified through learning, Pavlov (1927) observed what happened when a slight change was made in the classical conditioning procedure (discussed in Chapter 10). Instead of being preceded by a bell (the conditioned stimulus), the food (the unconditioned stimulus) was preceded by an aversive stimulus such as electric shock or a skin prick. Normally such stimuli presented alone will produce a variety of negative emotional responses. What Pavlov found was that after this conditioning, the dogs failed to demonstrate any emotional response to the aversive stimuli. Instead, these dogs began perceiving these stimuli as signals that food was on the way. They actually elicited salivation and approach behaviors!

Of course, such examples do not imply that all pain is learned. The point is that our pain perceptions and responses often have a significant psychological-learning component that directly and significantly contributes to the experiences of pain. Thus psychological variables play a direct role in the pain experience. How one reacts to pain sensations is as important an issue as the specific physiological mechanisms involved in transmitting and generating pain experiences. Pain is a complex behavior and not simply a sensory effect.

PAIN BEHAVIOR

Traditionally, in attempts to describe pain the focus was only on the physiological mechanisms underlying the report of pain and not on the verbalization of the patient himself or herself. However, Hilgard (1965) has reported that verbal self-report measures of pain tend to produce significantly greater levels of stimulus discrimination and are more closely associated with variation in stimulus presentations than are specific physiological measures. Other ways of measuring pain include use of observation of "pain behaviors" such as "lying down time," sighing, grimacing, rubbing, bracing, and the like (see Follick et al., 1980; Keefe and Block, 1982). The need for standardized or "objective" indices of pain has led to the development of taxonomies of pain behavior such as the one developed by Follick et al. (1985), shown in Table 11.1. Thus reliance on strictly physiological measures rather than verbal report indices does not necessarily yield a more valid or precise measure of an individual's pain than does verbal report. Again, pain is a complex behavior and not purely a sensory event. One needs to consider multiple behavioral components in the assessment and treatment of this behavior.

ORGANIC VERSUS PSYCHOGENIC PAIN

Together with the traditional attempt to describe pain in terms of the physiological mechanisms underlying the report of pain, there was a tendency to view organic pain as one type of pain and psychogenic pain as another kind of pain. The term **psychogenic** was used to imply that the pain was due to purely psychological causes, or that it was "all in the patient's mind," or that it was not "real" pain because an organic basis for it could not be found. This is an unfortunate myth. Psychogenic pain is not experienced any differently from that pain arising from some clearly delineated injury or physical disease. Psychogenic and organic pain both hurt the same. Moreover, the diagnosis of organically caused pain does not rule out the important role that psychological variables play for any particular patient. Indeed, in our discussion of the gate-control theory of pain we saw how the experience of pain may be produced by psychological factors through the hypothesized central control trigger mechanism.

Psychological factors are important not only to the experience of pain but also to response to treatment of the pain. For example, Blumetti and Modesti (1976) found that patients suffering from intractable back pain benefited significantly less from surgical intervention techniques if they scored high on the Hysteria and Hypochondriasis scales of the MMPI. In contrast, patients scoring within normal limits on these two scales were reported to gain greater benefits from surgery. Thus emotional and psychological variables again are shown to play a significant part in pain behavior.

TABLE 11.1   Operational Definitions for the Sixteen Pain Behaviors

1. *Asymmetry*
   Imbalance of 20 degrees from vertical in posture of body alignment, improper weight bearing during movement, favoring one side.

2. *Slow Response Time*
   Latency to initiate a response greater than or equal to 5 seconds following completion of a command or prior instruction.

3. *Guarded Movement*
   Slow, cautious movement relative to baseline; nonmethodical or jerky movement.

4. *Limping*
   Irregular, antalgic gait.

5. *Bracing*
   Pronounced use of extremity on body or object for support; assists movement by leaning on or pushing off chair, wall, body, and so forth; tension or rigidity evident in weight bearing extremity.

6. *Personal Contact*
   Rubs body or presses body with palm of hand or with three or more fingers placed flatly on body.

7. *Position Shifts*
   Changes in body alignment or in distribution of body weight.

8. *Partial Movement*
   Limited range of motivation, does not complete movement. Criteria for specific movements: straight and side leg raises less than 60 degrees, trunk rotation less than 75–80 degrees, lateral side bends less than 45 degrees, sit-up less than 90 degrees from vertical, toe touch—failure to extend palm below knee.

9. *Absence of Movement*
   Does not use body part, does not bend back, back rigid, does not attempt movement.

10. *Eye Movement*
    Rolls eyes; repetitive, rapid blinking; eyes closed for greater than 1 sec.

11. *Grimacing*
    Bites lips, grits teeth, pulls back corners of mouth.

12. *Quality of Speech*
    Monotone, flat.

13. *Pain Statements*
    Statements directly relating to pain, verbalizes pain complaints, states behavior is emitted to avoid pain, discusses pain medications.

14. *Limitation Statements*
    Statements relating to disability or impairment, expresses inability, verbalizes hesitation, or questions capacity to perform tasks.

15. *Sounds*
    Any pronounced utterance that is not language—moan, groan, or grunt.

16. *Pain-relief Devices*
    Transcutaneous electrical nerve stimulation (TENS), cane, brace on leg or back, crutches, and so forth.

From M. J. Follick, D. K. Ahern, and E. W. Aberger. Development of an audiovisual taxonomy of pain behavior. *Health Psychology,* 1985, *4,* 555–568.

ACUTE VERSUS CHRONIC PAIN

Before turning to a discussion of treatment approaches to pain, we must discriminate between acute and chronic pain. Acute pain is often the result of some specific and readily identifiable tissue damage (e.g., a broken leg, surgical lesion). With this type of pain, a physician usually prescribes a specific treatment that helps relieve the pain and results in its not persisting beyond the expected period of recovery. In contrast, while chronic pain usually begins with some specific acute episode, prescribed treatments do not result in any significant reduction of the pain. Traditional medical treatment fails to solve the patient's problem, and chronicity sets in.

Fordyce and Steger (1979) noted that an additional variable differentiating acute from chronic pain concerns the type of anxiety experienced by the patient. In acute pain experiences there is usually an increase in anxiety as pain intensity increases, which is then followed by a reduction in this anxiety once treatment begins. As we discussed earlier, a reduction in anxiety generally results in a decrease in pain sensation. Thus there is a cycle of pain reduction, followed by anxiety reduction, resulting in still more pain reduction, and so on. This cycle, however, is quite different for chronic pain patients. For these patients the initial anxiety associated with the pain persists and may eventually result in the development of feelings of greater anxiety, despair, and helplessness because of the failure of the health system's attempts to alleviate it.

There is evidence to suggest that chronic-pain patients develop specific psychological problems, because of the failure of attempts to alleviate their pain, that distinguish them from acute-pain patients. Sternbach et al. (1973) compared the MMPI profiles of a group of acute low back pain patients (pain present for less than six months) with those of a group of chronic low back pain patients (more than six months). The profile patterns are presented in Figure 11.2. As can be seen, there are significant differences between the two groups on the first clinical

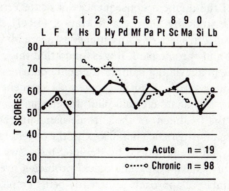

Figure 11.2 Comparisons of MMPI profiles of acute and chronic low back pain patients; major differences occurred on the first three clinical subscales: (Hs) Hysteria, (D) Depression, and (Hy) Hypochondriasis.

From R. A. Sternbach, S. R. Wolf, R. W. Murphy, and W. H. Akeson. Traits of pain patients: The low-back "loser." *Psychosomatics*, 1973, *14*, 226–229. Copyright © 1973, Academy of Psychosomatic Medicine. Reprinted by permission of the publisher.

scales (Hypochondriasis, Depression, and Hysteria). The combined elevation of these three scales is often referred to as the neurotic triad, since it is commonly found in neurotic individuals who are experiencing a great deal of anxiety. These results indicate that during the early acute stages of pain, there are not any major psychological problems produced by it. However, as the pain becomes chronic in nature, psychological changes begin to occur. These changes are most likely due to the constant discomfort, despair, and preoccupation with the pain that come to dominate the lives of these patients. As Sternbach (1974) noted in his description of chronic-pain sufferers:

> *Pain patients frequently say that they could stand their pain much better if they could only get a good night's sleep. They feel as though their resistance is weakened by their lack of sleep. They never feel rested. They feel worn down, worn out, exhausted. They find themselves getting more and more irritable with their families, they have fewer and fewer friends, and fewer and fewer interests. Gradually as time goes on, the boundaries of their world seem to shrink. They become more and more preoccupied with their pain, less and less interested in the world around them. Their world begins to center around home, doctor's office, and pharmacy. (p. 7)*

Similar results have also been found in research conducted with patients participating in a comprehensive treatment program for low back pain (to be discussed later in the chapter). Barnett (1986) found significant elevations on a variety of MMPI scales before the start of the treatment program in the chronic low back pain patients. At a six-month follow-up after successfully completing this treatment program, there was a significant *decrease* in these scales to normal levels. Thus these results suggest that the elevations of scores on psychological tests such as the MMPI seen in chronic low back pain patients are most likely due to the trauma and stress associated with their chronic condition and not due to some stable psychological traits. When successfully treated, these elevations disappear.

The importance of the different consequences of acute versus chronic pain is further illustrated by a study by Sheahy and Maurer (1974). These investigators evaluated the relative effectiveness of transcutaneous nerve stimulation as a treatment method for acute and chronic pain. It was found that this particular treatment was 80 percent effective in alleviating pain for the acute patients but only 25 percent effective for the chronic patients. Thus response to treatment is a factor that is significantly affected by this acute-chronic pain dimension.

It is obvious that the treatment of the chronic-pain sufferer will often have to deal not only with the pain experience but also with the psychological consequences such as anxiety and dysphoria produced by the long-term "wearing down" effects that produce a layer of behavioral-psychological problems over the original pain experience itself. A number of approaches currently being employed in various pain clinics have incorporated behavioral techniques to deal with such problems as part of a comprehensive treatment program. Before discussing comprehensive treatment programs for use with chronic-pain patients, we will briefly review a number of more specific therapeutic methods that have been suggested to be effective in relieving pain. As will be shown, although there is evidence for the effectiveness of some of these methods in alleviating acute pain, there is no evidence to support their effectiveness, when used alone, in significantly affecting chronic pain.

SPECIFIC PAIN TREATMENT METHODS

BIOFEEDBACK

In the last chapter we discussed biofeedback and its clinical applications. This procedure has been used with pain patients. Turk, Meichenbaum, and Berman (1979) reviewed the research literature on the application of biofeedback for the treatment of muscle tension and migraine headaches and other forms of chronic pain. They concluded that biofeedback was not found to be superior to other less expensive, less instrument-oriented treatments such as progressive muscle relaxation training and coping skills training. Moreover, the evidence for the effectiveness of biofeedback per se in reducing pain is marginal at best. The evidence rests mainly on case studies and poorly controlled research. Additional, more controlled research is greatly needed.

One problem with using biofeedback as the sole treatment is that one is in effect relying on the erroneous assumption that the etiological variables and pathophysiology of the pain to be controlled are known and can be voluntarily controlled. It is assumed that biofeedback training will provide subjects with information that will enable them to voluntarily control some aspect of their physiology that purportedly is causally linked to the pain experienced. However, as we have seen, pain is a complex behavior and not merely a pure sensory experience. One cannot expect that dealing solely with some physiological component of the pain process will totally eliminate the problem behavior. At best, it may serve as an adjunctive treatment in a comprehensive therapy regimen. Research is needed to determine for what individuals and for what types of pain biofeedback will prove to be a valuable adjunctive method. It may prove to have as its only active ingredient the ability to reduce anxiety. Indeed, Gatchel (1979) has reviewed the literature and concluded that biofeedback methods appear to be effective in reducing anxiety. Since anxiety and pain perception are closely related, biofeedback may have an impact on the pain process indirectly through reducing anxiety rather than through any pathophysiology per se. Future investigations are needed to more carefully delineate such issues.

HYPNOSIS

Hypnosis has a long history in clinical medicine. In 1843 James Braid discovered that the nervous system could be artificially induced into a state of "nervous sleep." He eventually named this state "hypnosis" after the Greek god of sleep. It was found that under this special state of sleep, individuals would be very responsive to verbal suggestions given by the hypnotist. Subsequently, during the middle and late nineteenth century, a number of prominent physicians including Hippolyte-Marie Bernheim and Jean-Martin Charcot began using hypnotism as a medical treatment. Between 1845 and 1853 James Esdaile, a Scottish surgeon working in India, performed nearly three hundred painless major operations, including amputations and cataract removals, with hypnosis as the only anesthetic.

Unfortunately, the discovery of ether and other anesthetic drugs led surgeons to prefer physical drug treatment to psychological treatment of hypnosis, even though hypnosis was shown to be equally effective and, in fact, led to fewer side effects and a lower mortality rate for many types of operations. However, hypnosis is currently experiencing a revival in clinical medicine, especially in the area of the control of pain, where traditional medical procedures have not proven to be totally effective. Currently there are numerous scientific reports documenting the effectiveness of hypnosis in alleviating pain (for reviews see Chaves and Barber, 1974; Shor, 1967). The procedure usually involves the induction of a hypnotic trance state and the suggestion of analgesia (imagining a part of the body to be numb or insensitive to pain). Relief from pain by hypnosis has been noted in the areas of obstetrics, surgery, dentistry, and even cancer treatment (Hilgard and Hilgard, 1975). For example, the use of hypnosis during childbirth has many benefits. In addition to reducing or totally eliminating the pain of labor and delivery, it can also reduce later back pain and facilitate rapid recovery. It has the added benefit of eliminating the possible negative effects of anesthesia on the newborn. One obstetrician successfully used hypnosis as the sole form of anesthesia in 814 out of 1,000 deliveries, including some caesarian deliveries (Hilgard and Hilgard, 1975). In the area of dentistry, Barber (1977) has reported the successful use of hypnosis as the sole source of anesthesia in dental procedures on 99 out of 100 patients, many involving extractions. Even with terminal cancer intense pain can be brought under patient's control so that they no longer have to depend heavily on morphine during the last phases of their lives (Sacerdote, 1966).

Hilgard (1975) concludes that there now is more than sufficient evidence demonstrating the usefulness of hypnosis in treating pain conditions. He does not propose that hypnosis be viewed as an alternative to chemical analgesics and anesthetics. However, it is a useful supplement in many cases where the anesthetics may be dangerous or where the patient is excessively anxious. It is a method that may prove beneficial on a short-term basis with many patients who are experiencing pain.

ACUPUNCTURE

Acupuncture, which originated in ancient China some two thousand years ago, was initially based on the theory that the vital organs of the body were connected through tubular systems or "meridians" that radiated underneath the skin. It was believed that life energy or *chi'i* flowed through these meridians; either an excess or a deficit of this life energy was believed to produce disease and pain. It was assumed that the insertion of needles into critical points along the meridian would correct the imbalance in the life energy. Not surprisingly, there has been no experimental support for this "meridian theory." Even the Chinese no longer consider it to be a reasonable explanation for the effectiveness of acupuncture therapy.

How does acupuncture actually work? Although there is still no clear understanding of the process, many believe some psychological mechanism is involved. Taub (1976) noted that in China the psychological state of the patient is taken into very serious consideration in determining who will and who will not receive acupuncture as a surgical anesthetic. Furthermore, Katz et al. (1974) reported that pain patients who benefit most from acupuncture are also highly hypnotizable. However, these authors do not believe that acupuncture and hypnosis operate through identical mechanisms, since the observable behaviors of patients undergoing hypnosis and acupuncture differ so markedly. The hypnotized patient is unresponsive to everything in the immediate environment, paying almost all attention to the hypnotist and suggestions to ignore the pain. The acupuncture patient, in contrast, is in complete contact with the environment and is totally aware of everything as treatment is being administered. Patients who have received both acupuncture and hypnosis have reported that they feel the two are totally different techniques. Thus, although there appears to be a relationship between hypnotizability and the effectiveness of acupuncture, the reason for the relationship is not known. Bakal (1979) suggests that possibly both acupuncture and hypnosis succeed in "closing the gating mechanism" in susceptible patients, but acupuncture exerts its effects primarily through one mechanism and hypnosis through another.

In support of the notion that acupuncture and hypnosis operate through different mechanisms, Mayer et al. (1976) conducted a study in which they compared the degree to which injections of the narcotic-antagonist drug naloxone reduced the analgesia provided through acupuncture and hypnosis. In this study experimental pain was induced by electrical stimulation of a tooth. One group of subjects was administered hypnosis, and the other group acupuncture. Pain estimates were then obtained. It was found that acupuncture increased the pain thresholds (i.e., the level of electrical stimulation perceived as painful) by 27 percent, whereas hypnosis increased pain thresholds by 85 percent. Thus hypnosis was found to be more effective than acupuncture for the induction of analgesia to the painful electrical stimulation. It was further found that following the subsequent injections of naloxone, the pain threshold of the acupuncture group fell drastically; naloxone had no effect on the pain threshold of the hypnosis group. The investigators therefore conclude that acupuncture probably achieves its effects by causing the release of endogenous opiatelike substances from central and periaqueductal gray matter (which the drug naloxone blocks). Hypnosis most likely achieves its analgesic effects through some higher cortical mechanisms.

In a more recent study Kiser et al. (1983) evaluated twenty patients with chronic pain syndrome of at least six months' duration who underwent nine sessions of acupuncture. Besides evaluating a host of psychological measures, blood samples were taken immediately before and after the acupuncture treatment regimen and radioimmunoassayed for two endorphins: beta-endorphin and met-enkephalin levels. Results indicated that this treatment resulted in significant improvement of both pain and psychiatric symptoms and *higher* plasma concentrations of met-enkephalin. Plasma beta-endorphin concentrations were unchanged. Moreover, the degree of symptom relief was highly correlated with degree of increase in plasma met-enkephalin. Thus these results again indicate that acupuncture relief of pain involves enhanced endorphin function.

Is acupuncture effective in reducing pain? Although additional evidence is needed, it appears that this technique is capable of producing some short-term anesthesia and analgesia, but it is not a proven technique for treating more chronic and persistent complaints of pain (Bakal, 1979). Levine, Gormley, and Fields (1976) evaluated the analgesic effects on patients with chronic pain (pain persisting for more than six months) associated with objective evidence of nerve damage and patients with chronic pain without evidence of nerve damage. It was found that for both types of chronic pain, the majority of patients, although demonstrating some initial relief from pain, eventually reported that the pain returned to pretreatment levels. Moreover, all patients eventually requested the termination of the acupuncture treatment. Other investigators have also reported that pain relief following acupuncture treatment tends to be short-lived (Murphy, 1976). Thus, like hypnosis, acupuncture may be beneficial for short-term relief of pain. However, it should not be viewed as an alternative to other forms of treatment for chronic pain.

COGNITIVE STRATEGIES

In recent years there has been a great increase in the use of cognitive strategies for the management of pain (Weisenberg, 1977a). Although many of these cognitive strategies have shown an ability to significantly modify the perception of experimentally induced pain, there have been only a few studies directly evaluating clinical pain. Moreover, of those studies of actual clinical pain, most have examined acute rather than chronic pain. Thus, although a number of cognitive strategies have shown promising results, one must avoid overgeneralizing from such studies. A great deal of additional investigation is needed to evaluate the effectiveness of these cognitive pain control procedures in dealing with clinical pain, especially of the chronic type.

In a clinical study of pain, Horan, Layng, and Pursell (1976) reported that those patients who were trained to engage in positive imagery (e.g., imagine that they were walking through a lush meadow or swimming in a clear blue lake) reported less discomfort and pain during dental treatment than patients who were administered no special training or who were instructed to visualize a series of two-digit numbers. Relatedly, Langer, Janis, and Wolfer (1975) found that patients who were instructed to selectively attend to the positive aspects of their hospitalization (e.g., relief from work responsibilities and stress) requested less analgesic pain medication for post-surgery pain than did patients who were merely given presurgery information.

In studies of experimentally induced pain, Barber and colleagues (Barber and Cooper, 1972; Chaves and Barber, 1974) also evaluated the cognitive strategy of distracting imagery. They trained subjects to use distracting imagery, such as imagining pleasant events, counting aloud, and attending to other stimuli in the environment (such as counting ceiling tiles). Subjects were also taught to attend selectively to ongoing sensations other than pain. For example, they were trained to imagine that the stimulated area was asleep or insensitive, or that it had been injected with novocaine. It was found that these cognitive strategies were effective in increasing the pain tolerance of subjects. Thus these results demonstrate that the performance of a variety of cognitive tasks in some way directs the subjects' attention away from the painful sensations. As subjects attend to stimuli that are unrelated to the pain, their tolerance for pain increases.

Meichenbaum and Turk (1976) have suggested the use of a "cafeteria style" approach to pain management. In their program, a form of **stress-inoculation training,** the individual is taught a variety of cognitive control strategies of the type just discussed, from which he or she may select when confronted with a painful stimulus. The individuals are also assisted in developing a plan to use when the pain becomes the most intense and are instructed to implement the plan at these critical moments. Such an approach shows promise in helping individuals better cope with their pain. However, as we noted at the beginning of this section, research is greatly needed to evaluate the effectiveness of such procedures in dealing with chronic clinical pain.

THE PAIN CLINIC: THE USE OF A COMPREHENSIVE OPERANT TREATMENT PROGRAM

As indicated by Fordyce and Steger (1979), the general inpatient strategies generally employed in pain clinics can be divided into two basic types: (1) "pure" operant or behavioral treatment programs in which reinforcement procedures for "well behavior" are the major components in treatment, and (2) "mixed" behavioral and other treatment programs in which treatment involves strategies other than reinforcement for "well behavior," such as group discussion with other patients, biofeedback techniques for relaxation and placebo, and family therapy that is not related to pain behavior management. The prototype of the "pure" operant pain treatment program was developed at the University of Washington Department of Rehabilitation Medicine by Fordyce and colleagues (Fordyce et al., 1968). This program involved a four- to eight-week inpatient period designed to gradually increase the general activity level and socialization of the patient and to decrease medication usage. The program is based on the assumption that, although pain may initially result from some underlying organic pathology, environmental consequences (such as attention of the patient's family and the rehabilitation staff) can modify and further maintain various aspects of "pain behavior," such as complaining, grimacing, slow and cautious body movements, requesting pain medication, and so on. Viewing pain as an operant behavior, Fordyce assumes that consequences, such as concern and attention from others, rest, medication, and avoidance of unpleasant responsibilities and duties, frequently reinforce the maladaptive pain behavior and hinder the patient's progress in treatment.

In their treatment program Fordyce and colleagues systematically controlled environmental events (e.g., attention, rest, medication) and made them contingent on adaptive behaviors. A major goal of the program is to increase behaviors such as participation in therapy and activity level while concomitantly decreasing or eliminating pain behaviors. Members of the patient's family are actively involved in the treatment program and work closely with the rehabilitation staff. They are taught to react to the patient's behavior in a manner that will reduce pain and to maximize the patient's compliance with, and performance in, the rehabilitation program. Through this operant approach the patient is taught to reinterpret the sensation of pain and tolerate it, while performing more adaptive behaviors that will gain the attention and approval of others. Such a program is initially conducted in the hospital and later continued on an outpatient basis.

An important feature of this program is the reduction in the amount of pain medication used by chronic-pain patients. This reduces the possibility of addiction and habituation to the analgesic medication and reduces the patient's general dependence on drugs. Often medication is provided on a p.r.n., or as needed, basis. Unfortunately, the medication is then contingent on the very pain behavior the rehabilitation staff would like to decrease (complaints of pain, requesting medication, etc.). Such a system may therefore increase various pain behaviors. In order to avoid this problem, the delivery of medication may be made contingent on the passage of time rather than the patient's pain behavior. The intervals between pain medication delivery are then gradually increased during the treatment program. Also, the medication itself may be presented to the patient in the form of a liquid that masks the color and taste of the medication (such as cherry syrup or Robitussin). Over a period of approximately two months, the dosage level of the medication in this "cocktail" is gradually decreased until the patient is given only the masking liquid without an active ingredient. The patient and his or her family are informed of this medication reduction procedure either before or after the medication has been eliminated.

This comprehensive program has been shown to produce significant decreases in the patient's complaints of pain and in the use of analgesic medication (see Fordyce and Steger, 1979). The following case history illustrates the type of individual for whom this operant procedure has been found to be effective:

> *Mrs. Y is a 37-year-old white administrator. Since 1948, approximately one year after her marriage, she had had virtually constant low-back pain, and had been decreasingly able to carry out normal homemaking activities. At the time of admission to the hospital, she complained of a continuous period of activity without an interval of reclining rest as approximately 20 minutes. Her husband reported she was active in the home an average of less than two hours daily. The remainder of her time was spent reclining; either reading, watching television, or sleeping. During Mrs. Y's 18-year history of back pain, she had undergone four major surgical procedures including removal of a herniated disc and a lumbosacral spine fusion. At the time of admission, Mrs. Y was taking four or five habit-forming analgesic tablets per day when she experienced pain. Physical and radiologic examination revealed a stable spine at the fusion site, with no evidence of neurologic deficit. (Fordyce et al., 1968, pp. 183–184)*

At the end of treatment the patient was able to walk almost one mile every day. (See Figure 11.3.) She was also actively participating in occupational therapy for approximately two hours a day. The narcotic component of the pain medication had been completely eliminated and her pain complaints had been virtually eliminated. Monthly follow-up visits on an outpatient basis indicated that she continued to increase her weekly activity level.

It is currently not known whether the long-term utilization of pain-incompatible behaviors as employed in these operant procedures will lead to a complete disappearance of pain. Patients may only be learning to avoid attending to and complaining about their pain. Indeed, the available data indicate that patients generally demonstrate only a certain degree of relief from their pretreatment pain levels following

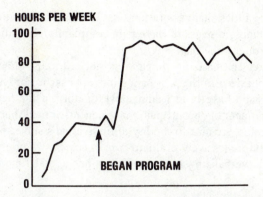

Figure 11.3   Changes in the total hours of activity per week for Mrs. Y during the course of treatment. Reprinted with permission from W. E. Fordyce, R. S. Fowler, J. R. Lehmann, and B. J. DeLateur. Some implications of learning in problems of chronic pain. *Journal of Chronic Diseases,* 1968, *21,* 179–190. Copyright © 1968, Pergamon Press, Ltd.

this behavioral intervention (Bakal, 1979). However, even if such procedures do not totally eliminate pain, they do make a significant difference between unbearable and bearable pain and between an unproductive, sedentary existence and a relatively normal life.

"FUNCTIONAL RESTORATION": A SPORTS MEDICINE APPROACH TO CHRONIC LOW BACK PAIN

In recent years there has been a newer and even more comprehensive behavioral approach to chronic low back pain termed functional restoration. The term **functional restoration** refers not merely to a treatment methodology for chronic low back pain but to a wider conceptualization of the entire problem, its diagnosis and management. Rather than accepting current limits in history-taking based solely through patients' self-report of pain and diagnosis through skeletal imaging technology, the methodology involves reliance on more objective information. Structured interviews and quantified self-report measures provide problem-oriented information for patient management. Moreover, objective assessment of physical capacity and effort, with comparison to a normative data base, add a new dimension to diagnosis. In keeping with a sports medicine philosophy, this permits the development of treatment programs of varied intensity and duration aimed primarily at restoring physical functional capacity and social performance. The previous goals of merely attempting to alter pain complaints, decreasing medications, and "improving the quality of life" are greatly enlarged by a focus on the vast societal problems associated with low back pain. This attention to realistic goals such as return to work and decreased use of the medical system increasingly has become the focus of treatment programs.

By no means, though, is self-reported pain ignored in this approach. Rather, such self-report data are interpreted only in the context of *overall* functioning. Adaptive, positive functioning is sometimes initially associated with an increase in pain complaints. Indeed, the phrase "no pain-no gain" is appropriately stressed to patients undergoing functional restoration. Rather than terminating and delaying further physical training because of these pain complaints, the patient may have to learn to "work through" the pain.

This orientation emphasizing *function* is not a totally radical or new one. Indeed, it was emphasized in the past pain clinic approach. Fordyce, Roberts, and Sternbach (1985), who have been leading investigators in the field of behavioral assessment and treatment of chronic pain, have cogently noted that it is not enough to simply evaluate and attempt to modify an individual's subjective experience of pain. One must comprehensively evaluate *pain behavior,* which involves not only what the patient is verbalizing but also his or her actual functioning. As they emphasize:

> . . . *behavioral methods for treating pain problems (chronic pain behaviorals) are not intended to "treat pain" in the traditional sense in which this implies directing attention to sources and mechanisms of noxious stimuli generating injury signals which lead to "pain." Behavioral pain methods do* not *have as their principal objective the modification of nociception, nor the direct modification of the experience of pain, although it very frequently happens that both are influenced by these methods. Rather,* behavioral methods *in pain treatment programs* are intended to treat excess disability and expressions of suffering . . . *The goal is to render chronic pain patients functional again and as normal in behavior as possible. (p. 115)*

Indeed, these investigators note that one of the major problems with past treatment and theoretical approaches to chronic pain, including some alleged behavioral ones, was that they focused too greatly on merely the subjective experience of pain. A distinction needs to be made between "pain" (the subjective experience) and **pain behavior,** or behavioral functioning. This is an extremely important point: The scientific literature tends to support the fact that the most appropriate goal is to modify excessive disability by focusing on *function.* The subjective component of pain (however it is assessed) also is often concurrently changed when functioning is changed. However, it has been found that there usually will be no major change in the subjective expression of "pain" without an improvement in functional activity and disability. This is the hallmark of the functional restoration approach. *One must focus on observable and objectively evaluated functioning along with self-report in order to comprehensively assess chronic pain behavior.*

The success of this functional restoration approach has been carefully documented in a number of recent studies involving the senior author (Mayer et al., 1985; Mayer et al., 1987). For example, in a recently completed two-year follow-up study of patients administered the functional restoration program (Mayer et al., 1987), significant changes in a number of important realistic outcome measures were found. At the follow-up, 87 percent of the treatment group was actively working as compared to only 41 percent of a nontreatment comparison group. Moreover, about twice as many of the comparison group patients had both additional spine surgery and unsettled worker's compensation litigation relative to the treatment group. The comparison group continued with approximately a five-times higher rate of patient visits to health professionals, and had higher rates of recurrence or reinjury. Finally, the treatment group also had significant improvements in self-report measures and physical function measures such as back strength and range of motion. Thus the results demonstrate the striking impact that a functional restoration program can have on these important outcome measures.

SUMMARY

Pain is an extremely common complaint in medical settings. Traditional medical treatments have frequently proven ineffective because pain is a complex phenomenon that involves not only physiological sensations and mechanisms but also significant behavioral/psychological components. Therefore, a model of pain that integrates both physiological and psychological components has the best chance of allowing a comprehensive understanding of the pain process. The gate-control theory of pain proposed by Melzack and Wall is an early example of such a model. There has also been intense interest in recent years in the role of endogenous opiate-like substances that constitute a neurochemically-based pain-regulation system. We briefly discussed the physiology of pain as well as the psychological influences such as anxiety and sociocultural learning factors on pain perception. This has led to an emphasis on the assessment of pain behavior, and not just the physiological components of pain. We must consider pain in the same manner as any other form of complex behavior, consisting of multiple behavioral components.

A number of specific pain treatment methods were discussed, including biofeedback, hypnosis, acupuncture, and cognitive strategies. Although there is evidence that these techniques are somewhat effective in reducing acute pain, they should be viewed merely as adjunctive treatment methods in a more comprehensive therapy regimen. The initial prototype of the operant pain treatment clinic developed by Fordyce and colleagues is an example of a comprehensive treatment approach to pain management. We also discussed the functional restoration approach to the treatment of pain, which incorporates return to work and reduced use of the health-care system as primary goals of treatment.

RECOMMENDED READINGS

Akil, H., Watson, S. J., Young, E., Lewis, M. E., Khachaturian, H. and Walker, J. M. Endogenous opioids: Biology and function. *Annual Review of Neuroscience,* 1984, *7,* 223–255.

Fordyce, W. E., and Steger, J. C. Chronic pain. In O. F. Pomerleau and J. P. Brady (Eds.), *Behavioral medicine: Theory and practice.* Baltimore: Williams & Wilkins, 1979.

Hilgard, E. R., and Hilgard, J. R. *Hypnosis in the relief of pain.* Los Altos, Calif.: William Kaufmann, 1975.

Turk, D. C., Meichenbaum, D. H., and Berman, W. H. Application of biofeedback for the regulation of pain: A critical review. *Psychological Bulletin,* 1979, *86,* 1322–1338.

Weisenberg, M. Pain and pain control. *Psychological Bulletin,* 1977, *84,* 1004–1008.

12

APPETITIVE BEHAVIORS: OBESITY, ALCOHOLISM, AND SMOKING

|||||||||||||||||||||||||||||||||||||||||||||||||||||||||||||||||||||||||||||||||||||||||||||||||||||||||||||||||||||

In this chapter we shall discuss three common appetitive problem behaviors that have significant health consequences and for which behavioral analysis and treatment techniques have been systematically employed and evaluated—obesity, problem drinking/alcoholism, and smoking. They represent areas in which health psychology has had a significant and practical impact on public health. Obesity was chosen because it occupies a central position in the area of behavioral medicine. It was one of the first major medical concerns to be successfully subjected to systematic behavioral analysis and treatment. Alcoholism was selected because it is a major national public health problem. There have been some encouraging efforts recently by behaviorally oriented investigators to better understand this problem behavior and develop possible methods of treatment. Smoking, too, is a major health problem that has received a great deal of behavioral research attention.

OBESITY

Obesity has become an important area of study in health psychology because it is a highly prevalent, chronic condition that is directly or indirectly associated with medical disorders such as hypertension, diabetes, and certain cancers (Powers, 1980). Although the relationships between obesity and certain health risks are not simple and linear ones (Andres, 1980), being overweight is a socially stigmatized condition. Many people want to lose weight, and many who are overweight feel bad about themselves.

As Stunkard (1979) has suggested, the area of obesity occupies a central position in the field of behavioral medicine because, historically, it was one of the first major health concerns dealt with by use of behavioral principles. Currently, more individuals are receiving some form of behavioral treatment for obesity than are receiving such treatment for all other types of conditions combined. Behavioral scientists have been interested not only in the treatment of obesity but also in developing a better understanding of the psychological mechanisms involved in the problem of food regulation. We will discuss these two interrelated areas.

ETIOLOGY OF OBESITY

Obesity is a complex phenomenon with biological, social, and psychological variables involved in its causes and consequences (Rodin, 1981). Despite extensive research, there are still large gaps in knowledge concerning the biological and behavioral factors that cause obesity. As a result, relatively little of the research on the etiology of obesity has, as yet, been translated into specific treatment techniques. Research on biological causes of obesity has considered the role of particular brain centers (e.g., in the hypothalamus) and certain hormones that are involved in eating behavior and hunger regulation (Rodin, 1981). Explanations for obesity have also been based on the notion of *set point,* that is, the concept that the body regulates its weight to maintain a certain amount of body fat (Nisbett, 1972). In addition, research has also considered that weight regulation is based on the number and size of fat cells or adipocytes. In this regard, it appears that the number of fat cells is determined by genetics or early nutrition (Hirsch and Knittle, 1970; Faust, 1980), and once an individual matures past childhood, the number of fat cells is determined and impossible to decrease. Therefore, whenever possible, it is important to prevent childhood obesity and the increased number of fat cells that results, because the individual may then live with a weight problem for the rest of his or her life.

The important contribution of genetic factors to obesity is illustrated by a recent adoption study by Albert Stunkard and colleagues (Stunkard et al., 1986). By examining relationships between parents and adoptees reared apart or in the same family, they found a sizeable relation between body weight of adoptees and their biological parents, and little relationship between weight status of offspring and their adopted parents. Thus obesity could be substantially predicted as a result of genetic factors, regardless of the familial environmental circumstances.

However, the role of genetic factors in determining obesity and body weight does not negate or trivialize the significant effect that social factors, such as cultural norms and attitudes toward thinness, play in determining body weight. For example, the Midtown Manhattan Study surveyed a large number of individuals in New York City and found an inverse relationship between the prevalence of obesity and socioeconomic status, with lower class individuals more likely to be overweight (Stunkard, 1975). In addition, this study found that the longer an individual's family had been in the United States, the less likely they were to be obese. Thus, obesity becomes less common as individuals become acculturated to the American norm disapproving of overweight.

PSYCHOLOGICAL ASPECTS OF FOOD REGULATION

Stanley Schachter conducted some of the earliest and most systematic research on psychological aspects of food regulation in humans. His research was prompted by the observation that obese individuals did not appear to regulate their eating behavior according to internal physiological needs. Schachter's (1968, 1971) initial research on obesity was stimulated by the results of a study reported by Stunkard

(1959). In this investigation obese and nonobese women who were patients in a medical clinic were requested to swallow a gastric balloon that allowed the measurement of gastric motility (gastric motility is a measure that is frequently used as an internal physiological cue or index of hunger). Each subject was then asked whether or not she was hungry and was requested to answer simply yes or no. The obese women reported being hungry significantly *less often* than the nonobese women. This difference was found to be largely accounted for by the fact that the nonobese women usually reported hunger during periods of gastric motility, while obese subjects reported no hunger during these periods. Thus the obese appeared to be insensitive to the internal cues of gastric motility.

Stunkard (1959) and others (e.g., Krantz, 1978) have interpreted these results as suggesting that, because of the social stigma associated with being obese in our society, the obese women may have been overly self-conscious and reluctant to admit they were hungry. However, Schachter (1971) noted: "For the obese . . . there is little correspondence between gastric motility (i.e., stomach contractions) and self-reports of hunger. Whether or not the obese subject describes himself as hungry seems to have almost nothing to do with the state of his gut" (p. 129). Schachter (1971) interpreted these findings as suggesting that obese persons are generally less responsive than nonobese individuals to internal physiological cues of hunger (stomach contractions) and more responsive to external environmental food cues such as the smell or sight of food. This concept of "external responsiveness" was assessed by Schachter and his colleagues in a number of experiments evaluating whether the obese regulate food intake as well as normals.

In one such experiment Schachter, Goldman, and Gordon (1968) recruited a group of obese and a group of nonobese subjects and requested that they have lunch or dinner prior to reporting to the experiment (which was advertised as a study of taste preferences). Immediately before the experimental procedure, half of the subjects in each group were fed roast beef sandwiches; the other half of the subjects were given nothing to eat. This experimental manipulation was a means of varying internal physiological cues of hunger. The subjects who were fed would obviously have fewer physiological cues of hunger, whereas such cues would remain and even increase in those subjects who were not fed.

All subjects were then requested to evaluate the taste characteristics of different types of crackers that were available in great abundance. Subjects were urged to sample as many or as few of the various crackers as they wished in making their judgments. This was to ensure that no subjects would feel inhibited to sample the crackers. The major dependent measure assessed was the number of crackers eaten by each subject. The results, presented in Figure 12.1, demonstrated that normal nonobese subjects ate significantly more crackers when their stomachs were empty than when they were full. In contrast, the fact that obese subjects were "preloaded" with roast beef sandwiches did not reduce the number of crackers they ate. They consumed as many as the obese subjects who were not initially fed the sandwiches.

A number of other studies have reported that the amounts of food eaten by obese individuals and their self-reports of hunger do not covary with food deprivation (Pliner, 1974; Schachter, 1971). Several other studies of fasting behavior have also

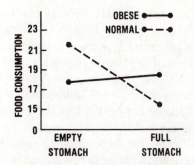

Figure 12.1   The effects of "preloading" with roast beef sandwiches on the number of crackers eaten by normal and obese subjects. The normal subjects, unlike the obese subjects, ate considerably more crackers when their stomachs were empty than when they were full.
From S. Schachter. *Emotion, Obesity, and Crime.* New York: Academic Press, 1971.

suggested that obese persons are relatively insensitive to the physiological concomitants of food deprivation.

Research also indicates that food intake of obese individuals is influenced by external factors (presence or absence of readily available food) significantly more than the food intake of normals (Decke, 1971; Nisbett, 1968). This concept of external responsiveness associated with obese individuals has been shown to be related also to other behaviors such as time perception (Pliner, 1973) and reactions to emotional stimuli (Rodin, Elman, and Schachter, 1974). Rodin (1977) and Schachter and Rodin (1974) have reviewed much of this research. These results indicate that overweight persons are significantly affected by external stimuli—not only those relevant to food but other stimuli as well, such as emotionally arousing events. They appear to be more **stimulus-bound,** being constrained and affected more than normals by stimuli in their immediate environment (e.g., distracted on proof-reading and reaction-time tasks by the emotional stimuli presented). Schachter and colleagues view this as a general personality trait or response style commonly found in the obese.

Schachter and his associates have speculated that the greater propensity toward external responsiveness and stimulus-bound behavior may be explained at the physiological level as due to the possibility that the ventromedial hypothalamus (VMH) portion of the brain may be functioning differently in obese and nonobese individuals. They base this speculation on certain similarities between VMH-lesioned animals and the obese human.

The ventromedial portion of the hypothalamus was isolated by Hetherington and Ransom (1940) as the main area involved in hunger control and regulation. In studies with animals it was shown that damage of this area caused extreme obesity. When lesions were made in rats' ventromedial hypothalami, the rats ate huge amounts of food, which increased their body weights to two or three times the normal level. This condition is termed **hyperphagia.** Such findings prompted researchers to speculate that this portion of the hypothalamus functions as a "satiation center." If this area is damaged, the animal can no longer detect satiation and will thus overeat.

In noting similarities between VMH-lesioned animals and the obese human, Schachter and Rodin (1974) wrote: ". . . Both the VMH-lesioned rat and the obese human appear to share a pattern of hyposensitivity to the internal or physiological cues associated with eating and hypersensitivity to the external cues associated with food proper" (p. 2). They go on to review a number of other striking similarities between the two that strongly implicate VMH functioning in the production of these differences. Thus hypothalamic misregulation may be involved in obesity in some humans. However, at present care must be taken in drawing any firm conclusions on the basis of these similarities. Future research is needed to more clearly delineate the precise biological mechanisms that may be involved in various differences found between obese and nonobese individuals.

It should be pointed out that a number of studies challenged Schachter's view of obesity and have failed to find these obese-normal differences in responsiveness to external cues (e.g., Nisbett and Temoshok, 1976; Rodin and Slochower, 1976). Several reasons have been offered to explain these equivocal results. An especially cogent argument is that the early studies primarily used populations such as college students and selected out moderately obese subjects from these. The average degree of obesity drawn from such a population was rather small. Indeed, Rodin (1978) noted that the very obese are different from the moderately obese in responsiveness to external cues: the very obese do not seem to attend to them as much. Thus among the obese there appear to be individual differences in degree of obesity and external-internal responsiveness. Future studies will have to take such differences into account. This is related to the general problem of defining obesity. How many pounds over normal weight should be considered as defining obesity? Also, if an obese person loses weight, can his or her responsiveness to external cues be expected to change completely? Such issues need to be carefully considered in research of this type.

In addition, more recent studies suggest that external responsiveness may be more a function of dieting than of obesity per se (Herman and Polivy, 1980; Rodin, 1981). In a series of studies (Herman and Polivy, 1980) it was noted that subjects who indicated that they regularly exerted efforts to diet and control their food intake behaved as though they were externally responsive—regardless of whether they were obese or normal weight. Such weight control efforts were called **dietary restraint,** and the health and behavioral consequences of dieting have become an area of study in health psychology.

BEHAVIORAL TREATMENT OF OBESITY

Ferster, Nurnberger, and Levitt (1962) produced the earliest systematic report of the behavioral analysis and treatment of eating behavior. Although the therapeutic results of this program were never published and were thought to have been only modest (Stunkard, 1975), the report did stimulate subsequent research on the application of operant conditioning techniques to the treatment of obesity.

A classic report by Stuart (1967) was a hallmark study responsible for the widespread investigation and subsequent use of behavioral treatment of obesity. In Stuart's (1967) program, mentioned in Chapter 10, the principle of stimulus control was employed in the treatment of obesity. The reader will recall that operant psychologists such as Ferster and Skinner view the majority of behavior as under stimulus control—that is, under the control of environmental stimuli events. Behavior is thus viewed as a function of external events. Stuart's program consisted of gradually restricting and eliminating stimuli that had come to elicit the maladaptive eating behavior. For example, the program involved guidelines such as restricting eating to specified times and places; not eating while engaged in other enjoyable activities such as watching television, listening to the radio, and so on; ridding the house of fattening foods; avoiding passing a restaurant or going grocery shopping when hungry. Using this stimulus control approach, Stuart's program produced remarkable success. At one-year follow-up, clients in the program had lost from twenty-six to forty-six pounds. Although weight losses of this magnitude have not been consistently found in studies conducted since Stuart's initial report, the behavioral treatment of obesity has been found, on the whole, to be effective (Stunkard, 1979).

In Chapter 10 we also reviewed the behavioral treatment study by Mahoney, Moura, and Wade (1973) in which principles of positive reinforcement were employed in helping individuals gain self-control over eating. The reader is referred to work by Ferguson (1975), Mahoney and Mahoney (1976), and Stunkard and Mahoney (1976) for a more detailed description of specific behavioral treatment methods.

In passing it should be noted that stimulus control approaches such as that employed by Stuart fit well with the concept of external responsiveness to food cues found by Schachter and colleagues to be associated with obese individuals. In a sense, external responsiveness is dealt with in these operant-behavioral programs by restricting eating to appropriate times and places and eliminating eating cues from the environment.

Through the years research designs have been refined to rule out the effect of nonspecific treatment and placebo factors in weight-reduction programs. One such noteworthy study was that conducted by Wollersheim (1970). We will briefly review this study in order to illustrate the quality of many treatment-evaluation studies.

Wollersheim's study involved the assessment of four experimental conditions: (1) behavioral treatment; (2) nonspecific therapy based on traditional psychotherapy techniques; (3) social pressure, modeled after lay weight-control programs using group support and pressure; and (4) a no-treatment control group.

Groups 2 and 3 were included to control for the nonspecific placebo effects produced by attention and interest that might be created by any form of treatment. In order to control for possible therapist effects, the four therapists employed in the study each treated a different group of five patients in each of the three treatment groups. Treatment consisted of ten sessions over a three-month period. Results of this study are presented in Figure 12.2. As can be seen, at the end of the treatment, as well as at an eight-week follow-up, subjects in the behavioral treatment group had lost significantly more weight than those in the no-treatment group. Moreover, they had lost significantly more weight than those in the other two treatment groups (who, in turn, lost more weight than no-treatment-group subjects). Thus the change produced by behavioral treatment was greater than the usual effects of treatment, as represented by changes in groups 2 and 3.

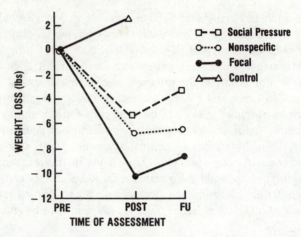

Figure 12.2   Mean weight loss of the focal (behavioral) treatment group, the two alternative treatment control groups, and the no-treatment control group.
From J. P. Wollersheim. Effectiveness of group therapy based upon learning principles in the treatment of overweight women. *Journal of Abnormal Psychology,* 1970, *76,* 462–474. Copyright © 1970 by the American Psychological Association. Reprinted by permission of the author.

Not only did behavioral treatment produce the greatest weight loss, it also produced the greatest changes in self-reports related to eating behavior. Compared to the other three groups, the behavioral treatment group showed significantly more improvement on four of six factors assessed by a questionnaire: "emotional and uncontrolled eating," "eating in isolation," "eating as a reward," and "between-meal eating."

APPLICATION OF BEHAVIORAL TREATMENT TO LARGE GROUPS

It is estimated that approximately 400,000 people in the United States are exposed each week to behavioral methods for the control of obesity administered through commercial clinics. Unfortunately, there has not been much controlled research of these programs. The first attempt at a controlled assessment of behavioral methods with a large group was conducted in collaboration with TOPS (Take Off Pounds Sensibly). TOPS is a thirty-year-old self-help group for obesity consisting of over 12,000 chapters throughout the United States with over 300,000 members. Levitz and Stunkard (1974) evaluated 298 female members of sixteen TOPS chapters in Philadelphia. Four treatment conditions were administered over a twelve-week period (each consisting of four matched TOPS chapters): (1) behavior modification administered by psychiatrists; (2) behavior modification administered by TOPS chapter leaders (who were laypersons); (3) nutrition education administered by TOPS chapter leaders; or (4) continuation of the standard TOPS program.

Results of the study demonstrated that the two behavior modification groups produced significantly more weight loss than did the other two groups, both at the end of treatment and at a one-year follow-up. Moreover, the dropout rate of the two behavior modification groups was lower during treatment, and significantly lower one year later, than that of the other two groups. Thus at follow-up 39.5 percent of subjects who received behavior modification had dropped out of the chapters, compared to 55 percent in the nutrition education group and 67 percent in the standard TOPS program group. This differential attrition rate, which biases against the behavior modification groups, makes the weight loss results even more impressive.

More recently, Hall and Hall (1982) reviewed seven large-scale uncontrolled clinical series that used behavioral treatment methods to produce weight loss. Results were somewhat different depending on whether "live-in" or community clinics were evaluated. In the live-in clinics, the percentage of patients falling into a twenty- to forty-pound weight-loss category surpassed the clinical figures originally reported by Stunkard and McClaren-Hume (1958). The latter study, which reviewed approximately 1,400 clinical cases (in which patients were provided with a variety of treatments including low-calorie diets, psychotherapy, chemotherapy, and various combinations), is often used as a "benchmark" against which other statistics are compared. This classic study found that only 25 percent of patients were able to lose as much as twenty pounds and only 5 percent lost as much as forty pounds. The losses at the live-in clinics reported by Hall and Hall (1982) surpassed this. In terms of outpatient clinics, the outcomes were not as impressive—only near or slightly below the Stunkard and McClaren-Hume statistics. As Hall and Hall (1982) note, however, in summarizing these results, the low dropout rates and absence of negative side effects and therapy risks make behavioral methods the treatment of choice in most clinical settings.

CONCLUSIONS

Unfortunately, there have not been additional evaluation studies to further demonstrate the effectiveness of behavioral treatment methods. However, together with the results of the small group studies discussed earlier, these results indicate quite clearly that behavioral treatment methods are extremely effective in helping individuals to lose weight. Indeed, most of the current commercial weight-reduction clinics employ behavioral methods as a core ingredient in their treatment package. The one important question that requires further attention, however, is the following: Once an individual has lost weight, what is the best way to aid him or her to avoid gaining it back? Although behavioral programs are effective in producing weight loss, the data on helping people maintain the weight loss are not as impressive (Stunkard, 1979). Future treatment programs will need to develop more effective methods for ensuring maintenance of weight loss.

The problem of self-selection of subjects in these treatment program evaluation studies must also be addressed. Are those individuals who seek out professional help representative of the general population of overweight people? Or do they represent only a small proportion of this population, whereas the majority of individuals can effectively lose weight on their own by developing their own diet/exercise weight-reduction programs? If individuals who seek out professional help are "hard-core" cases who have been unable to lose weight on their own by other means, then treatment improvement rates need to be interpreted with this fact in mind. The problem of self-selection of subjects must be considered in almost any treatment evaluation study, including the smoking and alcohol treatment investigations that we discuss later in this chapter. Information is greatly needed concerning the role such a factor plays in decreasing or increasing treatment success rates.

Finally, it should be pointed out that many current public health efforts on behalf of increased health are employing behavioral principles in educating the public to avoid becoming overweight. It is beyond the scope of this chapter to review such programs. The reader is referred to a review by Stunkard (1979) of the Stanford Heart Disease Prevention Program, the Swedish Diet and Exercise Program, and the German Television Weight Reduction Program. Also, Hollis, Connor, and Matarazzo (1982) have recently presented their Family Heart Alternative Diet Program as one means of preventing cardiovascular disease. Programs such as these highlight the important possibility of future application of behavioral control of eating behavior to large populations. Indeed, as Stunkard (1979) notes: ". . . the greatest importance of obesity for behavioral medicine may well be in the future. For current development and future trends in the behavioral control of obesity may foreshadow developments in all of behavioral medicine. Foremost among these trends is the application of behavioral measures to larger and larger populations" (p. 296).

PROBLEM DRINKING/ALCOHOLISM

Approximately 100 million people in the United States use alcoholic beverages moderately and without harmful effects. Another approximately 5 to 10 million abuse the use of alcohol and are labeled alcoholics or problem drinkers because of the harm they do to themselves, others, and/or society. The National Institute on Drug Abuse and Alcoholism has estimated that excessive problem drinking on and off the job is costing U.S. industry approximately 15 billion dollars a year. Besides these significant economic consequences, it also presents a significant health hazard. It is second only to heroin as an addiction that can cause death. Finally, it has been estimated by the National Highway Institute that 68 percent of the nation's highway fatalities are alcohol-related.

The precise statistics on the incidence of alcoholism vary depending on one's definition of alcoholism. There is as yet no one clear, precise, and totally accepted definition of alcoholism. In any consideration of alcoholism, one must be aware of the variety of possible drinking patterns and the possible complex of determinants—physiological, psychological, and cultural/situational—of maladaptive drinking behavior. More and more mental health professionals are using patterns of behavioral criteria that occur together in making judgments concerning the severity of the problem drinking.

PERSONALITY CHARACTERISTICS AND ALCOHOLISM

There have been a number of attempts to delineate specific personality characteristics associated with susceptibility to alcoholism. A widely cited longitudinal study called the Oakland Growth Study was started in the 1930s in Oakland, California.

In this study a group of children were extensively studied and then carefully followed through life. Information was collected concerning family behavior patterns, school behavior, and personality characteristics as assessed on personality tests and in interviews. In the 1960s many of the individuals in the initial sample, who were now in their mid-thirties, were contacted and interviewed to determine their alcohol drinking patterns (Jones, 1968, 1971). On the basis of the interview these persons were classified into one of five categories according to their drinking behavior, and then the developmental information collected earlier in their lives was examined to determine any associations. It was found that although certain characteristics in adolescent males that may index social difficulties that serve as a source of stress (sensitive to social criticism, less productive and industrious, less socially perceptive) do appear related to future problem drinking, these same characteristics are found in other forms of psychopathology. That is, they appear to predict future psychopathology in general, not specifically alcoholism. Indeed, research has consistently failed to find "alcoholic personality" characteristics that differentiate between alcoholics and nonalcoholics (Bandura, 1969; Miller, 1975).

There has, however, been a continuation of the search for specific personality traits. For example, McClelland, et al. (1972) have suggested that a need for power is linked to both social and excessive drinking. They propose that certain men drink in order to increase their sense of power, especially the perception of their sexual and aggressive conquests. Even though there are certain methodological deficiencies associated with this formulation (e.g., the reliance on projective personality tests such as the TAT, which have been demonstrated to have limited reliability and validity), it is an interesting formulation that warrants additional investigation.

BEHAVIORAL EXPLANATIONS OF ALCOHOLISM

The first influential behavioral explanation of the etiology of alcoholism was the **tension-reduction hypothesis.** This hypothesis assumes that alcohol is a tension reducer and that it is reinforcing for alcoholics because it reduces their tension and anxiety. A variety of evidence was accumulated to support this hypothesis. For example, it was demonstrated that increased anxiety and increased alcohol intake are associated (McNamee, Mello, and Mendelson, 1968). In animal studies, moreover, it was demonstrated that alcohol consumption helped to decrease fear and conflict (Freed, 1971), thus lending credence to the contention that alcohol reduces anxiety. Anxiety reduction due to alcohol consumption by human subjects was also demonstrated in numerous studies (Coopersmith, 1964).

These studies suggest a rather simple model of alcoholism development: some individuals may learn to cope with tension-producing life situations by drinking alcohol. But despite the array of research tending to support this tension-reduction hypothesis, it has not received universal support. Numerous research studies apparently contradict it. In a study by Nathan and O'Brien (1971), for example, a group of male alcoholics and a matched group of nonalcoholics were compared on a variety of behavior dimensions. It was found that after an initial twelve- to twenty-four-hour period of drinking during which anxiety level does decrease, there is a period during which anxiety and depression levels *increase*. These investigators concluded that alcoholism is much more complex than a simple tension-reduction model would assume. Comprehensive reviews with humans also suggest the inadequacy of the simple tension-reduction view of alcohol effects (Cappell, 1974; Marlatt, 1975; Mello, 1972; Nathan and Goldman, 1979).

In another study Steffen, Nathan, and Taylor (1974) examined the relationship between self-respect measures of tension and physiological measures of tension (muscle tension level) in alcoholics over a period of twelve days in which they had free access to alcohol. Although subjects became physiologically relaxed (reflecting a pharmacological effect of the drug) as they drank more, they became subjectively less comfortable. Similar results have been found for light social drinkers by Polivy, Scheuneman, and Carlson (1976). Despite the physiological tension-reducing properties of alcohol use, there seems to be a concomitant increase in the cognitive or self-report component of anxiety. It therefore appears that although the tension-reduction model may partly explain why the alcoholic initiates a new episode of drinking, it cannot explain why self-reported anxiety increases following alcohol ingestion. A more comprehensive learning theory model needs to be developed to take into account results such as these as well as expectancy effects of alcohol, to be discussed next.

ALCOHOL AND EXPECTANCY EFFECTS

In recent years methodologically sophisticated research has assessed the pharmacological effects of alcohol independently of expectancy effects. This research has demonstrated that what has long been considered simply the pharmacological effect of alcohol is actually the result of a complex interaction of a number of factors: the person's expectancy of what the effects of alcohol will be, his or her past history of alcohol use, the environment in which alcohol use occurs, and the specific actions of alcohol on physiological functioning.

A study by Marlatt, Demming, and Reid (1973) was the first to clearly demonstrate the significant impact of alcohol expectancy effects. In this study it was shown that the drinking of alcoholic subjects was determined by the *belief* that they were drinking alcohol rather than the pharmacological effects of drinking itself. Marlatt and colleagues manipulated the type of beverage consumed (alcohol or a tonic water placebo). All subjects were informed that they were participating in a taste-testing experiment on alcohol. Half of the subjects were further told that they would receive alcohol; the other half were told that they were in the "control" condition and would not receive alcohol but only tonic water. In reality, half of the subjects in each of these two groups received alcohol, while the other half received tonic water. All subjects were then allowed to regulate on their own the amount of beverage consumption during a fifteen-minute period. Results indicated that the actual amount of consumption was determined by whether the subjects thought they were drinking alcohol and not by the actual alcohol content of the drinks. Thus expectancy factors appear to play a significant role in determining beverage consumption by alcoholics.

There have also been studies demonstrating that the effects of alcohol are determined in part by situational cues. For example, Pliner and Cappell (1974) administered either alcohol or a placebo to nonalcoholic subjects. These subjects were then required to complete a "creativity" task, either in a small group or alone. It was found that subjects in the small groups revealed a more positive mood (as assessed by both self-report and observational measures) when they had consumed alcohol. In contrast, those subjects who completed the task alone demonstrated no significant differences in affect between the alcohol and placebo conditions. Examination of self-reported physical symptoms, though, revealed opposite effects: subjects performing the task alone reported more symptoms while drinking alcohol, while subjects in the small groups reported no differences between alcohol and placebo conditions. Pliner and Cappell (1974) interpret these findings as indicating that the actual behavioral effects of alcohol consumption depend on situational or cognitive factors, and not just on pharmacological factors.

There have been numerous other studies indicating the complex interaction of factors involved in determining the effect of alcohol on behaviors such as aggression, anxiety, pain, and sexual arousal. For example, in a series of studies Wilson and Lawson (1976a,b) found that both men and women reported higher levels of sexual arousal when they believed they had consumed alcohol (whether or not they had actually done so) than when they believed they had consumed tonic water. These results, combined with the findings that alcohol consumption actually *decreases* both penile and vaginal responses to erotic stimuli (Buddell and Wilson, 1976; Wilson and Lawson, 1976b), again nicely demonstrate that the subjective or psychological effects of alcohol consumption are many times relatively independent of the physiologically induced effects. The reader is referred to excellent reviews by Lang and Marlatt (1982) and Nathan and Goldman (1979) of other research of this type on expectancy factor. Nathan and Goldman (1979) provided an apt summary of the results of research in this area:

> In sum, the behavioral effects of alcohol clearly result from a complex interaction of factors. Among those factors are the expectancies one holds about alcohol's effects on behavior. Although we know that these expectancies influence the behavioral effects of alcohol, there remains the question of whether expectancies only produce effects when they interact with alcohol . . . or whether they can produce certain effects in the absence of alcohol. . . . Expectancy itself is as complex; it is related to belief symptoms, prior drinking experience, the immediate physical and social setting of drinking, dosage levels. . . . Such complexity suggests that the potential reinforcing capabilities of alcohol, manifold indeed, still remain to be clarified. (pp. 258–259)

A NEUROPSYCHOGENETIC MODEL OF ALCOHOLISM

In recent years a number of research findings have provided some new insights into the possible causes of alcohol craving. Blum (1984) has provided a summary of studies demonstrating a relationship between the action of alcohol and processes that operate in the brain, including an association between the craving for alcohol and a deficiency of naturally occurring opiatelike substances (the most important of which are endorphins and met-enkephalins). Animals with low levels of met-enkephalin in the brain were found to consume greater amounts of ethanol than animals with normal levels. Moreover, this same negative correlation between endogenous met-enkephalin levels and amount of ethanol consumed was found in alcohol-preferring and alcohol-nonpreferring inbred mice strains. Thus the close relationship and interaction between alcohol and opiates in the brain is an important neurophysiological component of drinking behavior. In terms of a genetic involvement, Blum (1984) has also reviewed research demonstrating that laboratory mice could be bred to prefer alcohol over water. In addition, these alcohol-preferring mice exhibited subnormal levels of met-enkephalins. This link between alcohol preference and opioid deficiency suggests a genetic factor as another major component in alcoholism.

Finally, Blum (1984) also emphasized the important role that psychological/environmental factors can play in alcoholism. He pointed out how chronic environmental stress can produce deficiency of met-enkephalins and endorphins. Thus psychological stress can lead to opioid deficiency, which, in turn, can lead to a growing craving for alcohol.

Obviously this neuropsychogenetic model emphasizes a number of different components that may be involved in the development of problem drinking. Combined with other psychological factors such as early modeling and conditioning experiences, this makes the study of alcoholism a quite complex endeavor. Moreover, it emphasizes the importance of taking a comprehensive treatment approach to this problem appetitive behavior.

TRADITIONAL BEHAVIORAL TREATMENTS OF PROBLEM DRINKING/ALCOHOLISM

Traditional behavioral techniques were basically unidimensional in nature, aimed primarily at eliminating only the maladaptive consumptive drinking behavior. A major method employed was **aversion therapy**. There are three basic varieties of aversion therapy methods, which use different aversive stimuli:

1. Chemical therapy, including chemical nausea agents such as Antabuse, Apomorphine, and Emetine and drugs that produce muscular paralysis such as Scoline.

2. Electric shock.

3. Verbal descriptions of nauseating scenes (**covert sensitization**).

A study by Thimann (1949) provides an example of an early chemical aversion procedure reported to be successful. Thimann gave patients an injection and an oral dosage of Emetine. Immediately prior to the expected emesis, the alcoholic was exposed to the sight, smell, and taste of a favorite alcoholic beverage. The unpleasant negative reaction produced by the chemical was in this way classically conditioned to alcohol. Conditioning sessions lasted from twenty to thirty minutes each day and were repeated daily for five to six days. Booster treatment sessions of one day each were given at intervals ranging from four to twelve weeks. In one of the most comprehensive and long-term follow-ups on this type of treatment, Lemere and

Voegtlin (1950) assessed the follow-up data on over four thousand patients. They found that one year after completion of treatment, 60 percent of this group remained abstinent from alcohol. They also found that periodic booster treatments administered on an outpatient basis were essential for treatment success.

A more widely known form of chemical aversion treatment uses Antabuse. Antabuse is a chemical that is taken in pill form by alcoholics each day, and two days after ingestion it interferes with the metabolic processing of alcohol by the body. If the Antabuse patient drinks alcohol, an extremely unpleasant reaction occurs, including nausea and other physiological discomforts. One of the problems with this type of treatment is that the patient can discontinue the use of Antabuse after leaving the hospital. Also, like other forms of aversion therapy, it cannot be used for patients with certain physical disorders because of the stressful nature of the chemical aversive treatment.

The drug succinylcholine (Scoline) has been used to induce muscular paralysis in aversion therapy. The usual procedure is first to inform the patient about the method and the effects of the drug. A saline drug apparatus is then attached to a vein in the patient's arm. The patient is given a glass of his or her favorite alcoholic beverage and told to grasp it, look at it, smell it, and taste it. The patient then gives it back to the clinician. After a number of such "familiarization" trials, the Scoline is put into the patient's bloodstream via the drug apparatus. The patient is then handed the beverage again to smell and sip, at which time the paralysis occurs. The patient becomes totally paralyzed, with the paralysis lasting from sixty to ninety seconds. During this time the patient is not able to move or breathe. If he or she starts to suffocate or if the paralysis lasts for more than about a minute, the patient is treated with a respirator. After a number of such trials, many patients develop a conditioned aversion to alcohol. It is assumed that the very powerful aversive sensation of respiratory paralysis makes this type of conditioning procedure especially effective in reducing drinking. However, research has shown that this technique is no more effective than less drastic procedures for reducing drinking in alcoholics (Miller and Eisler, 1976).

Aversion therapy employing electrical stimuli typically involves instructing the patient to sip a sample of his or her favorite drink but not to swallow it, at which time an electric shock is administered that can be terminated by spitting out the drink. This technique has been used with some success with alcoholics (see Blake, 1967; Miller and Hersen, 1972).

Finally, verbally induced aversion (covert sensitization), first developed by Cautela (1970), involves inducing aversive stimuli in the patient's own thoughts. The alcoholic may be asked to imagine a scene such as follows:

You are walking into a bar. You decide to have a glass of beer. You are now walking toward the bar. As you are approaching the bar, you have a funny feeling in the pit of your stomach. Your stomach feels all queasy and nauseous. Some liquid comes up your throat and it is very sour. You try to swallow it back down, but as you do this, the food particles start coming up your throat to your mouth. You are now reaching the bar and you order a beer. As the bartender is pouring the beer, vomit comes to your mouth. . . . As you run out of the barroom, you start to feel better and better.

When you get out into the clean, fresh air you feel wonderful. You go home and clean yourself up. (Cautela, 1970, p. 87)

The goal of this procedure is to pair unpleasant associations with drinking and pleasant associations with the absence of drinking.

The systematic evaluation of the various aversive therapy techniques has only recently begun. In reviews of such techniques, Davidson (1974) and Miller and Eisler (1976) note that they appear to effectively reduce the immediate reinforcing properties of drug intake. On the basis of these early results, aversion therapy has become widely available to patients in different hospitals in different states. Wiens and Menustik (1983) reported follow-up data from 685 patients treated with aversion therapy in a hospital. Results indicated that 63 percent of the patients treated maintained continuous abstinence for one year. Moreover, approximately one-third of the patients reported continuous abstinence for three years. Planned aftercare contact was a very important component of the treatment program for these patients.

More such research evidence of this type is needed to evaluate the long-term effectiveness of aversion therapy. Although a number of different aversive stimuli have been used, the most effective aversive stimulus has not been identified conclusively. Moreover, research addressing the issue of what patients respond best to this type of therapy is also needed.

CONTINGENCY CONTRACTING–OPERANT PROCEDURES

Operant procedures employing contingency contracting have been shown to have promise as a method of managing the behavior of alcoholics. The essential ingredient in such programs is that the reinforcement used to maintain sobriety is more powerful than the alcohol itself. Bigelow and his associates have conducted a number of studies demonstrating the potential value of such programs.

One of their first studies assessed the ability of four hospital employees, who were in danger of being fired, to abstain from drinking (Bigelow, Liebson, and Lawrence, 1973). These employees were required, on the basis of a contract, to report on a daily basis to the hospital's Alcoholism Treatment Unit to receive Antabuse. It was agreed that failure to report would result in no work and no pay. This contingency contract program was found to produce significant improvements in the job performance and attendance of all four employees. Similar results have been reported in studies employing both inpatients and outpatients (Griffiths, Bigelow, and Liebson, 1978). A wide variety of other such operant-contingency studies demonstrate that alcoholics can be helped to moderate or terminate their drinking in this manner (Lang and Marlatt, 1982; Nathan and Goldman, 1979).

MULTIMODAL BEHAVIORAL APPROACHES

Unidimensional techniques such as aversion therapy show promise for eliminating maladaptive drinking, the consumptive response (see box). However, treating only the consumptive behavior without simultaneously dealing with the situational variables that may be contributing to the maintenance of this drinking behavior lessens

"FROM ALCOHOLIC TO SOCIAL DRINKER?"

Through the years, a controversial question has been whether alcoholics can be treated and retrained to become controlled social drinkers. A common viewpoint, propounded by Alcoholics Anonymous (AA), is that alcoholism is an irreversible "disease" and so the alcoholic must totally abstain from drinking. If not, he or she will "lose control" and not be able to stem the "craving" or stop drinking until totally intoxicated. Some recent research questions the notion that total abstinence is needed in the treatment of alcoholism. Techniques have been developed that show great promise for teaching alcoholics to become controlled social drinkers.

In one of the first studies assessing the possibility of controlled drinking, Lovibond and Caddy (1970) trained alcoholics how to estimate their blood-alcohol level (BAL) on the basis of subjective feelings of intoxication. Patients then were requested to drink an alcoholic beverage to produce moderate BALs. When they drank and reached BALs above a predetermined cut-off point, electric shocks were administered to the chin, face, and neck. A control group of alcoholics was selected and treated in an identical manner *except* that these patients were administered random electric shock instead of shock contingent on their BALs. The first group demonstrated significant changes in drinking behavior, in addition to reporting dramatic improvements in overall health and well-being.

A number of studies were stimulated by these encouraging preliminary results (see Nathan and Goldman, 1979). One important finding of this research was that alcoholics appear to have a deficit in the ability to discriminate BAL on the basis of internal, subjective feelings or cues. The alcoholics' shifting tolerance levels apparently prevent them from using internal cues of BAL that nonalcoholics can effectively use over a long time period. As a consequence, BAL discrimination procedures that use external cues (e.g., learning to calculate BALs from a booklet that teaches alcohol dose–strength–metabolism relationships) have been developed to help alcoholics make accurate estimates of BAL in the natural environment (see Huber, Karlin, and Nathan, 1976; Lipscomb and Nathan, 1980). Although much more systematic long-term evaluation research of such procedures is needed, they show promise for the possibility of retraining some alcoholics to become controlled social drinkers.

This retraining possibility has been voiced in the literature during recent years (see Orford, Oppenheimer, and Edwards, 1976; Pattison, Sobell, and Sobell, 1977). A study published in 1975 by the Rand Corporation, a West Coast "think tank," generated a great deal of controversy because it suggested the possibility of "controlled" drinking and questioned the dogma of complete abstinence for some alcoholics (Armor, Polick, and Stambul, 1976). Opponents of the controlled drinking approach, primarily AA, argue that public acceptance of this Rand report position may give reformed alcoholics an "excuse" to take a few drinks in an attempt to become controlled drinkers. This might start them on the road back to alcoholism. These opponents have generated a great deal of public and political pressure against the Rand report, and attempts were made to force a retraction. This was unfortunate since the report did not advocate "controlled" drinking as a possibility for all alcoholics but suggested that this goal *might* be possible with certain alcoholics. The report emphasized that much additional research is needed to determine whether this is a viable approach. Indeed, comprehensive reviews of this "controlled social drinking" literature conclude that, because of conceptual and methodological short-comings of much of the past research in this area, a great deal of additional investigation is needed to determine the viability of this possibility (see Emrick, 1975; Lloyd and Salzberg, 1975; Nathan and Lansky, 1978).

Another important event that "fueled the fire" of this controversy was a study by Penderay, Maltzman, and West (1982). This investigation presented evidence based on a ten-year follow-up of the same patients originally treated in a study by Sobell and Sobell (1973). This latter study was frequently cited as an example of how controlled drinking behavior could be produced in alcoholics. Penderay and colleagues, after contacting the patients who were administered this form of controlled drinking treatment, significantly cast doubt on the validity of the original findings. They found that some of the treated patients had seriously relapsed, and they also questioned whether some of the original results may have been fabricated. These discrepancies were aired on the television show *60 Minutes*, which suggested to the audience that the data were in fact seriously flawed. A great deal of negative publicity was thus generated for the controlled drinking approach, and a blue-ribbon panel of independent investigators was formed to review Sobell and Sobell's experimental results. The investigators concluded that there was no reasonable cause to doubt the scientific or personal integrity of Sobell and Sobell. Subsequently, a Committee on Science and Technology of the U.S. Congress supported this conclusion.

Marlatt (1983) has provided a more detailed account of this controversy and has noted that the debate has continued, often on a very emotional level. The continuing focus on the validity of Sobell and Sobell's original work has seriously clouded the results of more recent research on this topic and has limited a more objective evaluation of the important underlying issues involved in this approach.

What, then, is the most constructive view to take at the present time on the issue of treatment goals (complete abstinence or controlled drinking)? Taking into account both sides of the issue, Nathan and Goldman (1979) suggest the following:

1. Abstinence should be considered the initial goal of treatment for alcoholism.

2. Sober alcoholics should not be led to believe that they can ever drink in a controlled manner. There are currently no unequivocal data to support the validity of this goal.

3. Alcoholics who have repeatedly attempted and failed to stop drinking, who regret having done so, and who are physically able to drink moderately should be considered as possible candidates for controlled-drinking treatment. This view is based on the assumption that controlled social drinking, while less desirable than complete abstinence, is nevertheless more desirable than uncontrolled alcoholism.

4. Additional research comparing the relative long-term effectiveness of abstinence-oriented versus controlled drinking-oriented drinking is greatly needed before any confident decision on treatment goals can be made for anyone.

the probability of long-lasting improvement. For example, if alcohol is being used to help cope with a stressful life situation, the alcoholic needs to learn alternative means of more adaptively dealing with the stress. If not, he or she may start to misuse other drugs, such as tranquilizers, or eventually return to the use of alcohol. Miller and Eisler (1976) suggest that a comprehensive behavioral treatment program should have three major objectives:

1. To decrease the immediate reinforcing properties of the drug. This can be accomplished through the use of aversion therapy or operant techniques.

2. To teach the person to perform new behaviors that are incompatible with drug abuse. For example, if the person is drinking in order to reduce stress, he or she can be taught more appropriate ways of dealing with stress—through relaxation training or learning more effective social skills to handle stressful situations.

3. To modify the individual's social environment so that he or she receives maximum reinforcement for activities that do not include the use of drugs; for example, by providing positive reinforcement such as praise, attention, or other pleasurable responses during periods of sobriety and not during periods of intoxication.

Such a comprehensive treatment program shows the greatest promise for bringing about long-term improvement but needs to be individualized for each patient.

CIGARETTE SMOKING AND TOBACCO USE

Nicotine, which is found in tobacco, is a stimulant that increases the general activity level of the central nervous system. This drug is usually not included in discussions of drug abuse because it is popular, legal, and widely used. It usually does not distort one's perceptions, decrease mental functioning, or cloud one's memory. However, tobacco addiction is the most common type of drug dependency in this country. Evidence indicates that nicotine can be an extremely addictive substance (Russell, 1976). If its use is suddenly discontinued, a period of depression may result. This period of depression in part accounts for the difficult time many individuals encounter when attempting to "kick the habit."

Although nicotine produces no apparent psychological damage, the means by which it is ingested—smoking—creates physiological damage. Chronic smoking is considered a major contributor to a variety of diseases: lung cancer; a number of other cancers, as of the larynx and esophagus; bronchitis; emphysema; and coronary artery disease. Indeed, the January 1979 report of the Surgeon General highlights the health implication of the smoking habit. As Joseph Califano, then Secretary of Health, Education and Welfare, pointed out when he forwarded the Surgeon General's report to Congress, smoking is "slow motion suicide." Overall, the mortality ratio for male cigarette smokers is 70 percent above that for nonsmokers. As a result of documentation of the health hazard, legislation was passed banning tobacco advertisements from television and radio. Also, each pack of cigarettes sold in this country is required to include an advertisement indicating its potentially lethal effects. But despite growing social disapproval of smoking, widely advertised medical dangers of smoking, and the rising cost of cigarettes, the annual consumption rate is still over two hundred packs of cigarettes per person over eighteen years of age (Standard and Poor, 1975). This statistic attests to the potent habit-forming effects of the stimulant.

Despite the many health hazards of smoking and public awareness of these, many smokers either cannot quit or, if they do manage to do so, relapse and return again to the habit (Bernstein and Glasgow, 1979; Krantz, Grunberg, and Baum, 1985; Leventhal and Cleary, 1980). Because of the frightening list of health dangers associated with cigarettes, health psychologists have sought to determine the reasons why people initiate and maintain the smoking habit.

INITIATION OF SMOKING

Research suggests that it is predominantly social and psychological factors that influence people to begin to smoke. Adolescents often begin to smoke as a response to social pressures to imitate peers, family members, or role models in the media (e.g., actors, athletes, etc.). Some youths begin the smoking habit as an expression of adolescent rebellion (Jessor and Jessor, 1977; Pomerleau, 1979). Occasionally, misconceptions about the health risks of smoking and of the fact that smoking is a powerful addiction can further contribute to initiation of the habit. There is also some evidence that certain personality characteristics, such as extraversion, are associated with increased likelihood of beginning smoking (Eysenck, 1973). In addition, it has recently been proposed that there are biological factors that affect the quality of the individual's initial experiences with cigarettes. That is, if early experiences include intense nausea, a person is less likely to become a habitual smoker (Silverstein et al., 1982).

Several psychological and sociological theories have been advanced to explain the initiation of the smoking habit. In fact, many of the major theories of psychological development (psychoanalytic, psychosocial, and social learning) have been invoked to explain why people smoke (Krantz et al., 1985). Approaches to the prevention of smoking (see Chapter 13) have considered and applied some of the psychological theories discussed as being important for initiation.

The psychoanalytic approach emphasizes the importance of oral fixation: a psychological arresting of development that leads to a need to seek oral gratification. Erikson's (1963) theory of psychosocial development maintains that two of the eight stages of psychosocial crises are most relevant to the initiation of smoking: the struggle to overcome inferiority (ages six to eleven) and the effort to establish an identity (ages twelve to eighteen). The theory of social learning (Bandura, 1977) emphasizes the fact that smoking has immediate socially reinforcing qualities (peer approval, imitation of media stereotypes and models) compared to delayed aversive consequences such as health dangers. Thus the advertising industry seeks to exploit this influence by emphasizing images of beauty, athletic prowess, and popularity as being associated with smoking.

Another theory used to explain why people become habitual smokers is the **affect management model**. As proposed by Tomkins (1966, 1968), it focuses on the fact that individuals seek to regulate internal emotional states. It was assumed that many people smoke in order to create positive emotional states or to reduce negative emotional states. Although initial research yielded results in support of this model, more recent work has raised doubts as to the validity of the affect management model for accurately predicting smoking behavior (Adesso and Glad, 1978; Leventhal and Avis, 1976).

Figure 12.3 presents some of the positive and negative factors that influence the development of smoking behavior, from initiation through maintenance of a habitual behavior. This diagram is designed to illustrate the array of social, psychological, and biological factors that affect smoking and to indicate at what point in the process they operate and whether they generally act to increase (+) or decrease (−) the likelihood of smoking.

MAINTENANCE OF SMOKING

Many of the same psychological factors that influence the initiation of smoking also act to maintain this behavior, but additional biological and psychological factors are extremely important. Research evidence leaves little doubt that for heavy smokers, smoking is an addictive process, with nicotine being the active drug in this process (Jarvik, 1979; Krasnegor, 1979). Some researchers argue that habitual smokers self-administer tobacco to obtain physiological effects of nicotine that produce psy-

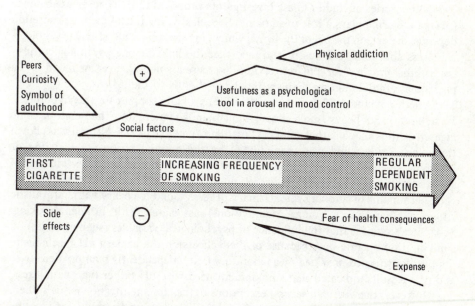

Figure 12.3   Factors affecting different stages in the development of smoking.
Reproduced by permission from R. Stepney. Smoking behavior: A psychology of the cigarette habit. *British Journal of Diseases of the Chest*, 1980, *74*, 325–344.

chological rewards such as increased attention or decreased stress (Ashton and Stepney, 1982). This explanation is known as the psychological tool model.

A more commonly held biological model for smoking maintenance is that repeated administration of some component of tobacco (probably nicotine or one of its metabolites) results in physical dependence (Jarvik, 1979). Support for this viewpoint derives from evidence that rats will self-administer nicotine and that human smokers smoke less when they are given chewing gum that contains nicotine (which is often prescribed to aid heavy smokers in quitting) or intravenous administration of nicotine. After physical dependence has been established, a smoker must continue to smoke to avoid unpleasant symptoms (irritability, sleep loss, weight gain, etc.; see the next section) that accompany withdrawal (Russell, 1979; Schachter, 1978).

However, biological factors alone cannot completely account for the characteristics of the smoking habit: maintenance of smoking involves the interacting of learning mechanisms with the biochemical and physiological effects of smoking (Hunt and Matarazzo, 1970). Research has shown that the physical effects of smoking may be linked, via conditioning mechanisms, to social and environmental events. So, for example, heavy smokers may light up a cigarette, even though their previous cigarette is still burning in the ashtray, and smokers may have a stronger urge to smoke in situations where they are used to smoking (e.g., parties).

A perspective on the complex interplay between biological and psychological processes was recently offered by Schachter and colleagues in what was termed the **nicotine-titration model**. This model is based on the notion that smokers smoke to maintain a certain level of nicotine, and that heavy smokers adjust their smoking rate to keep nicotine at a roughly constant level (Schachter, 1978; Schachter et al., 1977). In a series of studies, these investigators proposed that the acid-base balance (pH) of the urine plays a role in smoking. Specifically, the rate of nicotine excretion depends, in part, on the pH of the urine, which, in turn, can be altered by psychological stress and anxiety. Thus it is argued that the links among psychological processes, the craving for cigarettes, and increased smoking are mediated by a physiological addiction mechanism involving the pH of the urine.

A series of studies (Schachter et al., 1977) provides support for this hypothesis. First, a sample of heavy smokers consistently smoked more low- than high-nicotine cigarettes, thus showing that smokers "regulate" nicotine intake. Next, it was shown that when urinary pH was manipulated by the administration of alkalizing or acidifying agents, smokers smoked more when urine was acidified. A third set of studies examined the urinary pH-excretion mechanism as a mediator of psychological determinants of smoking rate. Urinary pH was found to covary with naturalistic situations (e.g., party going, examinations) associated with heavier smoking. Schachter's point is that the influence of psychological variables (such as stress) on smoking rate operate only because of their effects on the urinary pH mechanism. Support for this was provided by a laboratory that independently manipulated stress and pH. Results indicated that smoking covaried with pH rather than with stress.

However, there remain several exceptions to the nicotine-titration model. There are different types of smokers, some of whom do not appear to smoke for nicotine content (Schachter et al., 1977). In addition, the Schachter model makes the provocative prediction that smoking cigarettes with a lower nicotine content will *increase* the number of cigarettes smoked as heavy smokers seek to obtain their required nicotine levels, and data in this regard are contradictory (Garfinkel, 1979).

EFFECTS OF SMOKING CESSATION AND RELAPSE

Because of the health risks of cigarette smoking, most research has concentrated on the effects of this behavior rather than on the effects of cessation. However, as of 1980, nearly 30 percent of men and 16 percent of women in this country were former smokers, compared to a much smaller number in 1965 (USDHHS, 1983). Clearly, a sizable and increasing number of Americans were former smokers. These ex-smokers may experience irritability, sleep disturbances, and other psychological and physical problems (Grunberg, 1986). In addition, many ex-smokers gain weight—a situation that discourages some people from trying to quit and that can result in new health hazards for those who quit and gain large amounts of weight (Grunberg, 1982; 1986; Wack and Rodin, 1982).

Research by Grunberg (1982, 1986) suggests that weight gain accompanying withdrawal from nicotine may result from increased preferences for sweet-tasting foods. In these studies, smokers allowed to smoke ate fewer sweets than did non-smokers or deprived smokers. The three groups did not differ in consumption of nonsweet foods. A parallel study with animals showed that nicotine administration retarded normal growth-associated body-weight increases in young rats. Cessation of nicotine was accompanied by marked increases in body weight and concomitant increases in consumption of sweet foods. Moreover, these effects could not be explained by changes in total food consumption or activity level (Grunberg, 1986).

Ability to tolerate the withdrawal syndrome is crucial to the maintenance of smoking cessation. Therefore, further investigations of psychological and biological mechanisms responsible for symptoms accompanying withdrawal may suggest techniques for controlling the high relapse rate among those who quit smoking (see Chapter 13).

BEHAVIORAL TREATMENT OF SMOKING

Through the years a variety of approaches ranging from hypnosis to traditional group therapy have been used in an attempt to treat chronic smoking behavior. Such approaches usually show an initial period of abstention followed by relapse. They have produced an estimated long-term abstinence rate (greater than one year) of less than 15 percent (Pomerleau and Pomerleau, 1977). Recently developed behavior therapy techniques, however, show greater promise for producing lasting change. We briefly review the various behavioral procedures.

Aversion strategies

Aversion strategies have been the most common behavioral approach used to decrease smoking behavior. Aversive stimuli such as electric shock, noise, warm smoky air, and the consequences of rapid smoking have been used and paired with either actual or imagined smoking. Research reviews of the initial and long-term effectiveness of aversive conditioning procedures have been mixed (Bernstein and Glasgow, 1979). One approach, however, that showed some promise is the **rapid smoking** method. This method, initially used with good success by Lichtenstein and colleagues, involves the smoking of cigarettes at an extremely rapid rate until no additional smoking can be tolerated. The rapid smoking treatment sessions are repeated until the smokers indicate no additional desire to smoke. "Booster" sessions are subsequently administered if the desire should return. Lichtenstein and Penner (1977) reported an outcome evaluation study which found that 34 to 47 percent of all subjects who entered this type of treatment were still abstinent two to six years after treatment.

Even though the rapid smoking technique appears to have a good degree of long-term success, it is associated with some problems that limit its use. For example, smokers with cardiovascular or pulmonary diseases (obviously an important target population requiring treatment) are not likely to be able to tolerate such intense rapid smoking without demonstrating some ill effect (McAlister, 1975). Even for healthy individuals rapid smoking may be dangerous (Hauser, 1974). However, if safeguards are followed (e.g., excluding high-risk subjects and individuals over fifty-five, requiring physician approval for participation, and limiting the duration of exposure to rapid smoking), safety can be maintained (Sachs, Hall, and Hall, 1978).

Tension Reduction Strategies

Procedures such as systematic desensitization and relaxation training have been employed in an attempt to deal with stress and tension that causes smoking and/or that is associated with attempts at quitting. Results of controlled studies, however, either have failed to find such interventions superior to other approaches or have produced unimpressive success rates (Bernstein and Glasgow, 1979). Thus this major tension-reduction approach has not been shown to be useful in promoting cessation of smoking.

Stimulus Control

Earlier in this chapter we discussed the concept of stimulus control and how it was employed in the treatment of obesity. Such an approach has also been used in the treatment of smoking, with the goal being to gradually narrow the stimuli or cues that are associated with smoking (e.g., smoking only during certain situations or time periods). Results of various studies generally indicate that such stimulus-control procedures do not produce results that are superior to general control group conditions (Bernstein and Glasgow, 1979). An interesting finding of these studies is that subjects generally do quite well in decreasing smoking until they reach ten to twelve cigarettes a day. However, they then have great difficulty reducing their consumption rate below this level. Some have suggested that this is because the gradual reduction increases the reinforcement value of each cigarette and makes the remaining cigarettes harder and harder to give up (Flaxman, 1978).

Reinforcement of Nonsmoking

Another operant procedure attempts to eliminate smoking "indirectly" by reinforcing nonsmoking behavior. The most frequently employed approach has been to use some type of monetary reward, such as part of an initial deposit made by the subject, for nonsmoking during specified periods of time. Although early reviews of the research literature on this technique indicated generally unimpressive results, later research has demonstrated that it may be an effective means of *initiating* changes in smoking behavior (Bernstein and Glasgow, 1979). It may thus prove to be a useful component in a more elaborate and comprehensive treatment package.

Multimodal Treatment Approaches

As we indicated in Chapter 10, there is a current trend among behavior therapists to use several treatment techniques for a specific disorder in order to deal effectively with all the important controlling or causal variables. Multimodal behavior therapy techniques developed to treat smoking involve procedures such as the identification of situations that precipitate smoking, the training of new habits incompatible with smoking, aversion techniques, group support, and extensive follow-up. A number of controlled studies have produced some very encouraging results (see Delahunt and Curran, 1976; Lando, 1977). However, additional evaluative research is needed to more carefully document effectiveness. The multimodal technique is a promising approach that, as recently noted by Glasgow and Bernstein (1981), appears to offer the greatest potential for producing improved treatment outcomes.

THE PROBLEM OF RELAPSE

Some effective techniques to help people quit smoking have been developed. However, in the past investigators have not been concerned with the important problem of relapse. We know that up to 80 percent of smokers who initially succeed at quitting smoking will relapse over a twelve-month follow-up period (Hunt and Bespalec, 1974; see Chapter 13). Smoking relapse has recently received increased research attention. A National Working Conference on Smoking Relapse sponsored by the National Institutes of Health (Shumaker and Grunberg, 1987) took an important first step in addressing this significant health concern.

One major suggestion made by this conference was the use of a "stages-of-change" conceptualization of relapse prevention. Simply providing booster sessions to treatment programs is usually not successful in preventing relapse. Rather it was suggested that relapse-prevention programming be initiated in the early stages of the behavior-change process rather than after the individual has remained abstinent for a certain period of time. The major stages are: preparation and quitting, during which efforts are made to change how smokers view their smoking behavior; early maintenance of change; late maintenance of change; and recycling after a temporary relapse has occurred.

At each of these stages, a number of intervention techniques can be used, including cognitive-behavioral coping skills, social support, cue exposure, pharmacotherapy, and simple motivation. In addition, different modalities can be used, such as self-help, clinics, health providers, and the mass media. The challenge confronting future research is to determine the best method for tailoring these smoking-cessation strategies and stages of change to produce the most long-term results. In passing, it should also be noted that such a comprehensive relapse-prevention approach can also be applied to the other maladaptive behaviors reviewed earlier—obesity and alcoholism. The problem of relapse is as great a problem in these behaviors, and is discussed more fully in Chapter 13.

SMOKING EDUCATION AND PREVENTION PROGRAMS

As we noted earlier in this chapter, many current public health efforts are now employing behavioral principles in educating the public to increase good health habits (see Chapter 13). For many years school and health organizations have been providing education about the dangers of smoking, but only in recent years has attention been directed at modifying the behavioral and social factors involved in the smoking-initiation process. For example, there have been a number of impressive studies demonstrating the use of prevention strategies to discourage children and adolescents from initiating smoking (Evans, 1979; McAlister, Perry, and Macoby, 1979; see Chapter 13).

In a recent evaluative overview of research directed at the control of smoking behavior, Hunt and Matarazzo (1982) conclude that although the results of treatments are quite varied, pro and con, there are encouraging signs that changes are being made in smoking behavior. They point out that the prevailing "zeitgeist" is one of increasing public intolerance of smoking and increased legislation against smoking. This has been in large part due to the extensive education and prevention programs presented through the years. The nonsmoking ethos is a motivating factor important in accounting for recent statistics indicating a decline in the consumption rate of cigarettes. This nonsmoking ethos and the declining consumption rate, together with the conservative estimate that 25 percent of subjects achieve long-term abstinence after behavioral treatment (a figure that does not include those individuals who voluntarily quit on their own), provide reason for optimism about changing smoking behavior.

SUMMARY

This chapter describes how psychological analysis and treatment techniques have been systematically employed and evaluated with problem behaviors that have significant health consequences. Three common appetitive behaviors—obesity, problem drinking/alcoholism, and smoking were discussed. The area of obesity occupies a central position in the field of behavioral medicine–health psychology because, historically, it was one of the first major medical concerns to be dealt with by behavioral intervention techniques. We discussed biological and psychosocial factors in the etiology of obesity including genetics, the concept of set-point, and social norms. Next, we considered psychological aspects of food regulation, including Schachter's notion of "external responsiveness," as well as the behavioral treatment of obesity. The general conclusion was that behavioral treatment methods are the method of choice to aid people to lose weight. One important question requires further attention, though: Once an individual has lost weight, what is the best method to aid him or her to avoid gaining it back? Although behavioral programs are effective in producing weight loss, the data on helping people maintain weight loss are not as impressive.

In our discussion of alcoholism, we noted that there is no one clear, precise, and totally accepted definition of it. In any consideration of alcoholism, one must be aware of the variety of possible drinking patterns and the possible complex of determinants—physiological, psychological, and cultural/situational—of maladap-

tive drinking behavior. We reviewed recent evidence for neurophy
ences on the craving for alcohol and the interaction of physiological
cal factors in this process (the neuropsychogenetic model). In additi
the various cognitive-behavioral treatment techniques employed
including aversion techniques and contingency contracting–operant methods. Although unidimensional techniques such as aversion therapy show promise for eliminating the maladaptive drinking or consumptive response, one must also
simultaneously deal with the situational variables that may be contributing to the
maintenance of this drinking behavior. Multimodal behavioral approaches need to
be developed to deal with all the important contributing factors.

Finally, we discussed the problem of chronic smoking and the social, psychological, and biological factors that contribute to this habit. Initiation of smoking is
largely determined by social factors such as peer pressure and social modeling. The
nicotine-titration model proposes to explain the maintenance of smoking by suggesting that smokers smoke to keep nicotine at a roughly constant level in the body. In
this regard, we reviewed research by Schachter that implies that nicotine levels in
the body are affected by the acid-base balance (pH) of the urine. Also reviewed in
this chapter was research on the consequences of smoking cessation, including
weight gain, that impede many people from giving up the smoking habit.

We also noted that multimodal treatment techniques show some promise in
effectively reducing smoking behavior. Moreover, there are encouraging signs that
social pressures are having an effect on smoking behavior. The prevailing "zeitgeist"
is one of increasing public intolerance of smoking and increased legislation against
smoking. This nonsmoking ethos is a motivating factor important in accounting for
recent statistics indicating a decline in the consumption rate of cigarettes.

RECOMMENDED READINGS

Grunberg, N. E. Behavioral and biological factors in the relationship between tobacco use and
body weight. In E. S. Katkin and S. B. Manuck (Eds.), *Advances in behavioral medicine,* vol.
2. Greenwich, Conn.: JAI, 1986.

Hunt, W. A., and Matarazzo, J. A. Changing smoking behavior: A critique. In R. J. Gatchel,
A. Baum, and J. E. Singer (Eds.), *Behavioral medicine and clinical psychology: Overlapping
areas.* Hillsdale, N.J.: Elbaum, 1982.

Lang, A. R., and Marlatt, G. A. Problem drinking: A social learning perspective. In R. J.
Gatchel, A. Baum, and J. E. Singer (Eds.), *Behavioral medicine and clinical psychology:
Overlapping areas.* Hillsdale, N.J.: Erlbaum, 1982.

Mahoney, M. J., and Mahoney, K. *Permanent weight control: A total solution to the dieter's
dilemma.* New York: Norton, 1976.

Schachter, S., and Rodin J. *Obese humans and rats.* Hillsdale, N.J.: Erlbaum, 1974.

Schachter, S., Silverstein, B., Kozlowski, L. T., Perlick, D., Herman, C. P., and Liebling, B.
Studies of the interaction of psychosocial and pharmacological determinants of smoking.
Journal of Experimental Psychology: General, 1977, *106,* 3–40.

Stunkard, A. J. Behavioral medicine and beyond: The example of obesity. In O. F. Pomerleau
and J. P. Brady. (Eds.), *Behavioral medicine: Theory and practice.* Baltimore: Williams &
Wilkins, 1979.

13 PREVENTION AND HEALTH PROMOTION

||||||||||||||||||||||||||||||||||||||||||||||||||||||||||||||||||||||||||||||||||||||||||||||||||||||||||||||||||||||||||||||||||||

In the introductory chapter of this book, we described how at the turn of the century the leading causes of morbidity and mortality were the infectious diseases such as pneumonia and influenza. Today the leading causes of death are chronic diseases such as coronary heart disease and cancers—diseases that are strongly affected by behavioral and environmental factors. In recent years there has been an enormous increase in attention to behavioral factors in preventive medicine and health promotion. A recent Surgeon General's report on health promotion and disease prevention (USDHEW, 1979), increasing public and media interest in healthy lifestyles, and the growth of health-promotion programs in industry are but a few manifestations of this interest in behavioral aspects of prevention. All this attention to behavioral factors and health is certainly fashionable, but is it justified? The overwhelming weight of evidence suggests that it is (Grunberg, 1988).

LIFESTYLE RISK FACTORS AND MORTALITY: BEHAVIORAL IMMUNOGENS AND PATHOGENS

It has been estimated that 50 percent of the mortality from the ten leading causes of death may be attributed to lifestyle (Hamburg, Elliott, and Parron, 1982; USDHEW, 1979). Those habits that are health-impairing have been called **behavioral pathogens** (Matarazzo, 1984a, b), and beneficial or health-protective behavioral practices called **behavioral immunogens** (Matarazzo, 1984b). For example, in the United States cigarette smoking is linked with 350,000 deaths a year from heart disease, cancers, and chronic lung diseases (Grunberg, 1988). About 200,000 deaths a year have been attributed to excessive consumption of alcohol, and fatal injuries (many alcohol-related or caused by driver error and preventable by use of seat belts) claim 100,000 lives each year in the United States (USDHEW, 1979). Add to this list the recent public concerns about the AIDS epidemic—a disease that has become one of the leading killers of young adults and that can be prevented only through behavioral means. According to the 1979 Surgeon General's report on health promotion, ". . . a wealth of scientific research reveals that the key to whether a person will be healthy or sick, live a long life or die prematurely, can be found in several simple personal habits: smoking and drinking; diet, sleep and exercise; whether one obeys speed laws and wears seat belts; and a few other simple measures" (p. viii). Other estimates suggest that seven of the ten leading causes of death in this country (heart disease, cancer, stroke, automobile accidents, diabetes, cirrhosis of the liver, and arteriosclerosis) could be reduced significantly if vulnerable individuals would change just five behaviors: smoking, alcohol abuse, nutrition, exercise, and adherence to medications to control hypertension (Departmental Task Force Prevention, 1978).

These statements are, in part, derived from research such as a longitudinal study conducted by Belloc and Breslow (1972). They examined the relationship between personal health practices and subsequent health status and death rates among nearly seven thousand adults. Their survey identified seven specific personal health practices that were highly correlated with physical health. Sleeping seven to eight hours per day, eating breakfast almost every day, never smoking cigarettes, rarely eating between meals, being at or near prescribed weight, moderate or no use of alcohol, and regular physical activity were associated with good health. Those individuals who followed most or all of these seven simple practices were found in an initial survey to be in better general health compared to those who followed none or few of these practices (Belloc and Breslow, 1973). In a five-and-one-half year follow-up study of these individuals, the initial health practices were compared to subsequent mortality (see Figure 13.1). Summing the number of practices for each individual showed a strong relationship to mortality: the more positive behavioral health practices, the lower the mortality at each age group. These findings were subsequently confirmed after nearly ten years of follow-up (Breslow and Enstrom, 1980).

LIFESTYLE AND BEHAVIORAL CHARACTERISTICS THAT PREDICT LONGEVITY

Looking more closely at the protective behavioral immunogens, just what is the potential impact of adopting a healthy lifestyle? Other than preventing disease, one obvious answer is a long, healthy, and enjoyable life. To examine the potential consequences of health-promoting behavior, researchers interested in how to maximize human life expectancy have studied characteristics of people around the world who live long lives, with the idea that perhaps they are doing something right.

For example, in areas of the Soviet Republic of Georgia, between the Caucasus Mountains and the Black Sea, live the Abkhasians, individuals who claim to live to very old ages—sometimes as old as 120 to 170 years. In our society, about three individuals over age 100 per 100,000 people is considered normal (Santrock, 1986). However, the much higher percentage of about 400 centenarians per 100,000 people has been reported among the Abkhasians (Benet, 1976). Moreover, these people stay active, vigorous, and mentally and physically healthy into old age. Most of the elderly have good hearing and vision, have good posture, and are physically active, walking more than two miles a day and swimming regularly (Benet, 1976).

HEALTH PRACTICES AND MORTALITY

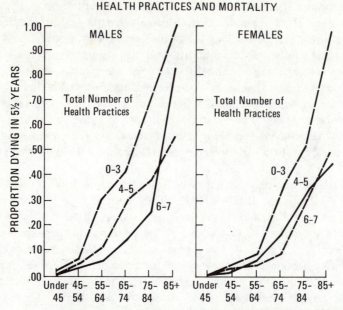

Figure 13.1   Age-specific mortality rates by number of health practices followed by subgroups of males and females.

Adapted from N. B. Belloc. Relationship of health practices and mortality. *Preventive Medicine,* 1973, 2, 67–81.

We now know that the Abkhasian claims of longevity are exaggerated, partly because no accurate birth records are kept and partly because old people have higher status in their society. It is also believed that the actual upper limits of human life span are about 110 to 120 years (Fries, 1976). The argument can convincingly be made that by avoiding or postponing the onset of chronic disease through preventive activities, it is possible for individuals to live longer and have healthier older years.

Despite exaggerated claims, the Abkhasians do appear to be especially long-lived. This is likely due to their genetic family history of longevity as well as their unique lifestyle (Weg, 1983). The Abkhasians lead predictable lives, and people stay physically and mentally active, maintaining vigorous work roles and habits as long as possible. Their staple diet is low in saturated fat and meat products and high in fruit and vegetables, with no or small amounts of alcoholic beverages and nicotine. Overeating is considered dangerous and obesity is greatly discouraged. These behavioral characteristics are strikingly similar to the behavioral immunogens described by Matarazzo.

However, the Abkhasians' longevity and vigorous old age cannot be understood without considering other psychosocial and cultural features of their environment. The most important of these factors are the well-defined cultural roles and uniformity and predictability of individual and group behavior. The integration of the elderly into an extended family and into community life as full, functioning members gives them a sense of belonging in work, decision making, and recreation. These social structures also provide them with a sense of personal control that helps reduce and avoid stress, and gives them social support and encouragement to maintain their zest for life. In sum, these lifestyle and psychosocial conditions combine to protect these older individuals against the chronic diseases that often accompany old age, and encourage a vigorous, active life that helps them maintain optimal psychological and physical functions (Fries, 1976; Weg, 1986). Indeed, research has made it possible to estimate one's own predicted life expectancy based on a variety of personal habits, in conjunction with some biological factors such as the longevity of one's parents (see box).

THE SCOPE OF PREVENTION IN HEALTH PSYCHOLOGY

The substantial relationships between major chronic diseases and modifiable behavioral factors that are under the individual's control have fostered prevention-oriented research and practice in health psychology. It is possible to classify preventive efforts into three types. **Primary prevention** refers to the modification of risk factors before disease develops. In many respects, this is a highly cost-effective and beneficial strategy, for in the long term the potential costs in lives and dollars of treating disease are likely to outweigh the costs of preventing unhealthy habits. Examples of primary prevention efforts include educational campaigns to prevent adolescents from smoking or to encourage "safer sex" practices to prevent AIDS. Although it has many long-term effects, primary prevention is particularly challenging since it is often difficult to motivate otherwise healthy people to make changes in their behavior that may not have immediate benefits, despite the promise of long-term health gains (Miller, 1983).

The terms **secondary prevention** and **tertiary prevention** refer, respectively, to interventions taken to arrest the progress of illness already in early asymptomatic stages and rehabilitation and treatment interventions to stop the progression of a clinically manifest disease (Institute of Medicine, 1978). While less cost effective and perhaps less beneficial in the long run, secondary and tertiary prevention activities may be easier to accomplish in that appropriate target groups (e.g., those that are ill) can be easily identified and are more motivated to change their behavior.

FACTORS AFFECTING PREVENTIVE HEALTH BEHAVIORS

As we discussed in Chapter 8, health behaviors can be defined as those actions people undertake to maintain or enhance their health (Kasl and Cobb, 1966). According to Leventhal, Prohaska, and Hirschman (1985), health behaviors are affected by social factors, emotional factors, symptoms, and cognitive factors. Social factors are important because health-related habits and lifestyles develop in the context of the family and society. As children become socialized, they develop attitudes toward themselves and their bodies. Among individuals raised in middle- and upper-class environments, proper nutrition, exercise, periodic medical checkups, immunizations, and so on are considered to be important, so children learn and incorporate these values as they grow up. Peer pressure is another important social influence on the acquisition or maintenance of health habits, particularly for adolescents and children (Evans et al., 1981).

Health and risk behaviors are also regulated by the presence or absence of bodily sensations or symptoms (Leventhal et al., 1985). For example, many smokers decide

HOW LONG WILL YOU LIVE?

This is a rough guide for calculating your personal longevity. The basic life expectancy for males is age 67 and for females it is age 75. Write down your basic life expectancy. If you are in your 50s or 60s, you should add ten years to the basic figure because you have already proven yourself to be quite durable. If you are over age 60 and active, add another two years.

Basic Life Expectancy   _____
Decide how each item below applies to you and add or subtract the appropriate number of years from your basic life expectancy.

1. Family history
   Add 5 years if 2 or more of your grandparents lived to 80 or beyond.   _____
   Subtract 4 years if any parent, grandparent, sister, or brother died of heart attack or stroke before 50. Subtract 2 years if anyone died from these diseases before 60.   _____
   Subtract 3 years for each case of diabetes, thyroid disorders, breast cancer, cancer of the digestive system, asthma, or chronic bronchitis among parents or grandparents.   _____

2. Marital status
   If you are married, add 4 years.   _____
   If you are over 25 and not married, subtract 1 year for every unwedded decade.   _____

3. Economic status
   Subtract 2 years if your family income is over $40,000 per year.   _____
   Subtract 3 years if you have been poor for greater part of life.   _____

4. Physique
   Subtract one year for every 10 pounds you are overweight.   _____
   For each inch your girth measurement exceeds your chest measurement deduct two years.   _____
   Add 3 years if you are over 40 and not overweight.   _____

5. Exercise
   Regular and moderate (jogging 3 times a week), add 3 years.   _____
   Regular and vigorous (long distance running 3 times a week), add 5 years.   _____
   Subtract 3 years if your job is sedentary.   _____
   Add 3 years if it is active.   _____

6. Alcohol
   Add 2 years if you are a light drinker (1–3 drinks a day).   _____
   Subtract 5 to 10 years if you are a heavy drinker (more than 4 drinks per day).   _____
   Subtract 1 year if you are a teetotaler.   _____

7. **Smoking**
   Two or more packs of cigarettes per day, subtract 8 years.   _____
   One to two packs per day, subtract 4 years.   _____
   Less than one pack, subtract 2 years.   _____
   Subtract 2 years if you regularly smoke a pipe or cigars.   _____

8. **Disposition**
   Add 2 years if you are a reasoned, practical person.   _____
   Subtract 2 years if you are aggressive, intense, and competitive.   _____
   Add 1–5 years if you are basically happy and content with life.   _____
   Subtract 1–5 years if you are often unhappy, worried, and often
   feel guilty.   _____

9. **Education**
   Less than high school, subtract 2 years.   _____
   Four years of school beyond high school, add 1 year.   _____
   Five or more years beyond high school, add 3 years.   _____

10. **Environment**
    If you have lived most of your life in a rural environment, add
    4 years.   _____
    Subtract 2 years if you have lived most of your life in an urban
    environment.   _____

11. **Sleep**
    More than 9 hours a day, subtract 5 years.   _____

12. **Temperature**
    Add 2 years if your home's thermostat is set at no more than
    68°F.   _____

13. **Health Care**
    Regular medical check ups and regular dental care, add 3
    years.   _____
    Frequently ill, subtract 2 years.   _____

Reprinted, by permission of the publisher, from R. Schulz. *The Psychology of Death, Dying, and Bereavement.* Reading, Mass.: Addison-Wesley, 1978, pp. 97–98.

to stop smoking cigarettes when they begin to notice ill effects that they feel from smoking (e.g., shortness of breath, coughing). However, in heavy smokers, the short-term symptoms associated with nicotine withdrawal (weight gain, irritability, sleep loss, etc.) may be sufficiently unpleasant that they relapse and resume smoking again (Grunberg, 1982).

Whether or not people engage in healthy behaviors also depends on their emotional state. For example, some individuals may overeat when they feel bored, lonely, or tense—all emotions they have learned to cope with by eating. Smokers may also not wish to stop smoking because of the unpleasant feelings they will experience as they give up the smoking habit. A final set of determinants of whether individuals engage in health-promoting behavior are their beliefs and attitudes about the benefits and dangers of performing or not performing such behaviors. Health beliefs and attitudes form the core of research on health promotion and disease prevention in health education and health psychology, with the **health belief model** (see Chapter 8) being the most extensively studied approach to why people do or do not engage in health behavior.

BARRIERS TO MODIFYING HEALTH BEHAVIORS

Given the compelling evidence that an individual's personal behaviors play such an important role in determining his or her health, why is it that people still smoke, eat improperly, fail to get adequate exercise, and so on? Unfortunately, unhealthy behaviors are stubbornly resistant to change and highly subject to relapse. Two broad sets of causes are considered to be major obstacles to lifestyle modification. The first is the learning theory notion called the **gradient of reinforcement**. This refers to the fact that immediate rewards and punishments are much more effective than delayed ones (Miller, 1983). Thus, if engaging in a behavior (e.g., eating a particular food) provides immediate relief or gratification, or if failing to engage in this behavior provides immediate discomfort, the behavior should be easily acquired and difficult to extinguish. Thus a smoker may derive gratification and avoid unpleasant withdrawal symptoms each time he or she smokes a cigarette, making smoking difficult to give up. Furthermore, the health threats posed by smoking, poor diet, overweight, and not exercising seem remote compared to the immediate pleasures of indulging, and the inconvenience and effort involved in adopting more healthful preventive behaviors also act as barriers to behavior change. The relative influence of remote or delayed reinforcement may also be a reason why the strategy of prevention receives less attention from physicians, patients, and the health care system in general compared to that afforded treatment of diseases after they become problems (Miller, 1983).

Forces in the social and physical environment comprise a second major set of barriers to lifestyle modification. Healthy or unhealthy habits are developed and maintained by social and cultural influences deriving from the family and society (Syme, 1978). In the last twenty years Americans have made significant progress in changing their attitudes toward exercise and proper nutrition and have become well informed about the modifiable risk factors for cancers and cardiovascular disorders. However, there are still powerful social pressures that lead teenagers to smoke and economic pressures such as the lack of insurance reimbursement for helping patients prevent illness that lead physicians and other health care providers to put less energy into prevention (Leventhal and Hirschman, 1982; Stachnik et al., 1983). Moreover, further economic and physical barriers are found in the higher cost and lower availability of healthier foods and in the lack of time and opportunity for exercise at many worksites (Grunberg, 1982).

CHANGING HEALTH-RELEVANT BELIEFS AND BEHAVIORS

What are some of the strategies used to help people acquire and practice health-promoting behaviors? Intervention research on prevention has used a variety of approaches ranging from small-scale efforts employing behavior modification to change single risk factors via face-to-face instruction, to large-scale public education efforts to change multiple habits using media communication techniques.

Educational Approaches

A basic premise of health education efforts is that three sets of factors—predisposing factors, enabling factors, and reinforcing factors—influence health behavior and are modifiable by educational interventions. According to Green (1984), **predisposing factors** are those factors that motivate the decisions to take particular health actions. They include the traditional aims of education such as awareness, understanding, attitudes, and beliefs about health-promoting and health-damaging behavior. **Enabling factors** are the types of skills needed to carry out an action, whether the action is motivated or not. Examples of enabling factors would be skills in self-care and the ability to conduct a breast self-examination. **Reinforcing factors** include the rewards the person obtains for performance of the health behavior in question (Green, 1984). Examples of reinforcing factors include social and peer approval and stress reduction. These are the kinds of reinforcers that often lead adolescents to smoke or use drugs, and recent school-based health education campaigns have used the concept of inoculation against peer pressure to counter these influences. In administering these inoculations, students are reinforced for acquiring skills that help them resist or decline cigarettes or drugs (e.g., Evans et al., 1981).

Clearly, the most effective health education campaigns combine learning experiences appropriately targeted at all three sets of factors that influence health behavior. As Green (1984) and others have noted, a behavior that is highly reinforced and motivated will not succeed unless enabling factors are also present. Similarly, an enabled and motivated behavior that is socially punished or ridiculed will also not endure.

Despite well-formulated health education models and intensive efforts, many health education campaigns have not reached the goals they set out to achieve. There are several reasons why health-related educational efforts can go awry. One reason for their lack of success is that the campaigns may not be directed or targeted optimally to the appropriate audience. A second reason is that they arouse too much fear, which can *inhibit* behavioral changes. A third reason is that peoples' naive theories of illness tell them things that are at odds with the health education message they receive. Later in this chapter we shall discuss the influence of fear communications and naive theories of illness in modifying preventive behavior. We discuss the importance of appropriate targeting of health education campaigns later in the discussion of AIDS prevention.

Effects of Fear Communications

Early laboratory studies examined the role of fear in motivating health attitude and behavior change (Janis, 1967; Leventhal, 1970). One might think that the more fearful a person is about the possible consequences of engaging in a particular behavior, the more likely he or she would be to change the behavior in question. Instead, these studies found that fear communications had limited effects. For example, Janis and Feschbach (1953) studied three groups of subjects who received messages designed to produce high, medium, or low levels of fear about what would happen to their teeth and gums if they failed to brush their teeth. Results of the study indicated that self-reported occurrence of tooth brushing was increased least effectively by the high fear appeal, with low and moderate fear appeals producing greater change. The high-fear group exhibited more signs of being aroused and vigilant after hearing the messages, but seemed motivated not to accept the messages presented—instead they minimized and denied the importance of the threat. These and similar results led Janis (1967) to hypothesize that two processes—vigilance and defensive avoidance—affected the outcome of fear communications. At lower and moderate levels of fear, subjects become increasingly vigilant and interested in the information conveyed and more motivated to incorporate the information into appropriate behavior. (See Figure 13.2-A) However, at high levels of fear—particularly when the recommendations presented do not fully relieve the fear—individuals tend to avoid the message as a defense against the anxiety produced. Janis's (1967) model of fear and attitude change is closely related to effects of fear in coping with surgery discussed in Chapter 8.

However, a large number of studies have subsequently found that higher levels of fear lead to somewhat more attitude change and slightly more behavioral change over a wide range of health issues, including use of seat belts, dental hygiene, quitting or reducing cigarette smoking, and taking tetanus inoculations (Leventhal and Hirschman, 1982). These studies also showed that the effects of fear-arousing, threatening messages tended to be short-lived, with behavioral changes dissipating within one week of the communication. In addition, when high fear messages fail to persuade, the failure generally reflects the target individual's feelings that they are unable to cope with the danger conveyed by the message. Thus, if fear is to lead to a change in behavior in addition to attitude change, instructions as to how to take appropriate action must be added to the threat message (Leventhal, 1970). (See Figure 13.2-B.)

In this regard, Leventhal (1970) has proposed the *parallel process model* of fear and attitude change. In this model the subject copes with the fear communication by two means: fear control and danger control. Danger control refers to coping behavior directed at reducing the threat—directly manipulating the situation to reduce or eliminate the source of danger. Fear control, on the other hand, refers to coping aimed at making one feel better regardless of the presence of threat. If a health communication is so threatening that people become preoccupied with reducing fear, they may do this to the point of ignoring the information, not coping with the danger, and not changing their health-related attitudes or behavior. Thus this model explains why, under certain circumstances, high fear messages may fail to persuade.

Common-Sense Models of Illness and Their Effects
Leventhal et al. (1982) have noted that people form personal cognitive models or "representations" of health and illness, models that are used to guide their interpretation of illness and bodily states. These cognitive models may or may not correspond to medical reality as defined by the physician or by an outside observer. As we noted in Chapter 8, it is clear that these representations play an important role in determining much of health and illness behavior.

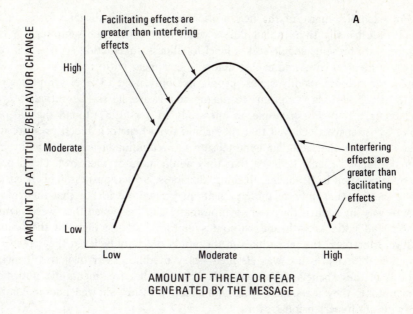

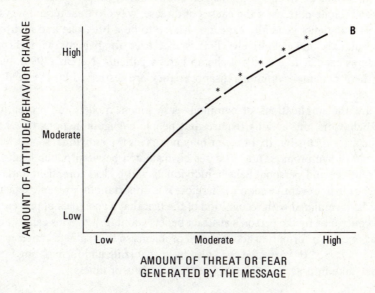

Figure 13.2   Hypothesized relations between fear and attitude-behavior change. (A) Curvilinear relationship between threat and attitude and behavior change suggested by fear-drive model of Janis (1967).
(B) Positive relationships between threat and attitude and behavior change under particular conditions
suggested by Leventhal's (1970) parallel response model.

Adapted with permission from J. C. Brigham. *Social Psychology.* Boston: Little-Brown, 1986, p. 488.
Copyright © 1986 by John C. Brigham. Reprinted by permission of Scott Foresman and Company.

For example, many of the health-oriented actions people take focus on illness. People usually think about illness when they experience symptoms. When symptoms are present, people seek a label for illness, take action such as self-care or seeking medical care, and expect illness to disappear with treatment. However, in order to interpret bodily states, people not only need to label symptoms but also to attach various symptoms to diagnosed disease states (Leventhal, Meyer, and Nerenz, 1980). For example, in one study Meyer (1981) found that 90 percent of hypertensives believed that they could tell when their blood pressure was elevated, despite the fact that hypertension is predominately asymptomatic. Yet the majority of patients believed that they could monitor their own blood pressure by signs such as headache, flushing, dizziness, or nervousness. This occurred despite the fact that none of these patients had definite evidence that their blood pressure was high when they were symptomatic and low when they were asymptomatic, and patients with and without symptoms did not differ in their blood pressure. Moreover, the individuals in this study not only believed they could tell when their blood pressure was elevated—they modified their own treatment on the basis of these beliefs. Those patients who felt that treatments did not affect the symptoms they associated with high blood pressure showed poorer compliance with antihypertension treatment.

Other than links between symptoms and bodily states, people's representations of health also include notions of the causes of disease, ways to treat it, and ways to prevent illness. Patients generally expect a disease to be a brief one and a cure to be achieved quickly and definitively. This is true even for patients with chronic diseases such as cancer. In a study of chemotherapy patients, Nerenz (1980) found that when these patients' symptoms disappear they are distressed by the need for continued treatment.

What are the implications of common-sense illness models for prevention? Preventive behaviors and actions require that people engage in actions that have long-term health benefits but that may or may not affect the individual's experience or explanation of symptoms. Thus, in cases of mismatch between public health or practitioner advice and personal beliefs, individuals will be less compliant and less likely to engage in a preventive action. Therefore it is important for preventive health messages to be formulated with recognition of the fact that a good deal of preventive behavior is controlled by the person's abstract beliefs about health. This can be done by providing enough information about health problems so that patients' misconceptions can be addressed or corrected, and also by recognizing and formulating interventions that take into account peoples' representations of illness.

BEHAVIOR MODIFICATION AND COGNITIVE APPROACHES TO PREVENTION

As described in Chapter 10, a variety of cognitive-behavioral treatment procedures, based in learning theory, have been applied in medical settings. Several of these techniques have applicability to promoting healthy behavior. Some examples of these applications are presented here.

Applied behavioral analysis is a behavioral change strategy based on the operant conditioning principle that behavior is determined by its antecedents and consequences (Chesney, 1984). This strategy involves identifying a particular target behavior to be modified (e.g., increasing physical exercise levels) and observing the current status of the behavior, along with its antecedents and consequences. After the period of observation, the environmental antecedents and consequences are changed accordingly in order to modify the rate of occurrence of the behavior. One example of successful application of applied behavioral analysis is the control of obesity. So widespread is the application of behavioral approaches to this health problem that more people have been receiving behavioral treatments for obesity than for all other conditions combined (Stunkard, 1979).

The initial stage of behavior modification programs for obesity involves describing the behavior to be changed by keeping a diary record. Each time they eat, patients write down the food, time of day, the people they were with, and the feelings they were experiencing. Next, an analysis of the diary record identifies stimuli or events that may cue the eating (e.g., watching television, sight of high-calorie desserts). These environmental antecedents are then controlled by restricting eating to one place or working with families not to keep high-calorie foods on hand. In the next stage patients are instructed to modify their eating behavior by reducing their eating speed, not combining eating with other activities such as reading or television watching, and so on. Finally, the environmental consequences are modified by reinforcing patients for weight loss and for behavioral changes. This may be done by having them give themselves points or other tangible rewards.

In contrast to the applied behavioral analysis approach, the **cognitive-behavioral perspective** is based on the belief that a large portion of human learning is cognitively mediated. That is, rather than directly responding to their environment, humans react to their thoughts or conceptions of the environment. These approaches recognize the importance of irrational patterns of thinking in causing maladaptive patterns of behavior (Ellis, 1962). In addition, it is considered very desirable to combine and integrate cognitive-based treatment approaches with techniques based purely on performance (Kendall and Turk, 1984). Examples of successful health-promoting cognitive-behavioral intervention are programs for modification of the Type A behavior pattern described in Chapter 5. In one such program directed at healthy men, a cognitive-behavioral intervention involving regular group sessions was superior to programs of regular physical exercise in reducing the intensity of Type A behavior (Roskies et al., 1986).

Combinations of social learning, educational, and behavior modification approaches have also been utilized successfully in health-promotion efforts. For example, Foreyt et al. (1979) compared several strategies to induce changes in diet: an educational intervention involving a diet booklet, counseling about nutrition alone, and nutrition counseling plus a behavioral intervention involving group discussion. They found initial reductions in dietary cholesterol to be greatest in the combined behavioral plus discussion group. However, as is frequently the case with lifestyle modifications, there was a tendency for relapse to occur after six months. A combined cognitive-social learning intervention was also used (Friedman et al., 1986) to reduce Type A behavior in post-infarction coronary patients, with the beneficial result of decreasing the likelihood of recurrent heart attack in patients who underwent this treatment (see Chapter 5).

RELAPSE AND RELAPSE PREVENTION

Although health habits can be altered by behavioral, educational, or other means, it is often difficult to maintain these changes over a long period of time. The term **relapse** is used to refer to a more or less regular or sustained return to the original pattern of behavior or habit. A **slip** refers to an isolated episode of return to previous behavior. There is a characteristic pattern of relapse (see Figure 13.3) that appears to apply not only to the treatment of smoking, alcohol abuse, and heroin addiction (Hunt et al., 1971) but also to behaviors such as exercise habits (Dishman, 1982), diet modifications (Foreyt et al., 1979), and preventive dental care (Lund and Kegeles, 1982). Up to 80 percent of individuals who initially succeed at stopping smoking, losing weight, or otherwise modifying their behavior will relapse over a twelve-month period (Brownell et al., 1986).

An example of an important and growing application of cognitive-behavioral treatments to health promotion is the prevention of relapse. It has been shown, for example, that when people deviate from weight-control regimens, a majority of episodes were preceded by distorted or maladaptive thinking (Sjoberg and Persson, 1979). An illustration of these thoughts were "I've already lost a lot of weight, so I can indulge myself once," or "An extra sandwich now will help me eat less later." One slip or relapse episode preceded by these thoughts had the effect of leading to

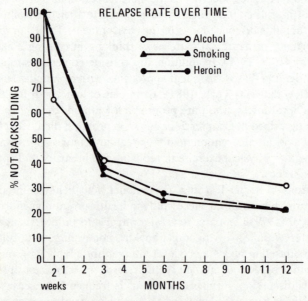

Figure 13.3   Relapse rates for addictive behaviors following treatment.
Reproduced with permission from W. A. Hunt, L. W. Barrett, and L. G. Ranch. Relapse rates in addiction programs. *Journal of Clinical Psychology,* 1971, *27,* 455–456.

subsequent slips. Similar cognitive distortions and maladaptive thinking have been shown to precede relapse from smoking cessation programs and from alcoholism treatments (Marlatt and Gordon, 1985).

These cognitive determinants of relapse have led to novel approaches to preventing relapse. The best-known approach, developed by Marlatt and Gordon (1985), is called **relapse prevention**. The goals of this method are to (1) teach subjects to anticipate and prevent the occurrence of relapse after a behavior change attempt (e.g., to prevent a recent ex-smoker from returning to habitual smoking) and (2) to help the individual recover from a lapse or slip before it intensifies into a full-blown relapse (Marlatt, 1985). To achieve these goals, relapse prevention involves training people in behavioral skills such as identifying situations that place them at a high risk for a slip, teaching them how to avoid or deal with these situations, and preparing them for coping with withdrawal symptoms. People also learn cognitive intervention skills that facilitate development of realistic expectations about the possibility of lapses and minimize reactions of guilt, frustration, or anxiety if these occur. Other lifestyle change procedures, such as training in relaxation, exercise regimens, and other techniques of coping with life stresses, are also taught. These cognitive-behavioral approaches have proven to be effective in several studies (Marlatt and Gordon, 1985).

PREVENTION OF SMOKING

In spite of a decrease in adult smoking since the release of the 1964 U.S. Surgeon General's Report on Smoking and Health, there has been a discouraging increase in smoking among adolescents—particularly teenage girls. Research has shown that adolescents begin smoking largely in response to social pressures. These social forces include the imitation of peers, family members, and role models (including actors, athletes, and adults in general) and peer pressures to be accepted (Evans et al., 1979). Some youths also begin smoking as an expression of adolescent rebellion or antisocial tendencies (Jessor and Jessor, 1977). Because of these psychosocial influences on the initiation of smoking, preventive interventions in schools have been attempted to deter smoking in adolescents. These studies have used, with some success, various social psychological techniques of peer modeling, attitude change, and other social learning and social-psychological procedures.

The most widely known of these studies is a three-year longitudinal study—the Houston project, conducted by Evans et al. (1981). This project used an intervention strategy based on Bandura's (1977) social learning theory. As applied to the initiation of smoking, this theory would suggest that by observing others, children acquire expectations and learned behaviors with regard to smoking. For example, by observing peers and role models smoking and experiencing positive consequences (e.g., social approval, pleasure from the cigarette), they would be likely to engage in the same behavior as the model. Based on this assumption, Evans et al. (1981) developed interventions to inoculate students against social influences to smoke.

The Houston project developed persuasive film messages and posters (see Figure 13.4) to teach grade school students about peer and media pressures to smoke and

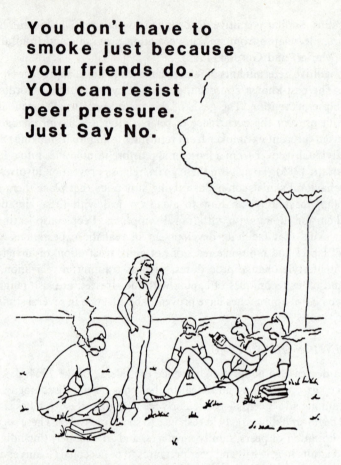

You don't have to smoke just because your friends do. YOU can resist peer pressure. Just Say No.

Figure 13.4   Poster used to counteract peer pressure.
Reprinted, by permission, from the Social Psychological Deterrents of Smoking in Schools Project, Richard I. Evans, University of Houston, Principal Investigator. Supported by the National Heart, Lung and Blood Institute, NIH Grant 17269.

to educate students about effective coping techniques to avoid accepting and trying cigarettes. The types of social pressures that influence the adolescent to begin smoking (e.g., peers, smoking parents, and cigarette advertisements) were presented along with a high-status, similar-aged model demonstrating ways to resist such pressures (e.g., stalling for time, putting counterpressure on the smoker by mentioning the health risks of smoking). These techniques were designed to give students the skills to resist the social pressures to smoke. Other films were also shown to demonstrate the immediate physiological consequences of smoking (e.g., carbon monoxide in the breath). In this study, hundreds of students in matched experimental and control groups were compared for cigarette smoking rates at the start of the project and during follow-up periods for three years. The results indicated a moderately successful impact of the films and posters, with the experimental groups smoking less frequently and rating lower intentions to smoke compared to a control group receiving no intervention (Evans et al., 1981).

Subsequent antismoking programs conducted by others have built on and expanded the use of these techniques, for example, by using older adolescent peer leaders to teach skills for resisting social pressures and teaching students more general social and life skills (Best et al., 1984; Botvin et al., 1980; Telch et al., 1982). These studies have reported similar or higher success rates, reducing smoking onset rates by about 50 percent, but it is important for studies to conduct long-term follow-ups of students to determine if interventions prevent or merely delay the onset of smoking. Design of these antismoking intervention studies in adolescents present a number of difficulties and challenges to health psychologists: difficulties in assigning students to conditions, low levels of smoking at entry into the study, and so on (Flay, 1985). However, social learning and attitude change techniques are now being widely used in the prevention of smoking and are a good example of how health psychology research can be used to address an important social and health problem.

MODIFYING CARDIOVASCULAR RISK FACTORS

As discussed in Chapter 5, potentially modifiable risk factors for cardiovascular disease include cigarette smoking, increased serum cholesterol levels, hypertension, stress and Type A behavior, lack of exercise and sedentary living, and obesity (Kannel, 1987). Therefore, a variety of intervention trials have been conducted to determine whether these behavioral risk factors can be altered and whether this reduces cardiovascular risk.

The range of prevention strategies includes interventions involving direct face-to-face interactions between therapists and patients and public health approaches consisting of mass communication (e.g., media advertising) to change attitudes and behavior. As noted earlier, behavioral treatments administered through face-to-face treatments have been used successfully in altering diet (Foreyt et al., 1979), smoking (Bernstein and Glasgow, 1976), and physical exercise (Dishman, 1982), but the typical pattern has been short-term success followed by relapse. Well-conducted mass media campaigns directed at large populations can effectively transmit information, alter some attitudes, and produce small shifts in behavior (Meyer et al., 1980). Despite small changes, these health-promotion campaigns are highly cost effective and practically significant because they reach very large numbers of people. Face-to-face and public health approaches have been combined in some intervention studies to maximize the effects obtained.

We shall describe three major preventive projects directed at cardiovascular risk modification: the North Karelia Project, the Stanford Heart Disease Prevention Project, and the Multiple Risk Factor Intervention Trial. The first study employed a media-only campaign, the second incorporated a combined media and face-to-face approach, and the third study used primarily a face-to-face approach.

The North Karelia Project
This project (Puska, 1984) was conducted in Finland—a country with very high rates of coronary heart disease. It began in 1972 as a campaign based in North

Karelia to prevent cardiovascular disease. The study used media educational efforts to stop cigarette smoking, encourage the early detection of hypertension, and decrease cholesterol levels by having people change to low-fat diets. Included in the interventions was a smoking cessation intervention involving televised counseling sessions emphasizing the prevention of relapse. After five years the study reported a decrease in estimated cardiovascular risk in the population that received education compared to a reference population group that did not receive education. Changes included a decrease in smoking, in butter consumption, and in the number of men with untreated high blood pressure. The rate of occurrence of heart attacks and strokes also decreased a significant amount. A later ten-year follow-up revealed a further decrease in risk factors (Puska, 1984).

The Stanford Heart Disease Prevention Project

One of the largest community-wide projects, which employed a combination of mass media and face-to-face approaches, is the Stanford Heart Disease Prevention Project (Farquhar et al., 1977; Meyer et al., 1980). Initially three communities similar in size and socioeconomic status were studied over a three-year period: one community served as a control; a second was exposed to a mass media campaign, including radio and television announcements, billboard and printed advertisements on heart disease risk factors including smoking, diet, and exercise; and a third community received the same mass media campaign plus face-to-face behavioral therapy for high-risk persons. The results indicated that the media campaign alone produced some modest reductions in smoking at three-year follow-up. These participants became more informed about cardiovascular risk factors and reported reduced intake of dietary fats and cholesterol. However, the reductions in cardiovascular risk factors were considerably larger when the media campaign was supplemented with face-to-face instruction. The Stanford study suggests that mass media efforts are most successful when incorporated in a more comprehensive program directed at the modification of health habits. Based on the early findings, the Stanford study has been expanded into a five-city project in which the targets are smoking, nutrition, hypertension treatment, and obesity (Farquhar et al., 1984). The Five City Project will also be able to determine if changes in cardiovascular risk factors induced by the interventions are paralleled by similar changes in cardiovascular morbidity and mortality.

The Multiple Risk Factor Intervention Trial (MRFIT)

The MRFIT study (MRFIT Group, 1982) was a large-scale longitudinal study organized to see whether heart disease mortality could be lowered by eliminating three major, correctable risk factors: smoking, hypertension, and elevated serum cholesterol. Subjects were over twelve thousand men who had elevated risk factors for coronary heart disease (smoking, hypertension, and/or having elevated serum cholesterol) but who had not yet had clinical evidence of heart disease (e.g., heart attack). The participants were randomly assigned to either a Special Intervention (SI) program that included treatment for hypertension, intensive counseling for cigarette smoking, and dietary advice for lowering blood pressure levels. The SI interventions were based in medical clinics and carried out by medical, nursing, or behavioral staff. Patients in the other group (Usual Care, or UC) were referred to their usual sources of medical care (in most cases private practitioners).

At the end of the study, the mortality results were not what the study designers had projected: instead of lowered coronary mortality in the SI group, there were *no* significant differences between the SI and UC groups. It appears that the UC "control group" and the SI experimental group changed their behaviors and decreased significantly in cardiovascular risk over the course of the study. The study's designers had originally anticipated no appreciable decline in risk factors in the UC group. This lowering of risk factors by individuals receiving "usual care" parallels the real reduction in cardiovascular mortality that has occurred in the United States over the last twenty years (see Chapter 5). Another reason why there may not have been significant differences between SI and UC groups is that some of the medical therapies used for hypertension were unexpectedly harmful for a subset of patients (MRFIT Group, 1982).

The unexpected results of the MRFIT study has sparked considerable controversy, and most proponents of the importance of behavioral factors in prevention probably have mixed reactions to these results. Despite their disappointment over the lack of significant group differences, they are pleased that Americans are avoiding high-fat and high-cholesterol foods, keeping their blood pressure controlled, stopping smoking, and increasing their regular physical activity (Grunberg, 1988).

MODIFYING CANCER RISK FACTORS

Cancer is the second leading cause of mortality in the United States today. In this country roughly 50 percent of cancer deaths result from lung, large intestine, colon and rectum, pancreas, and breast cancers (Grunberg, 1988; Roberts, 1984). Overall cancer rates have remained relatively stable except for lung and stomach cancer. The increase in lung cancer rates is largely attributed to smoking and tobacco use. Indeed, it has been estimated that more than three-quarters of cancer cases are tied to lifestyle factors (National Cancer Institute, 1984). Such factors as the foods people eat, whether or not they smoke, and the work they do all affect their likelihood of getting cancer.

The associations of smoking with a variety of cancers, especially cancer of the lung, are well known and well established. However, dietary factors are gaining increasing attention as cancer causes. For example, human epidemiological and animal laboratory studies indicate that consuming certain kinds of foods is associated with gastrointestinal, breast, ovary, and prostate cancer, and possibly with respiratory system and bladder cancer (Roberts, 1984). Excessive food intake, consumption of high-fat diets, and particular types of food preparation (smoking, frying) are associated with increased cancer rates, while reducing total food intake and consumption of low-fat diets, fruits, and vegetables may actually decrease the likelihood of various cancers (Grunberg, 1988).

There is consistent evidence of a relationship between fat intake and breast cancer, and also cancer of the large intestine, prostate, and possibly other organs (Roberts, 1984). Epidemiological studies also indicate that increased intake of dietary fiber from vegetables, fruits, and whole-grain cereals decreases risk of colorectal cancer. Consumption of vegetables such as broccoli, cabbage, brussels sprouts, and dark-green and yellow vegetables rich in carotene is associated with decreased risk of cancer at several sites (Roberts, 1984). Smoking, barbequeing, and charcoal broiling of foods can deposit carcinogenic substances on food surfaces and therefore can contribute to cancer risk (Grunberg, 1988). Knowledge and awareness of the relationships between what we eat and long-term health has spread, in part due to prevention-oriented educational campaigns conducted by public service–minded grocery chains.

The association of diet and breast cancer has led to intervention studies to determine if reducing dietary fat intake in women at risk for breast cancer by virtue of having benign breast disease will lower the incidence of their disease (Boyd et al., 1985). Similar dietary intervention studies to lower risk of breast cancer are ongoing in the United States and Canada, and the National Cancer Institute has made public education about the dietary antecedents of cancer an important prevention objective (National Cancer Institute, 1984).

WORKSITE HEALTH PROMOTION

People spend a large proportion of their time at work, and the occupational setting is therefore a convenient place for health-promotion interventions. Prevention activities conducted at work are nearby and accessible, and employers stand to benefit from healthier employees. In addition, the worksite is an environment where organizational and social structures can be used to design interventions that are effective.

Worksite health-promotion programs include hypertension screening and treatment, smoking cessation, weight loss, stress management, and supervised aerobic physical exercise (Fielding, 1984). Many corporations now offer at least some of these programs, with the justification for their cost being that employee morale will be enhanced, that productivity will be improved, and that health insurance and hospitalization costs will be reduced. However, evaluation research concerning these programs has been of uneven quality, and scientific proof of the efficacy of these programs remains unclear (Krantz et al., 1985; Nathan, 1984). However, such programs do appear to be feasible, and health psychologists are currently working on developing more effective, convenient, and cost-effective programs.

One example of a novel worksite health-promotion intervention has been tried in the area of weight loss. Typically, weight-loss interventions have not translated well from clinical to work settings: attrition is often higher and resultant weight loss is reported to be less for worksite programs. Brownell et al. (1984) evaluated several weight-loss competitions held in business-industrial settings. In a one such competition, a challenge to lose the most weight was issued by the presidents of three banks to see which bank could achieve the greatest average weight loss. Workers therefore were not only losing weight for the benefit of their own health but were part of a group competition. Nearly one-third of the workforce participated in a twelve-week program, and the results were most encouraging. The dropout rate in the competition was exceptionally low and average weight loss was high. Both employees and management reported positive changes in morale and employee-management relations, and the cost-effectiveness of the weight loss was the best ever reported. (See Figure 13.5.) This study demonstrated how motivation can be enhanced by harnessing the group loyalty and social support that can be engaged at the worksite. As a

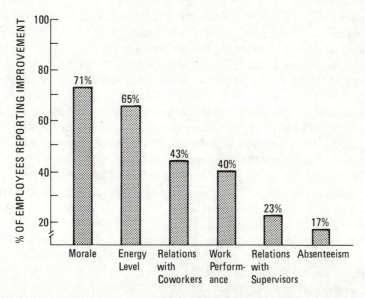

Figure 13.5   **Percentage of employees reporting improvement in work-related areas due to weight loss. All employees who did not report improvement in an area listed "no change" as a response.**
Reprinted by permission of the publisher from K. D. Brownell, et al. Weight loss competitions at the work site: Impact on weight, morale, and cost effectiveness. *American Journal of Public Health,* 1984, *74,* 1283–1285.

result of the success of this strategy with weight loss, it is currently being applied to other health habits such as smoking.

Worksite physical exercise programs are also becoming increasingly popular. A recent study evaluated the feasibility and effectiveness of an attempt to increase the exercise levels of all employees at four large companies (Blair et al., 1986). Employees at the intervention sites were exposed to a health-promotion program that provided a regular exercise program as well as resources and encouragement for smoking cessation, stress management, weight loss, and hypertension control. When compared to workers at other companies, there was a widespread and clinically significant increase in the number of regularly exercising employees and in employee fitness. The long-term maintenance of exercise habits over a two-year period was also encouraging. Thus large numbers of people can be encouraged to adopt healthier lifestyles through effective worksite interventions.

PREVENTION OF AIDS

As we discussed in Chapter 6, AIDS is a life-threatening disease caused by a virus, HIV, and spread by sexual contact or exposure to substantial amounts of infected blood. Currently there is no vaccine to protect us from AIDS, and, because HIV attacks and resides in the T-helper cells of the immune system, victims may be made more vulnerable to further infection and to other pathogens. Thus AIDS patients often exhibit other syndromes, particularly "opportunistic" diseases such as pneumonia. There is also no cure, and effective treatments are currently limited. Once a person is infected with HIV, he or she is likely to develop AIDS; there are no known ways of blocking or reversing this process. The key, then, is to prevent people from ever being infected with HIV, to reduce behaviors that put people at risk for HIV infection. Health psychologists and behavioral scientists play an important role in this effort.

We have discussed a number of obstacles to prevention of various diseases, and all apply to AIDS as well. Compounding the problem, however, is both the nature of the disease and its primary modes of transmission. AIDS is spread through sexual contact and by sharing needles in drug use, and behavior change in these areas has not been very successful in the past. Attempts to curtail teenage pregnancy have not fared particularly well, and the dependence involved in drug use makes this behavior very resistant to interventions. A number of different approaches to preventing the spread of the AIDS virus have been attempted, with some success.

Several approaches to preventing HIV infection through sexual contact exist, ranging from advocacy of abstinence from sex and monogamous sexual relationships to the use of condoms and the practice of "safer" sex. Limiting the number of different sexual partners can reduce the risk of infection, particularly if one's part-ners are from low-risk groups. The use of protection during sex is one of the more important alternatives to basic changes in one's sexual behavior. By preventing exchange of blood, semen, or vaginal fluid, protected sex can greatly reduce the risk of infection (Francis and Chin, 1987). Condoms have been shown to reduce the likelihood of HIV transmission (Conant et at., 1986). It has been difficult to change sexual behavior, however, as the use of condoms may be seen as negative and may meet with resistance from sexual partners. Part of prevention attempts has been teaching people how to handle resistance to safer sex practices.

A common assumption of many campaigns to reduce risky behaviors is that repetitive media presentation of information about the risks and alternative behav-iors will lead to reduction of risk. The findings of a number of studies indicate that this can occur, but often does not, depending on a range of factors (Leventhal and Cleary, 1980). Sometimes publicity that is not part of a deliberate campaign may lead to behavior change, as was the case when the media carried reports of the dangers associated with the use of birth control pills and intrauterine devices (IUDs). Use of these methods of contraception declined following this publicity (Jones et al., 1980). There is some evidence that publicity and information campaigns have had positive effects on behaviors that increase one's risk of HIV infection, but because those at risk are members of different groups, unfocused campaigns may not work as well as those aimed at smaller, homogenous groups.

Since 1983, when the Public Health Service suggested that members of groups at high risk for AIDS limit the number of sexual partners, gay men have shown behavior change and reduction of the number of partners they reported (Curran, 1985). Other researchers have also reported declines in risky sexual behavior among gay men (McKusick et al., 1985; Martin, 1986). Targeted and intensive interventions that respond to individual needs and that emphasize identification and modeling may be effective in further reducing behaviors that increase risk of HIV infection (Solomon and DeJong, 1986).

Targeting specific high-risk groups is an important aspect of prevention programs. This allows us to tailor the content of the program to specifically fit the needs, lifestyle, and risks of the group being addressed. By selecting target groups, one can address very specific fears, concerns, behaviors, and misconceptions. In designing prevention programs for AIDS, several high-risk groups are clear and have been targeted. Homosexuals, sexually active young people, and intravenous drug users are among these groups, but they may be crosscut by sex, culture, ethnic background, and so on. Though targeting increasingly smaller groups may not be economical, it makes sense that such an approach would be more effective. People who are at risk for AIDS are not all the same—some are young, others are older, some use drugs, some do not, and so on. Knowing whom one is speaking to and what his or her prevalent perceptions are should increase the effectiveness of resulting interventions.

Nevertheless, an important part of prevention of any illness is providing information about the illness, how one can "catch it," and so on. With a disease such as AIDS, information dissemination may take on even greater importance, owing to the fear surrounding it and distrust by some groups of "office" information. There has not been a great deal of research on knowledge about AIDS, but polls have suggested that people overestimate and underestimate their risk of getting AIDS and that people who report being most knowledgeable about the disease report the least fear of getting it (see Singer and Rogers, 1986). Familiarity appears to be an important aspect of one's ratings of how vulnerable people feel: in San Francisco, where the per-capita rate of AIDS is highest in the United States, only a third of respondents indicated that AIDS was a personal health concern, compared to 57 percent of respondents in New York, 50 percent in Miami, and 47 percent in Los Angeles (see Temoshok, Sweet, and Zich, 1987). This could be due to many reasons, but one explanation is that San Franciscans, who have had the most exposure to the disease and news about it and probably to prevention campaigns, therefore have more information on which to base risk estimates. Another explanation is simply that the greater fear in the San Francisco area causes many people to deny the threat.

In an attempt to assess knowledge and attitudes about AIDS, Temoshok, Sweet, and Zich (1987) administered a questionnaire in the late spring of 1985 to 399 people in San Francisco, New York, and London. One finding of this survey was the respondents categorized as being at greater risk by virtue of being gay or bisexual perceived AIDS as more important than did the rest of the sample. This group was also more knowledgeable about AIDS, had been concerned about AIDS for a longer period of time, viewed themselves as being more susceptible to the disease, and rated the risk of getting AIDS as higher than did others in any of the three cities. Knowledge about AIDS was negatively correlated with fear of the disease: those who indicated more knowledge about the disease tended to report less fear of it. Unfortunately, knowledge *was not associated with changes in sexual behavior.* Similarly, perceived risk of AIDS was not related to changes in sexual behavior. Among Londoners and New Yorkers who did not report themselves being gay or bisexual, fear and antigay attitudes were related to changes in sexual behavior (Temoshok, Sweet, and Zich, 1987).

These results suggest that education alone is not sufficient to produce the kinds of behaviors needed to prevent the spread of AIDS. While efforts designed to increase people's knowledge are important, they should be coupled with attempts to reduce fears and prejudice. Among London respondents, fear of AIDS was negatively correlated with knowledge as those who reported greater fear or antigay attitudes also had less knowledge of AIDS (Temoshok et al., 1987). This again suggests that fear of AIDS may encourage denial and avoidance of information about it. Since this group was the lowest risk group (at the time of the survey, AIDS had been evident for less time and was less prevalent in London than in New York or San Francisco), these data are of particular interest for early prevention efforts. Fear and prejudice were considerably less predictive of knowledge or behavior among San Francisco residents or among gays and bisexuals in any city, suggesting that the tactics for early and later stages of preventive interventions could emphasize different issues.

Knowledge about a disease and our theories about its causes and consequences are important factors in efforts to prevent illnesses. This is no different for AIDS, where fear and misconception abound. Since AIDS is a sexually transmitted disease, a number of groups that may not perceive themselves to be at risk are in fact in the higher risk groups: Sexually active adolescents, for example, are likely to come in contact with sexually transmitted diseases, and it is estimated that more than half of the 20 million victims of sexually transmitted diseases reported each year will be under twenty-five years of age (DiClemente, Zorn, and Temoshok, 1987). This means that teenagers, college students, and young adults, by virtue of their greater sexual activity and greater likelihood of having several sexual partners, may be at risk for HIV infection. Yet the level of knowledge of the disease in this group is poor: high school students do not know very much about AIDS, and they do not believe they are likely to get it (Price, Desmond, and Kukulka, 1985). College students have also been studied, and they too express little concern about getting AIDS and do not report changes in their sexual behavior (Simkins and Eberhage, 1984). In a study of 1,326 students from ten high schools in San Francisco, DiClemente et al. (1987) found that students knew that AIDS was spread through sexual contact and by sharing needles during drug use. What they did not know was how they could *not* get the disease—only 41 percent knew that one could not get the disease from kissing someone and 26 percent were not sure that the use of condoms would lower the risk of contracting AIDS. Most of those studied were interested in learning more about AIDS.

Drug users may be particularly resistant to behavior change and are difficult to reach with information or behavior change interventions. It appears that the media is effective in conveying basic information about AIDS, but it is not likely that this alone will change drug users' behavior sufficiently to reduce the incidence of the disease in this group (Des Jarlais and Friedman, 1987). It has been argued that, consistent with the idea of targeting groups, interventions should include very specific information about how the disease is spread and how it can be stopped. Thus detailed information about how drug users should or should not clean their needles and the like should be included in any attempt to change their behavior (Des Jarlais and Friedman, 1987).

SUMMARY

The leading causes of death today are chronic diseases that are strongly affected by behavioral factors. Awareness of the importance of personal lifestyle decisions for health and longevity has resulted in renewed interest in behavioral factors in preventive medicine. Health-impairing habits or *behavioral pathogens* have been identified and include such factors and smoking, excessive alcohol consumption, improper diet, and so on. *Behavioral immunogens,* or health-protective behaviors, include the converse or opposite of these practices. In a major study seven specific health practices were highly correlated with better health and lowered mortality: getting a good night's sleep, not smoking, eating breakfast every day, not eating between meals, being at or near prescribed weight, moderate or no use of alcohol, and regular physical activity. Similar behaviors have been shown to be characteristic of societies known for their longevity.

Barriers to modifying health behaviors include the fact that healthy lifestyles have long-term rewards but often do not provide immediate benefits. In addition, forces in the social and cultural environment often lead individuals to engage in unhealthy behaviors, despite knowledge of their health consequences (e.g., peer pressure leading teenagers to smoke).

Techniques for changing health beliefs and behaviors include educational approaches, including fear communications, and behavioral modification approaches, including applied behavioral analysis and cognitive-behavioral interventions. Despite the fact that health behaviors can be modified by various approaches, it is difficult to maintain these changes over a long period of time, and an important problem is that of relapse. Relapse prevention is an important application of cognitive-behavioral treatments to health promotion.

Health-promotion programs have been directed at preventing smoking in adolescents. Many of these programs (e.g., the Houston Project) are based on social learning theory and employ techniques of modeling and attitude change. Several programs have also been conducted to modify cardiovascular risk factors in large numbers of people. These projects, which have met with some success, have employed media campaigns sometimes supplemented by face-to-face therapy approaches. Examples of such programs include the Stanford Heart Disease Prevention Project and the Finnish North Karelia Project.

Another major study, the Multiple Risk Factor Intervention Trial (MRFIT), was designed to see if mortality could be lowered in high coronary risk men through intensive face-to-face efforts to modify hypertension, high serum cholesterol, and smoking. The results of the MRFIT were equivocal, with no significant differences between special intervention and control groups. Many people believe this resulted from the fact that members of the control group also lowered their cardiovascular risk more than anticipated.

Cancer risk may also be lowered by stopping or preventing smoking and eating a low-fat, high-fiber diet, and major efforts at cancer prevention through lifestyle modification are currently underway.

The occupational setting is a convenient place for health-promotion interventions. Such activities include worksite hypertension screening and antismoking, stress management, physical exercise, and weight-control programs. Novel approaches such as weight-loss competitions at the worksite have been used to increase employee motivation.

AIDS education is another important behavioral health-promotion activity. Several approaches to preventing infection from the AIDS virus exist, ranging from advocacy of sexual abstinence, to monogamous sexual relationships, to the use of condoms and the practice of "safer" sex. Because of the high AIDS infection risk in intravenous drug users, educational efforts directed at this group are also important.

RECOMMENDED READINGS

Grunberg, N. E. Behavioral factors in preventive medicine and health promotion. In W. Gordon, A. Herd, and A. Baum (Eds.), *Perspectives on behavioral medicine.* vol. 3. New York: Academic Press, 1988.

Matarazzo, J. D., et al. *Behavioral health: A handbook of health enhancement and disease prevention.* New York: Wiley, 1984.

U.S. Department of Health, Education, and Welfare. *Healthy people: The Surgeon General's report on health promotion and disease prevention (background papers).* USPHS Publication #79-55071A, 1979.

REFERENCES

Abramson, L. Y., Garber, J., Edwards, N. B., and Seligman, M. E. P. Expectancy changes in depression and schizophrenia. *Journal of Abnormal Psychology,* 1978, *87,* 102–109.

Abramson, L. Y., Seligman, M. E. P., and Teasdale, J. Learned helplessness in humans: Critique and reformulation. *Journal of Abnormal Psychology,* 1978, *87,* 49–74.

Ader, R. Plasma pepsinogen level as a predictor of susceptibility to gastric erosions in the rat. *Psychosomatic Medicine,* 1963, *25,* 221–230.

———. Behavioral influences on immune responses. In S. M. Weiss, J. A. Herd, and B. H. Fox (Eds.), *Perspectives on behavioral medicine.* New York: Academic Press, 1981a.

———. (Ed.). *Psychoneuroimmunology.* New York: Academic Press. 1981b.

Ader, R., and Cohen, N. Behaviorally conditioned immunosuppression. *Psychosomatic Medicine,* 1975, *37,* 333–340.

———. (1981). Conditioned immunopharmacologic responses. In R. Ader (Ed.), *Psychoneuroimmunology.* New York: Academic Press.

Adesso, V. J., and Glad, W. R. A behavioral test of smoking typology. *Addictive Behaviors,* 1978, *3,* 35–38.

Aiello, J. R., and Thompson, D. Personal space, crowding and spatial behavior in a cultural context. In I. Altman, A. Rappoport, and J. Wohlwill (Eds.), *Human behavior and environment,* vol. 4. New York: Plenum, 1980.

Akil, H., Watson, S. J., Young, E., Lewis, M. E., Khachaturian, H., and Walker, J. M. Endogenous opioids: Biology and function. *Annual Review of Neuroscience,* 1984, *7,* 223–225.

Alexander, A. B., and Smith, D. D. Clinical applications of EMG biofeedback. In R. J. Gatchel and K. P. Price (Eds.), *Clinical applications of biofeedback: Appraisal and status.* New York: Pergamon Press, 1979.

Alexander, F. *Psychosomatic Medicine: Its principles and applications.* New York: Norton, 1950.

Alloy, L. B., Peterson, C., Abramson, L. Y., and Seligman, M. E. P. Attributional style and the generality of learned helplessness. *Journal of Personality and Social Psychology,* 1984, *46,* 681–687.

Altmaier, E. M., and Happ, D. A. Coping skills training's immunization effects against learned helplessness. *Journal of Social and Clinical Psychology,* 1985, *3,* 181–189.

American Heart Association. *Heart facts.* Dallas, Tex.: American Heart Association, 1982.

American Psychiatric Association. *Diagnostic and statistical manual of mental disorders,* 3rd ed. Washington, D.C.: APA, 1980.

Andrés, R. Effect of obesity on total mortality. *International Journal of Obesity,* 1980, *4,* 381–386.

Andrew, J. M. Recovery from surgery, with and without preparatory instruction, for three coping styles. *Journal of Personality and Social Psychology,* 1970, *15,* 223–226.

Angarano, G., Pastore, G., and Monno, L. Rapid spread of HTLV-III infection among drug addicts in Italy. *Lancet,* 1985, *2,* 1302.

Annent, J. *Feedback and human behavior.* Baltimore: Penguin Books, 1969.

Antoni, M. H. Temporal relationship between life events and two illness measures: A cross-lagged panel analysis. *Journal of Human Stress,* 1985, *11,* 21–26.

Armor, D. J., Polich, J. M., and Stambul, H. B. *Alcoholism and treatment.* Santa Monica, Calif.: Rand Corporation, 1976.

Ashton, H., and Stepney, R. *Smoking: Psychology and pharmacology.* New York: Tavistock, 1982.

Atkinson, J. P., Sullivan, T. J., Kelly, J. P., and Parker, C. W. Stimulation by alcohols of cyclic AMP metabolism in human leukocytes. Possible role of cyclic AMP in the anti-inflammatory effects of ethanol. *Journal of Clinical Investigation,* 1977, *60*(2), 284–294.

Auerbach, S. M., Martelli, M. F., and Mercuri, L. G. Anxiety, information, interpersonal impacts, and adjustment to a stressful health care situation. *Journal of Personality and Social Psychology,* 1983, *44,* 1284–1297.

Averill, J. R. Personal control over aversive stimuli and its relationship to stress. *Psychological Bulletin,* 1973, *80,* 286–303.

Ax, A. R. The physiological differentiation between fear and anger in humans. *Psychosomatic Medicine,* 1953, *15,* 433–442.

Ayllon, T., and Azrin, N. H. *The token economy: A motivational system for therapy and rehabilitation.* New York: Appleton-Century-Crofts, 1968.

Baekeland, F., and Lundwall, L. Dropping out of treatment: A critical review. *Psychological Bulletin,* 1975, *82,* 738–783.

Baider, L., and Sarell, M. Coping with cancer among Holocaust survivors in Israel: An exploratory study. *Journal of Human Stress,* 1984, *10,* 121–127.

Bakal, D. A. Headache: A biopsychological perspective. *Psychological Bulletin,* 1975, *82,* 369–382.

———. *Psychology and medicine: Psychobiological dimensions of health and illness.* New York: Springer, 1979.

Baker, G. W., and Chapman, D. W. (Eds.). *Man and society in disaster.* New York: Basic Books, 1962.

Balint, M. *The doctor, the patient, and his illness.* London: Pitman, 1964.

Ballenger, J. J. Experimental effect of cigarette smoke on human respiratory cilia. *New England Journal of Medicine,* 1960, *263*(17), 832–835.

Ban, T. *Recent advances in the biology of schizophrenia.* Springfield, Ill.: Charles C. Thomas, 1973.

Bandura, A. *Principles of behavior modification.* New York: Holt, Rinehart & Winston, 1969.

———. Psychotherapy based upon modeling principles, In A. E. Bergin and S. L. Garfield (Eds.), *Handbook of psychotherapy and behavior change: An empirical analysis.* New York: Wiley, 1971.

———. Self-efficacy: Toward a unifying theory of behavioral change. *Psychological Review,* 1977a, *84,* 191–215.

———. *Social learning theory.* Englewood Cliffs, N. J.: Prentice-Hall, 1977b.

Bandura, A., Blanchard, E. B., and Ritter, B. The relative efficacy of desensitization and modeling approaches for inducing behavioral, affective, and attitudinal changes. *Journal of Personality and Social Psychology,* 1969, *13,* 173–199.

Bandura, A., Grusec, J. E., and Menlove, F. L. Vicarious extinction of avoidance behavior. *Journal of Personality and Social Psychology,* 1967, *5,* 16–23.

Bandura, A., Ross, D., and Ross, S. A. Imitation of film-mediated aggressive models. *Journal of Abnormal and Social Psychology,* 1963, *66,* 3–11.

Barber, J. Rapid induction analgesia: A clinical report. *American Journal of Clinical Hypnosis,* 1977, *19,* 138–147.

Barber, T. X., and Cooper, B. J. The effects on pain of experimentally induced and spontaneous distraction. *Psychological Reports,* 1972, *31,* 647–651.

Barefoot, J. C., Dahlstrom, W. C., and Williams, R. B. Hostility, CHD incidence, and total mortality: A 25-year follow-up study of 255 physicians. *Psychosomatic Medicine,* 1983, *45,* 59–63.

Barnett, J. The comparative effectiveness of the Millon Behavioral Health Inventory and the Minnesota Multiphasic Personality Inventory as predictors of treatment outcome in a rehabilitation program for chronic low back pain (Ph.D. diss. University of Texas Health Science Center, Dallas, 1986).

Baron, R., and Rodin, J. Personal control as a mediator of crowding. In A. Baum, J. E. Singer, and S. Valins (Eds.), *Advances in environmental psychology.* Hillsdale, N.J.: Erlbaum, 1978.

Bartrop, R. W., Lazarus, L., Luckhurst, E., Kiloh, L. G., and Penny, R. Depression lymphocyte function after bereavement. *Lancet,* 1977, *1,* 834–836.

Baum, A., Aiello, J. R., and Calesnick, L. Crowding and personal control: Social density and the development of learned helplessness. *Journal of Personality and Social Psychology,* 1978, *36,* 1000–1011.

Baum, A., Aiello, J. R., and Davis, G. E. Urban stress, withdrawal and health. Paper presented at the annual meeting of the American Psychological Association, New York, 1979.

Baum, A., Calesnick, L. E., Davis, G. E., and Gatchel, R. J. Individual differences in coping with crowding: Stimulus screening and social overload. *Journal of Personality and Social Psychology,* 1981.

Baum, A., Fisher, J. D., and Solomon, S. Type of information, familiarity, and the reduction of crowding stress. *Journal of Personality and Social Psychology,* 1981, *40* (1), 11–23.

Baum, A., and Gatchel, R. J. Cognitive determinants of reactions to uncontrollable events: Development of reactance and learned helplessness. *Journal of Personality and Social Psychology,* 1981, *40,* 1078–1089.

Baum, A., Gatchel, R. J., Aiello, J. R., and Thompson, D. Cognitive mediation of environmental stress. In J. Harvey (Ed.), *Environment, cognition, and social behavior.* Hillsdale, N.J.: Erlbaum, 1981.

Baum, A., Gatchel, R. J., Streufert, J., Baum, C. S., Fleming, R., and Singer, J. E. Psychological stress for alternatives of decontamination of TMI-2 reactor building atmosphere. Washington, D.C.: U.S. Nuclear Regulatory Commission (NUREG/CR-1584), 1980.

Baum, A., and Greenberg, C. I. Waiting for a crowd: The behavioral and perceptual effects of anticipated crowding. *Journal of Personality and Social Psychology,* 1975, *32,* 671–679.

Baum, A., and Koman, S. Differential response to anticipated crowding: Psychological effects of social and spatial density. *Journal of Personality and Social Psychology,* 1976, *34,* 526–536.

Baum, A., Lake, C. R., Gatchel, R. J., Fleming, R., Schaeffer, M. A., Collins, D. L., Gisriel, M. M., Singer, J. E., Baum, C. S., and Streufert, S. Chronic stress at Three Mile Island: Psychological, behavioral, physiological, and biochemical evidence.

Baum, A., Singer, J. E., and Baum, C. S. Stress and the environment. *Journal of Social Issues,* 1981, *37,* 4–35.

Baum, A., and Valins, S. *Architecture and social behavior: Psychological studies of social density.* Hillsdale, N.J.: Erlbaum, 1977.

———. Architectural mediation of residential density and control: Crowding and the regulation of social contact. *Advances in Experimental Social Psychology,* 1979, *12,* 131–175.

Beatty, J. Biofeedback in the treatment of migraine: Simple relaxation or specific effects. In L. White and B. Tursky (Eds.), *Clinical biofeedback: Efficacy and mechanisms.* New York: Guilford Press, 1982.

Beck, A. T. *Cognitive therapy and emotional disorders.* New York: International Universities Press, 1976.

Beck, S. J. *Rorschach's Test I: Basic processes,* 3rd ed. New York: Grune & Stratton, 1961.

Becker, M. H. *The health belief model and*

personal health behavior. Thorofare, N.J.: Charles B. Slack, 1974.

————. Sociobehavioral determinants of compliance. In D. L. Sackett and R. B. Haynes (Eds.), *Compliance with therapeutic regimens.* Baltimore: Johns Hopkins University Press, 1976.

Becker, M. H., and Maiman, L. A. Sociobehavioral determinants of compliance with health and medical care recommendations. *Medical Care,* 1975, *13,* 10–24.

Bedell, S., and Delbanco, T. L. Choices about cardiopulmonary resuscitation in the hospital—when do physicians talk with patients. *New England Journal of Medicine,* 1984, *310*(17), 1089–1093.

Beecher, H. K. Relationship of significance of wound to the pain experienced. *Journal of the American Medical Association,* 1956, *161,* 1609–1613.

Belgian-French Pooling Project. Assessment of Type A behavior by the Bortner scale and ischemic heart disease. *European Heart Journal,* 1984, *5,* 440–446.

Belloc, N. B. Relationship of health practices and mortality. *Preventive Medicine,* 1973, *2,* 67–81.

Belloc, N. B., and Breslow, L. Relationship of physical health status and health practices. *Preventive Medicine,* 1972, *1,* 409–421.

Benet, S. *Abkhasians: The long-living people of the Caucasus.* 1974. New York: Holt, Rinehart and Winston.

Bennik, C. D., Hulst, L. L., and Benthem, J. A. The effects of EMG biofeedback and relaxation training on primary dysmenorrhea. *Journal of Behavioral Medicine,* 1982, *5,* 329–342.

Benson, J. S., and Kennelly, K. J. Learned helplessness: The result of uncontrollable aversive stimuli? *Journal of Personality and Social Psychology,* 1976, *34,* 138–145.

Berger, B. G. Running toward psychological well-being: Special considerations for the female client. In M. L. Sachs and G. Buffone (Eds.), *Running as therapy: An integrated approach.* Lincoln: University of Nebraska Press, 1984.

Berkman, L. F., and Syme, S. L. Social networks, host resistance, and mortality: A nine-year follow-up study of Alameda County residents. *American Journal of Epidemiology,* 1979, *109,* 186–204.

Bernstein, D. A., and Glasgow, R. E. Smoking. In O. F. Pomerleau and J. P. Brady (Eds.), *Behavioral medicine: Theory and practice* Baltimore: Williams & Wilkins, 1979.

Best, J. A., Flay, B. R., Towson, S., Ryan, M. J., Perry, C. L., Brown, K. S., Kerssell, M. W., and D'Avernas, J. R. Smoking prevention and the concept of risk. *Journal of Applied Social Psychology,* 1984, *14,* 257–273.

Bettelheim, B. *The informed heart: Autonomy in a mass age.* Glencoe, Ill.: Free Press, 1960.

Bieliauskas, L. A. Life stress and aid-seeking. *Journal of Human Stress,* 1980, *6,* 28–36.

Bieliauskas, L. A., and Webb, J. T. The social readjustment rating scale: Validity in a college population. *Journal of Psychosomatic Research,* 1974, *18,* 115–123.

Bigelow, G., Liebson, I., and Lawrence, C. Prevention of alcohol abuse by reinforcement of incompatible behavior. Paper presented at the annual meeting of the Association for Advancement of Behavior Therapy, December 1973.

Bignami, G. Selection for high rates and low rates of avoidance conditioning in the rat. *Animal Behaviour,* 1965, *13,* 221–227.

Birk, L. (Ed.). *Biofeedback: Behavioral medicine.* New York: Grune & Stratton, 1973.

Black, J. L., Dolan, M. P., DeFord, H. A., Rubenstein, J. A., Penk, W. E., Robinowitz, R., and Skinner, J. R. Sharing of needles among users in intravenous drugs [letter]. *New England Journal Medicine,* 1986, *314*(7), 446–447.

Blair, S. N., Piserchia, P. V., Curtis, S. W., and Crowder, J. H. A public health intervention model for work-site health promotion: Impact on exercise and physical fitness in a health promotion plan after 24 months.

Journal of the American Medical Association, 1986, *255*(7), 921–926.

Blake, B. C. The application of behavior therapy to the treatment of alcoholism. *Behavior Research and Therapy,* 1967, *3,* 78–85.

Blanchard, E. B., Kolb, L. C., Pallmeyer, T. P., and Gerardi, R. J. Psychophysiological study of post-traumatic stress disorders in Vietnam veterans. *Psychiatric Quarterly,* 1981, *54,* 220–227.

Blum, K. Psychogenetics of drug seeking behavior. In E. E. Muller and A. R. Genezzani (Eds.), *Central and peripheral endorphins: Basic and clinical aspects.* New York: Raven, 1984.

Blum, L. H. *Reading between the lines: Doctor-patient communication.* New York: International Universities Press, 1972.

Blumenthal, J. A., Williams, R., Kong, Y., Schanberg, S. M., and Thompson, L. W. Type A behavior and angiographically documented coronary disease. *Circulation,* 1978, *58,* 634–639.

Blumetti, A. E., and Modesti, L. M. Psychological predictors of success or failure of surgical intervention for intractable back pain. In J. J. Bonica and D. Abbe-Fessard (Eds.), *Advances in pain research and therapy,* vol. 1. New York: Raven, 1976.

Bonica, J. J. *The management of pain.* Philadelphia: Lea & Febiger, 1953.

Bootzin, R. R. Stimulus control of insomnia. Paper presented at the American Psychological Association, Montreal, August 1973.

———. *Behavior modification and therapy: An introduction.* Cambridge, Mass.: Winthrop, 1975.

Borynsenko, M., and Borysenko, J. Stress, behavior, and immunity: Animal models and mediating mechanisms. *General Hospital Psychiatry,* 1982, *4*(1), 413–419.

Bott, E. Teaching of psychology in the medical course. *Bulletin of the Association of American Medical Colleges,* 1928, *3,* 289–304.

Botvin, G. J., Eng, A., and Williams, C. L. Preventing the onset of cigarette smoking through life skills training. *Preventive Medicine,* 1980, *9,* 135–143.

Bovbjerg, D., Ader, R., and Cohen, N. Behaviorally conditioned immunosuppression of a graft vs. host response. *Proceedings of the National Academy of Sciences,* 1982, *79,* 583–585.

Boyd, J. R., Covington, T. R., Stanaszek, W. F., and Coussons, R. T. Drug defaulting, II. Analysis of noncompliance patterns. *American Journal of Hospital Pharmacy,* 1974, *31,* 485–491.

Boyd, N. F., Fish, E. B., Fishnell, E., Cousins, M. L., Bayliss, S. E., and Bruce, W. R. Diet and breast disease: Evidence for the feasibility of a clinical trial involving a major reduction in dietary fat. In T. G. Burish, S. M. Levy, and B. E. Meyerowitz (Eds.), *Cancer, nutrition, and eating behavior: A biobehavioral perspective.* Hillsdale, N.J.: Erlbaum, 1985.

Boyle, C. M. Differences between patients' and doctor's interpretation of some common medical terms. *British Medical Journal,* 1970, *2,* 286–289.

Brady, J. V. Ulcers in "executive" monkeys. *Scientific American,* 1958, *199,* 95–100.

Brady, J. V., Porter, R. W., Conrad, D. G., and Mason, J. W. Avoidance behavior and the development of gastroduodenal ulcers. *Journal of Experimental Analysis of Behavior,* 1958, *1,* 69–73.

Brand, R. J. Coronary-prone behavior as an independent risk factor for coronary heart disease. In T. M. Dembroski, S. M. Weiss, J. L. Shields, S. G. Haynes, and M. Feinleib (Eds.), *Coronary-prone behavior.* New York: Springer-Verlag, 1978.

Brand, R. J., Rosenman, R. H., Jenkins, C. D., Sholtz, R. I., and Zyzanski, S. J. Comparison of coronary heart disease prediction in the Western Collaborative Group. Study using the Structured Interview and the Jenkins Activity Survey assessments of the coronary-prone Type A behavior pattern. *Journal of Chronic Diseases,* in press.

Brand, R. J., Rosenman, R. H., Sholtz, R. I., and Friedman, M. Multivariate prediction of coronary heart disease in the Western Collaborative Group Study compared to the findings of the Framingham Study. *Circulation,* 1976, *53,* 348–355.

Brehm, J. W. *A theory of psychological reactance.* New York: Academic Press, 1966.

Brende, J. O. Electrodermal responses in post-traumatic syndromes. A pilot study of cerebral hemisphere functioning in Vietnam veterans. *Journal of Nervous and Mental Disease,* 1982, *170*(6), 352–361.

Breslow, L., and Enstrom, J. E. Persistence of health habits and their relationship to mortality. *Preventive Medicine,* 1980, *9,* 469–483.

Brigham, J. C. *Social psychology.* Boston: Little, Brown, 1986.

Brooks, G. R., and Richardson, F. C. Emotional skills training: A treatment program for duodenal ulcer. *Behavior Therapy,* 1980, *11,* 198–207.

Brown, G. W., Bhrolchain, M. N., and Harris, T. Social class and psychiatric disturbance among women in an urban population. *Sociology,* 1975, *9,* 225–254.

Brown, J. D., and Lawton, M. Stress and well-being in adolescence: The moderating role of the physical exercise. *Journal of Human Stress,* 1986, *12,* 125–131.

Brownell, K. D. Public health approaches to obesity and its management. *Annual Review of Public Health,* 1986, *7,* 521–533.

Brownell, K. D., Cohen, R. Y., Stunkard, A. J., Felix, M. J., Cooley, N. B. Weight loss competitions at the work site: Impact on weight, morale, and cost-effectiveness. *American Journal of Public Health,* 1984, *74,* 1283–1285.

Bruns, C., and Geist, C. S. Stressful life events and drug use among adolescents. *Journal of Human Stress,* 1984, *10,* 135–139.

Buddell, D. W., and Wilson, G. T. The effects of alcohol and expectancy set on male sexual arousal. *Journal of Abnormal Psychology,* 1976, *85,* 225–234.

Bulman, R. J., and Wortman, C. B. Attribution of blame and coping in the "real world": Severe accident victims react to their lot. *Journal of Personality and Social Psychology,* 1977, *35,* 351–363.

Burch, J. Recent bereavement in relation to suicide. *Journal of Psychosomatic Research,* 1972, *16,* 361–366.

Burks, N., and Martin, B. Everyday problems and life change events: Ongoing versus acute sources of stress. *Journal of Human Stress,* 1985, *11,* 27–35.

Burstein, S., and Meichenbaum, D. The work of worrying in children undergoing surgery. Unpublished manuscript. Cited in B. Melamed, Psychological preparation for hospitalization, in S. Rachman (Ed.), *Contributions to medical psychology.* New York: Pergamon, 1977.

Buss, A. H. *Psychopathology.* New York: Wiley, 1966.

Buss, A. H., and Plomin, R. *A temperament theory of personality development.* New York: Wiley, 1975.

Byrne, D. Repression-sensitization as a dimension of personality. In B. Mayer (Ed.), *Progress in experimental personality research,* vol. 1. New York: Academic Press, 1964.

Caizza, A. A., and Ovary, Z. Ethanol intake and the immune system of guinea pigs. *Journal of Studies on Alcohol,* 1976, *37*(7), 959–964.

Calhoun, J. B. Ecological factors in the development of behavior anomalies. In J. Zubin and H. F. Hunt (Eds.), *Comparative psychopathology.* New York: Grune & Stratton, 1967.

———. Space and the strategy of life. *Ekistics,* 1970, *29,* 425–437.

Cameron, J. S., Glasgow, E. F., Ogg, C. S., et al. Membranoproliferative glomerulonephritis and persistent hypocomplemtaemia. *British Medical Journal,* 1970, *4,* 7–14.

Campbell, R. J., and Henry, J. P. Animal models of hypertension. In D. S. Krantz, A. Baum, and J. E. Singer (Eds.), *Handbook of psychology and health,* Vol. 3, *Cardiovascular disorders and behavior.* Hillsdale, N.J.: Erlbaum, 1983.

Cannon, W. B. The emergency function of

the adrenal medulla in pain and the major emotions. *American Journal of Physiology,* 1914, *33,* 356–372.

———. The James-Lange theory of emotions: A critical examination and an alternative. *American Journal of Psychology,* 1927, *39,* 106–124.

———. Neural organization for emotional expression. In M. L. Reymert (Ed.), *Feelings and emotions: The Wittenberg Symposium.* Worcester, Mass.: Clark University Press, 1928.

———. *Bodily changes in pain, hunger, fear and rage.* Boston: Branford, 1929.

———. Studies on the conditions of activity in the endocrine organs, XXVII. Evidence that the medulliadrenal secretion is not continuous. *American Journal of Physiology,* 1931, *98,* 447–452.

———. Stresses and strains of homeostasis (Mary Scott Newbold lecture). *American Journal of Medical Sciences,* 1935, *189,* 1–14.

Caplan, R. D., Cobb, S., and French, J. R. P., Jr. Relationships of cessation of smoking with job stress, personality, and social support. *Journal of Applied Psychology,* 1975, *60,* 211–219.

Cappell, H. An evaluation of tension models of alcohol consumption. In Y. Israel et al. (Eds.), *Research advances in alcohol and drug problems.* New York: Wiley, 1974.

Carlens, E. Smoking and the immune response in the airpassages. *Broncho-Pneumologie,* 1976, *26,* 322–323.

Carne, C. A., Weller, I. V., Sutherland, S., Cheingsong-Popov, R., Ferns, R. B., Williams, P., Mindel, A., Tedder, R., and Adler, M. W. Rising prevalence of human T-lymphotropic virus type III (HTLV-III) infection in homosexual men in London. *Lancet,* 1985, *1,* 1261–1262.

Cassem, N. H., and Hackett, T. P. Psychiatric consultation in a coronary care unit. *Annual Internal Medicine,* 1971, *75,* 9–14.

Cautela, J. R. The treatment of alcoholism by covert sensitization. *Psychotherapy: Theory, research, and practice,* 1970, *1,* 83–90.

Centers of Disease Control. *Acquired im-munodeficiency syndrome (AIDS) weekly surveillance report: United States,* September 26, 1986.

Chambers, W. N., and Reiser, M. F. Emotional stress in the precipitation of congestive heart failure. *Psychosomatic Medicine,* 1953, *15,* 38–60.

Chaves, J. F., and Barber, T. X. Cognitive strategies, experimenter modeling, and expectation in the attenuation of pain. *Journal of Abnormal Psychology,* 1974, *83,* 356–363.

Chen, E., and Cobb, S. Family structure in relation to health and disease. *Journal of Chronic Diseases,* 1960, *12,* 544–567.

Chesney, M. A. Behavior modification and health enhancement. In J. D. Matarazzo, S. M. Weiss, J. A. Herd, N. E. Miller, and S. M. Weiss (Eds.), *Behavioral health: A handbook of health enhancement and disease prevention.* New York: Wiley, 1984.

Chesney, M. A., Black, G. W., Chadwick, J. H., and Rosenman, R. H. Psychological correlates of the coronary-prone behavior pattern. *Journal of Behavioral Medicine,* 1981, *4,* 217–230.

Chesney, M. A., Sevelius, G., Black, G. W., Ward, M. M., Swan, G. E., and Rosenman, R. H. Work environment, Type A behavior, and coronary heart disease risk factors. *Journal of Occupational Medicine,* 1981, *23,* 551–555.

Chiriboga, D. A., and Cutler, L. Stress and adaptation: Life span perspectives. In L. W. Poon (Ed.), *Aging in the 1980's: Psychological issues.* Washington, D.C.: American Psychological Association, 1980.

Christopherson, V. Socio-cultural correlates of pain response. Final report of Project #1390, Vocational Rehabilitation Administration. Washington, D.C.: U.S. Department of Health, Education, and Welfare, 1966.

Clements, C. D., and Sider, R. C. Medical-ethics assault upon medical values. *Journal of the American Medical Association,* 250(15), 2011–2015.

Coates, D., and Wortman, C. Depression maintenance and interpersonal control. In A. Baum and J. E. Singer (Eds.), *Advances in environmental psychology,* vol. 2. Hillsdale, N.J.: Erlbaum, 1980.

Coates, R. A., Soskoline, C. L., Calzavara, L., Read, S. E., Fanning, M. M., Shepherd, F. A., Klein, M. M., and Johnson, J. K. The reliability of sexual histories in AIDS-related research: Evaluation of an interview-administered questionnaire. *Canadian Journal of Public Health,* 1987, *77*(5), 343–348.

Cobb, B., Clark, R., McGuire, C., and Hone, C. Patient-responsible delay of treatment of cancer: A social psychological study. *Cancer,* 1954, *1,* 920–926.

Cobb, S. Social support as a moderator of life stress. *Psychosomatic Medicine,* 1976, *38,* 300–314.

Cobb, S., Kasl, S. V., French, J. R. P., Jr., and Norstebo, G. The intrafamilial transmission of rheumatoid arthritis. Why do wives with rheumatoid arthritis have husbands with peptic ulcer? *Journal of Chronic Diseases,* 1969, *22,* 279–295.

Cobb, S., and Rose, R. M. Hypertension, peptic ulcer, and diabetes in air traffic controllers. *Journal of the American Medical Association,* 1973, *224,* 489–492.

Cohen, A. J., Li, F. P., Berg, S., Marchetta, D. J., Tsai, S., Jacobs, S. C., and Brown, R. S. Heredity renal-cell carcinoma associated with a chromosomal translocation. *New England Journal of Medicine,* 1979, *301,* 592–595.

Cohen, E. A. *Human behavior in the concentration camp.* New York: W. W. Norton, 1953.

Cohen, R. E., and Tennen, H. Self-punishment in learned helplessness and depression. *Journal of Social and Clinical Psychology,* 1985, *3,* 82–96.

Cohen, S. Environmental load and allocation of attention. In A. Baum, J. E. Singer, and S. Valins (Eds.), *Advances in environmental psychology,* vol. 1. Hillsdale, N.J.: Erlbaum, 1978.

———. Aftereffects of stress on human performance and social behavior. A review of research and theory. *Psychological Bulletin,* 1980, *88,* 82–108.

Cohen, S., and McKay, G. Social support, stress, and the buffering hypothesis: A theoretical analysis. In A. Baum, J. E. Singer, and S. E. Taylor (Eds.), *Handbook of psychology and health,* Vol. 4. Hillsdale, N.J.: Erlbaum, 1984.

Cohen, S., and Syme, S. L. *Social support and health.* Orlando, Fla.: Academic Press, 1985.

Cohen, S., and Wills, T. A. Stress, social support, and the buffering hypothesis: A critical review. Psychological Bulletin, 1985, *98,* 310–357.

Cohen, S., Evans, G., Krantz, D. S., and Stokols, D. Physiological, motivational, and cognitive effects of aircraft noise on children: Moving from the laboratory to the field. *American Psychologist,* 1980, *35,* 231–243.

Cohen, S., Evans, G. W., Stokols, D., and Krantz, D. S. *Behavior, health, and environmental stress.* New York: Plenum, 1986.

Cohen, S., Rothbart, M., and Phillips, S. Locus of control and the generality of learned helplessness in humans. *Journal of Personality and Social Psychology,* 1976, *34,* 1049–1056.

Collins, A., and Frankenhaeuser, M. Stress responses in male and female engineering students. *Journal of Human Stress,* 1978, *4,* 43–48.

Conant, M., Hardy, D., Sernatinger, J., Spicer, D., and Levy, J. A. Condoms prevent transmission of AIDS-associated retrovirus [letter]. *Journal of the American Medical Association,* 1986, *255*(13), 1706.

Conge, G. A., and Gouche, P. Effet de l'intoxication experimentale par l'alcool sur la reponse d'immunité à mediation cellulaire de la souris. *Food and Chemical Toxicology,* 1985, *23*(12), 1099.

Cook, W. W., and Medley, D. M. Proposed hostility and pharisaic virtue scales for the MMPI. *Journal of Applied Psychology,* 1954, *38,* 414–418.

Coopersmith, S. Adaptive reactions of alcoholics and nonalcoholics. *Quarterly Journal of Studies on Alcohol,* 1964, *27,* 262–278.

Corah, N. L., and Boffa, J. Perceived control, self-observation, and response to aversive stimulation. *Journal of Personality and Social Psychology,* 1970, *16,* 1–4.

Coser, R. L. *Life on the ward.* East Lansing: Michigan State University Press, 1962.

Costa, P. T., Jr. Is neuroticism a risk factor for CAD? Is Type A a measure of neuroticism? In T. Schmidt, T. Dembroski, and G. Blumchen (Eds.), *Biological and psychological factors in cardiovascular disease.* New York: Springer-Verlag, 1986.

Cox, D. J., and Hobbs, W. Biofeedback as a treatment for tension headaches. In L. White and B. Tursky (Eds.), *Clinical biofeedback: Efficacy and mechanisms.* New York: Guilford Press, 1982.

Cox, J. P., Evans, J. F., and Jamieson, J. L. Aerobic power and toxic heart rate responses to psychosocial stressors. *Personality and Social Psychology Bulletin,* 1979, *5,* 160–163.

Cox, T., and MacKay, C. Psychosocial factors and psychophysiological mechanisms in the etiology and development of cancer. *Social Science and Medicine,* 1982, *16,* 381–396.

Coyne, J. C., and Lazarus, R. S. Cognitive style, stress perspective, and coping. In J. L. Kutash and L. B. Schlesinger (Eds.), *Handbook on stress and anxiety.* San Francisco: Jossey-Bass, 1980.

Cromwell, R. L., Butterfield, E. C., Brayfield, F. M., and Curry, J. J. *Acute myocardial infarction: Reaction and recovery.* St. Louis: C. V. Mosby, 1977.

Croog, S. H. Problems of barriers in the rehabilitation of heart patients: Social and psychological aspects. *Cardiac Rehabilitation,* 1975, *6,* 27.

———. Recovery and rehabilitation of coronary patients: Psychological aspects. In D. S. Krantz, A. Baum, and J. E. Singer (Eds.), *Handbook of psychology and health,* vol. 3, *Cardiovascular disorders and behavior.* Hillsdale, N.J.: Erlbaum, 1983.

Curran, J. W., Morgan, W. M., Hardy, A. M., Jaffe, H. W., Darrow W. W., and Dowdle, W. R. The epidemiology of AIDS: Current status and future prospects. *Science,* 1985, *229,* 1352–1357.

Dahl, L. K., Heine, M., and Tassinari, L. Role of genetic factors in susceptibility to experimental hypertension due to chronic excess salt ingestion. *Nature,* 1962 *194,* 480–482.

Dahlstrom, W. G., and Welsh, G. S. *An MMPI handbook.* Minneapolis: University of Minnesota Press, 1960.

Dahlstrom, W. G., Welsh, G. S., and Dahlstrom, L. E. *MMPI handbook,* vol. 1, *Clinical interpretations.* Minneapolis: University of Minnesota Press, 1972.

Dalessio, D. J. *Wolff's headache and other head pain.* New York: Oxford University Press, 1972.

Dattore, P. J., Shontz, F. C., and Coyne, L. Premorbid personality differentiation of cancer and noncancer groups: A list of the hypotheses of cancer proneness. *Journal of Consulting and Clinical Psychology,* 1980, *48,* 388–394.

Davidson, W. S. Studies of aversive conditioning of alcoholics: A critical review of theory and research methodology. *Psychological Bulletin,* 1974, *81,* 571–581.

Davis, M. S. Variations in patients' compliance with doctors' orders: Analysis of congruence between survey responses and results of empirical investigations. *Journal of Medical Education,* 1966, *41,* 1037–1048.

———. Physiologic, psychological and demographic factors in patient compliance with doctors' orders. *Medical Care,* 1968, *6,* 115–122.

Davis, R. Stress and hemostatic mechanisms. In R. S. Eliot (Ed.), *Stress and the heart.* Mount Kisco, N.Y.: Futura, 1974.

Davidson, L. M., and Baum, A. Chronic stress and posttraumatic stress disorders. *Journal of Consulting and Clinical Psychology,* 1986, *54*(3), 303–308.

Decke, E. Effects of taste on the eating behavior of obese and normal persons. Cited in S. Schachter (Ed.), *Emotion, obesity, and crime.* New York: Academic Press, 1971.

Delahunt, J., and Curran, J. P. The effectiveness of negative practice and self-control techniques in the reduction of smoking behavior. *Journal of Consulting and Clinical Psychology,* 1976, *44,* 1002–1007.

Dembroski, T. M. Reliability and validity of methods used to assess coronary-prone behavior. In T. M. Dembroski, S. M. Weiss, J. L. Shields, S. G. Haynes, and M. Feinleib (Eds.), *Coronary-prone behavior.* New York: Springer-Verlag, 1978.

Dembroski, T. M., MacDougall, J. M., Herd, J. A., and Shields, J. L. Perspectives on coronary-prone behavior. In D. S. Krantz, A. Baum, and J. E. Singer (Eds.), *Handbook of psychology and health vol. 3: Cardiovascular disorders and behavior.* Hillsdale, N.J.: Erlbaum, 1983.

Department Task Force on Prevention. *Disease prevention and health promotion: Federal programs and prospects* (DHEW Publication No. 79-55071B). Washington, D.C.: U.S. Government Printing Office, 1978.

Derogatis, L. R., Abeloff, M. D., and Melisaratos, N. Psychological coping mechanisms and survival time in metastatic breast cancer. *Journal of the American Medical Association,* 1979, *242,* 1504–1508.

Derogatis, L. R., Lipman, R. S., and Covi, L. The SCL-90: An outpatient psychiatric rating scale. *Psychopharmacology Bulletin,* 1973, *9,* 13–28.

Derogatis, L. R., Rickels, K., and Rock, A. F. The SCL-90 and the MMPI: A step in the validation of a new self-report scale. *British Journal of Psychiatry,* 1976, *128,* 280–289.

Des Jarlais, D. C., Friedman, S. R., and Strug, D. AIDS and needle sharing within the IV drug use subculture. In D. Feldman and T. Johnson (Eds.), *The Social Dimensions of AIDS: Methods and Theory.* New York: Praeger, 1987.

Deutsch, C. P. Auditory discrimination and learning: Social factors. *The Merrill-Palmer Quarterly of Behavior and Development,* 1964, *10,* 277–296.

Diamond, S. *Personality and temperament.* New York: Harper & Row, 1957.

DiClemente, R. J., Zorn, J., and Temoshok, L. Adolescents and AIDS: A survey of knowledge, attitudes and beliefs about AIDS in San Francisco. *American Journal of Public Health,* 1986, *76*(12), 1443–1445.

Diener, C. I., and Dweck, C. S. An analysis of learned helplessness: Continuous changes in performance, strategy, and achievement cognitions following failure. *Journal of Personality and Social Psychology,* 1978, *36,* 451–461.

Dillard, C. O. *The family viewpoint.* Paper presented at the Cardiac Seminar Program, *Heart Disease, Stress and Industry,* The President's Committee on Employment of the Handicapped, New York, 1982.

Dimsdale, J. A perspective on Type A behavior and coronary disease. *New England Journal of Medicine,* 1988, *318,* 110–112.

Dimsdale, J. E., Hackett, J. P., Hutter, A. M., Block, P. C., and Catanzano, D. Type A personality and extent of coronary atherosclerosis. *American Journal of Cardiology,* 1978, *42,* 583–586.

Dishman, R. K. Compliance/adherence in health related exercise. *Health Psychology,* 1982, *1,* 45–59.

Doehrman, S. R. Psycho-social aspects of recovery from coronary heart disease: A review. *Social Science Medicine,* 1977, *11,* 199–218.

Dohrenwend, B. S., and Dohrenwend, B. P. *Stressful life events: Their nature and effects.* New York: Wiley, 1974.

Donovan, W. L., and Leavitt, L. A. Simulating conditions of learned helplessness: The effects of interventions and attributions. *Child Development,* 1985, *56,* 594–603.

Douglas, D., and Anisman, H. Helplessness or expectation incongruency: Effects of aversive consequence on subsequent performance. *Journal of Experimental Psychology: Human Perception and Performance,* 1975, *1,* 411–417.

Dunbar, F. *Psychosomatic diagnosis.* New York: Harper & Row, 1943.

Dutton, D. G., and Aron, A. P. Some evidence for heightened sexual attraction under conditions of high anxiety. *Journal of*

Personality and Social Psychology, 1974, *30,* 510–517.

Dweck, C. S. The role of expectations and attributions in the alleviation of learned helplessness. *Journal of Personality and Social Psychology,* 1975, *31,* 674–685.

Dweck, C. S., and Bush, E. S. Sex differences in learned helplessness: (1) Differential debilitation with peer and adult evaluators. *Developmental Psychology,* 1976, *12,* 147–156.

Dweck, C. S., and Gilliard, D. Expectancy statements as determinants of reactions to failure: Sex differences in persistence and expectancy change. *Journal of Personality and Social Psychology,* 1975, *32,* 1077–1084.

Dweck, C. S., and Reppucci, N. D. Learned helplessness and reinforcement responsibility in children. *Journal of Personality and Social Psychology,* 1973, *25,* 109–116.

Eales, L. J., Nye, K. E., Parkin, J. M., Weber, J. N., Forster, S. M., Harris, J. R. W., and Pinching, A. J. Association of different allelic forms of group-specific component with susceptibility to and clinical manifestation of human immunodeficiency virus infection. *Lancet,* 1987, *1,* 999–1002.

Edwards, A. L. *Edwards personal preference schedule.* New York: Psychological Corporation, 1959.

Egbert, L. D., Battit, G. E., Welch, C. E., and Bartlett, M. K. Reduction of postoperative pain by encouragement and instruction of patients. *New England Journal of Medicine,* 1964, *270,* 825–827.

Einhorn, H. J., and Hogarth, R. M. Confidence in judgment: Persistence of the illusion of validity. *Psychological Review,* 1978, *85,* 395–416.

Elling, R., Whittemore, R., and Green, M. Patient participation in a pediatric program. *Journal of Health and Human Behavior,* 1960, *1,* 183–189.

Ellis, A. *Reason and emotion in psychotherapy.* New York: Lyle Stuart, 1962.

Emrick, C. D. A review of psychologically oriented treatment of alcoholism. *Journal of Studies on Alcoholism,* 1975, *36,* 88–108.

Engel, G. L. A psychological setting of so-matic disease: The giving up–given up complex. *Proceedings of the Royal Society of Medicine,* 1967, *60,* 553–563.

Engel, G. L. A life setting conducive to illness: The giving up–given up complex. *Bulletin of the Menninger Clinic,* 1968, *32,* 355–365.

Erichsen, J. E. *On concussion of the spine: Nervous shock and other injuries of the nervous system in their clinical and medicolegal aspects.* London: Longmans, Green, 1882.

Erikson, E. H. *Childhood and society.* New York: Norton, 1983.

Erlenmeyer-Kimling, J., and Jarvik, L. F. Genetics and intelligence: A review. *Science,* 1963, *14a,* 1477–1479.

Euler, U. S. von. *Noradrenaline.* Springfield, Ill.: Charles C. Thomas, 1956.

———. Twenty years of noradrenaline. *Pharmacological Review,* 1966, *18,* 29.

Evans, G. W. Human spatial behavior: The arousal model. In A. Baum and Y. M. Epstein (Eds.), *Human response to crowding.* Hillsdale, N.J.: Erlbaum, 1978.

Evans, G. W., and Jacobs, S. V. Air pollution and human behavior. *Journal of Social Issues,* 1981, *37,* 95–125.

Evans, R. I. Smoking in children and adolescents: Psychosocial determinants and prevention strategies. In *Smoking and health: A report of the Surgeon General* (DHEW Publication No. [PHS] 79-50066). Washington, D.C.: U.S. Government Printing Office, 1979.

Evans, R. I., Henderson, A. H., Hill, P. C., and Raines, B. E. Smoking children and adolescents: Psychosocial determinants and prevention strategies. In *Smoking and health: A report of the Surgeon General* (DHEW Publication No. [PHS] 79-50066). Washington, D.C.: U.S. Government Printing Office, 1979.

Evans, R. I., Rozelle, R. M., Maxwell, S. E., Raines, B. E., Dill, C. A., et al. Social modeling films to deter smoking in adolescents: Results of a three year filed investigation. *Journal of Applied Psychology,* 1981, *66,* 399–414.

Exner, J. E., Jr. *The Rorschach systems.* New York: Grune & Stratton, 1974.

Eysenck, H. J. Personality and the maintenance of the smoking habit. In W. L. Dunn (Ed.), *Smoking behavior: Motives and incentives.* New York: Wiley, 1973.

Farquhar, J. W., Breitrose, H., Haskell, W. L., Meyer, A. J., Maccoby, N., et al. Community education for cardiovascular health. *Lancet,* 1977, *1,* 1192–1195.

Farquhar, J. W., Wood, P. D., Breitrose, H., Haskell, W. L., Meyer, A. J., Maccoby, N., Alexander, J. K., Brown, B. W., McAlister, A. L., Nash, J. D., and Stern, M. P. Community education for cardiovascular health. *Lancet,* 1977, *1,* 1192–1195.

Faust, I. M. Nutrition and the fat cell. *International Journal of Obesity,* 1980. *4,* 314–321.

Ferguson, J. M. *Learning to eat: Behavior modification for weight control.* Palo Alto, Calif.: Bull Publishing Co., 1975.

Ferster, C. B., Nurnberger, J., and Levitt, E. B. Behavioral control of eating. *Journal of Mathetics,* 1962, *1,* 87–109.

Field, P. Effects of tape-recorded hypnotic preparation for surgery. *International Journal of Clinical and Experimental Hypnosis,* 1974, *22,* 54–61.

Fielding, J. D. Health promotion and disease prevention at the worksite. *Annual Review of Public Health,* 1984, *5,* 237–266.

Fink, R., Shapiro, S., and Roester, R. Impact of efforts to increase participation in repetitive screenings for early breast cancer detection. *American Journal of Public Health,* 1972, *62,* 328–336.

Finkelman, J. M., and Glass, D. C. Reappraisal of the relationship between noise and human performance by means of a subsidiary task measure. *Journal of Applied Psychology,* 1970, *54,* 211–213.

Finklea, J. F., Sandifer, S. H., and Smith, D. D. Cigarette smoking and epidemic influenza. *American Journal of Epidemiology,* 1969, *90*(1), 390–399.

Fisher, C. L., Gill, C., Daniels, J. C., Cobb, E. K., Berry, C. A., and Ritzman, S. E. Effects of the space flight environment on man's immune system. *Aerospace Medicine,* 1972, *43,* 856–859.

Fiske, S. T., and Taylor, S. E. *Social cognition.* Reading, Mass.: Addison-Wesley, 1984.

Flanders, W. D., and Rothman, K. J. Interaction of alcohol and tobacco in laryngeal cancer. *American Journal of Epidemiology,* 1982, *115*(3), 371–379.

Flaxman, J. Quitting smoking now or later: Gradual, abrupt, immediate, and delayed quitting. *Behavior Therapy,* 1978, *9,* 260–270.

Flay, B. R. Psychosocial approaches to smoking prevention: A review of findings. *Health Psychology,* 1985, *4,* 449–488.

Flay, B. R., d'Avernas, J. R., Best, J. A., Kersell, M. W., and Ryan, K. B. Cigarette smoking: Why young people do it and ways of preventing it. In P. Firestone and P. McGrath (Eds.), *Pediatric behavioral medicine.* New York: Springer-Verlag, 1985.

Fleming, R., Baum, A., Gisriel, M. M., and Gatchel, R. J. Mediating influences of social support on stress at Three Mile Island. *Journal of Human Stress,* 1982, *8*(3), 14–22.

Flynn, C. B. Three Mile Island telephone survey. Washington, D.C.: U.S. Nuclear Regulatory Commission (NUREG/CR-1093), 1979.

Folkins, C. H., and Sime, W. E. Physical fitness training and mental health. *American Psychologist,* 1981, *36,* 373–389.

Ford, C. E., and Neale, J. M. Learned helplessness and judgments of control. *Journal of Personality and Social Psychology,* 1985, *49,* 1330–1336.

Fordyce, W. E., and Steger, J. C. Chronic pain. In O. F. Pomerleau and J. P. Brady (Eds.), *Behavioral medicine: Theory and practice.* Baltimore: Williams & Wilkins, 1979.

Fordyce, W. E., Fowler, R. S., Lehmann, J. F., and DeLateur, B. J. Some implications of learning in problems of chronic pain. *Journal of Chronic Diseases,* 1968, *21,* 179–190.

Foreyt, J. P., Scott, L. W., Mitchell, R. W.,

and Gotto, A. M. Plasma lipid changes in the normal population following behavioral treatment. *Journal of Consulting Clinical Psychology,* 1979, *47,* 440–452.

Fosco, E., and Geer, J. H. Effects of gaining control over aversive stimuli after differing amounts of no control. *Psychological Reports,* 1971, *29,* 1153–1154.

Fox, B. H. Behavioral issues in prevention of cancer. *Preventive Medicine,* 1976, *5*(1), 106–121.

Fox, P. E., and Oakes, W. F. Learned helplessness: Noncontingent reinforcement in video game performance produces adversement on performance on a lexical decision task. *Bulletin of the Psychosomatic Society,* 1984, *22,* 113–116.

Fox, W. Problem of self-administration of drugs; with particular reference to pulmonary tuberculosis. *Tubercle,* 1958, *39,* 269–274.

Francis, D. P. and Chin, J. The prevention of acquired immunodeficiency syndrome in the United States. An objective strategy for medicine, public health, business, and the community. *Journal of the American Medical Association,* 1987, *257*(10), 1357–1366.

Francis, V., Korsch, B. M., and Morris, M. J. Gaps in doctor–patient communication. *New England Journal of Medicine,* 1969, *280,* 535–540.

Frankenhaeuser, M. Behavior and circulating catecholamines. *Brain Research,* 1971, *31,* 241–262.

———. Biochemical events, stress, and adjustment. Reports from the Psychological Laboratories, University of Stockholm, 1972 (368).

———. Experimental approaches to the study of catecholamines and emotion. Reports from the Psychological Laboratories, University of Stockholm, 1973 (392).

———. The role of peripheral catecholamines in adaption to understimulation and overstimulation. In G. Serban (Ed.), *Psychopathology of human adaptation.* New York: Plenum, 1976.

———. Quality of life: Criteria for behav-

ioral adjustment. *International Journal of Psychology,* 1977, *12,* 99–110.

———. Coping with job stress: A psychobiological approach. Reports from the Department of Psychology, University of Stockholm, 1978 (532).

———. Psychoneuroendocrine approaches to the study of emotion as related to stress and coping. In H. E. Howe and R. Dienstbier (Eds.), *Nebraska symposium on motivation 1978.* Lincoln: University of Nebraska Press, 1979.

Frankenhaeuser, M. The sympathetic-adrenal and pituitary-adrenal response to challenge: Comparison between the sexes. In T. M. Dembroski, T. H. Schmidt, and G. Blumchen (Eds.), *Biobehavioral bases of coronary heart disease.* Basel: Karger, 1983.

Frankenhaeuser, M., Jarpe, G., and Mattell, G. Effects of intravenous infusions of adrenaline and noradrenaline on certain psychological and physiological functions. *Acta Physiologica Scandinavia,* 1961, *51,* 175–186.

Frankenhaeuser, M., and Johansson, G. Stress at work: Psychobiological and psychosocial aspects. Paper presented at the 20th International Congress of Applied Psychology, Edinburgh, 1982.

Frankenhaeuser, M., Nordheden, B., Myrsten, A. L., and Post, B. Psychophysiological reactions to understimulation and overstimulation. *Acta Psychologia,* 1971, *35,* 298–308.

Frankenhaeuser, M., and Rissler, A. Effects of punishment on catecholamine release and efficiency of performance. *Psychopharmacologia,* 1970, *17,* 378–390.

Franklin, M., Krauthamer, M., Razzak Tai, A., and Pinchot, A. *The heart doctors' heart book.* New York: Grosset & Dunlap, 1974.

Franks, J. D. *Persuasion and healing.* New York: Schocken Books, 1961.

Freed, E. The effect of alcohol upon approach-avoidance conflict in the white rat. *Quarterly Journal of Studies on Alcoholism,* 1971, *28,* 236–254.

Friedland, G. H., Harris, C., Butkus-Small,

C., Shine, D., Moll, B., Darrow, W., and Klein, R. S. Intravenous drug abusers and the acquired immunodeficiency syndrome (AIDS). Demographic, drug use, and needle-sharing patterns. *Archives of Internal Medicine,* 1985, *145*(8), 1413–1417.

Friedman, M., Byers, S. O., Diamanti, J., and Rosenman, R. H. Plasma catecholamine response of coronary-prone subjects (Type A) to a specific challenge. *Metabolism,* 1975, *4,* 205–210.

Friedman, M., and Rosenman, R. H. *Type A behavior and your heart.* New York: Knopf, 1974.

Friedman, M., Rosenman, R. H., Straus, R., Wurm, M., and Kositcheck, R. The relationship of behavior pattern A to the state of the coronary vasculature: A study of 51 autopsied subjects. *American Journal of Medicine,* 1968, *44,* 525–538.

Friedman, M., Thoresen, C. D., Gill, J. J., Powell, L. H., Ulmer, D., Thompson, L., Price, V. A., Rabin, D. D., Breall, W. S., Dixon, T., Levy, R., and Bourg, E. Alterations of Type A behavior and reduction in cardiac recurrences in post myocardial infarction patients. *American Heart Journal,* 1984, *108,* 237–248.

Friedman, M., Thoresen, C., Gill, J., Ulmer, D., Powell, L., Price, V., Brown, B., Thompson, L., Rabin, D., Breall, W., Bourg, E., Levy, R., and Dixon, T. Alteration of Type A behavior and its effects on cardiac recurrences in post myocardial infarction patients: Summary results of the recurrent coronary prevention project. *American Heart Journal,* 1986, *112,* 653–665.

Friedman, R., and Iwai, J. Genetic predisposition and stress-induced hypertension. *Science,* 1976, *193,* 161–192.

Friedman, S. B., Glasgow, L. A., and Ader, R. Psychosocial factors modifying host resistance to experimental infections. *Annals of the New York Academy of Sciences,* 1969, *164* (Art. 2), 381–392.

Fries, J. F. Aging, natural death, and the compression of morbidity. *New England Journal of Medicine,* 1976, *303,* 130–135.

Froese, A., Hackett, T. P., Cassem, N. H.,

and Silverberg, E. L. Trajectories of anxiety and depression in denying and nondenying acute myocardial infarction patients during hospitalization. *Journal of Psychosomatic Research,* 1974, *18,* 413–420.

Fromm, E. *The sane society.* New York: Rinehart, 1955.

Galton, F. *Hereditary genius: An inquiry into its laws and consequences.* London: Macmillan, 1869.

Garcia, J., Hankins, W. G., and Rusinak, K. W. Behavioral regulation of the milieu interne in man and rat. *Science,* 1974, *185,* 825–831.

Garrity, T. F. Social involvement and activeness as predictors of morale six months after myocardial infarction. *Social Science and Medicine,* 1973a, *7,* 199–207.

———. Vocational adjustment after first myocardial infarction: Comparative assessment of several variables suggested in the literature. *Social Science and Medicine,* 1973b, *7,* 705–717.

Garrity, T. F. Morbidity, mortality, and rehabilitation. In W. D. Gentry and R. B. Williams (Eds.), *Psychological aspects of myocardial infarction and coronary care.* St. Louis: C. V. Mosby, 1975.

Garrity, T. F., and Marx, M. B. Critical life events and coronary disease. In W. D. Gentry and R. B. Williams, Jr. (Eds.), *Psychological aspects of myocardial infarction and coronary care,* 2nd ed. St. Louis: C. V. Mosby, 1979.

Garrity, T. F., McGill, A., Becker, M., Blanchard, E., Crews, J., Cullen J., Hackett, T., Taylor, J., and Valins, S. Report of the task group of cardiac rehabilitation. In S. M. Weiss (Ed.), *Proceedings of the National Heart and Lung Institute working conference on health behavior* (DHEW Publication No. 76-868). Washington, D.C.: U.S. Government Printing Office, 1976.

Garrity, T. F., and Ries, J. B. Health status as a mediating factor in the life change-academic performance relationship. *Journal of Human Stress,* 1985, *11,* 118–124.

Garfinkel, L. Changes in the cigarette consumption of smokers in relation to changes in tar/nicotine content of cigarettes smoked. *American Journal of Public Health,* 1979, *69,* 1274–1276.

Gatchel, R. J. Biofeedback and the treatment of fear and anxiety. In R. J. Gatchel and K. P. Price (Eds.), *Clinical application of biofeedback: Appraisal and status.* Elmsford, N.Y.: Pergamon, 1979.

————. Effectiveness of two procedures for reducing dental fear: Group-administered desensitization and group education and discussion. *Journal of the American Dental Association,* 1980, *101,* 634–637.

————. Clinical effectiveness of biofeedback in reducing anxiety. In H. Wagner (Ed.), *Social psychophysiology: Theory and clinical applications.* London: Wiley, 1988.

Gatchel, R. J., Deckel, A. W., Weinberg, N., and Smith, J. E. The utility of the Millon Behavioral Health Inventory in the study of chronic headaches. *Headache,* 1985, *25,* 49–54.

Gatchel, R. J., McKinney, M. E., and Koebernick, L. F. Learned helplessness, depression, and physiological responding. *Psychophysiology,* 1977, *14,* 25–31.

Gatchel, R.J., Mayer, T.G., Capra, P., Diamond, P., and Barnett, J. Millon Behavioral Health Inventory: Its utility in predicting physical function in low back pain patients. *Archives of Physical Medicine and Rehabilitation,* 1986, *67,* 878–882.

Gatchel, R. J., and Price, K. P. (Eds.). *Clinical applications of biofeedback: Appraisal and status.* Elmsford, N.Y.: Pergamon, 1979.

Gatchel, R. J., and Proctor, J. D. Physiological correlates of learned helplessness in man. *Journal of Abnormal Psychology,* 1976, *85,* 27–34.

Geer, J. H. Biofeedback and the modification of sexual dysfunctions. In R. J. Gatchel and K. P. Price (Eds.), *Clinical applications of biofeedback: Appraisal and status.* Elmsford, N.Y.: Pergamon, 1979.

Geer, J. H., Davison, G. C., and Gatchel, R. J. Reduction of stress in humans through nonveridical perceived control of aversive stimulation. *Journal of Personality and Social Psychology,* 1970, *16,* 731–738.

Geer, J. H., and Messé, M. Sexual dysfunctions. In R. J. Gatchel, A. Baum, and J. E. Singer (Eds.), *Behavioral medicine and clinical psychology: Overlapping areas.* Hillsdale, N.J.: Erlbaum, 1982.

Gentry, W. D., and Matarazzo, J. D. Medical psychology: Three decades of growth and development. In L. A. Bradley and C. K. Prokop (Eds.), *Medical psychology: Contributions to behavioral medicine.* New York: Academic Press, 1981.

Gilberstadt, H. A modal MMPI profile type in neurodermatitis. *Psychosomatic Medicine,* 1962, *24,* 471–476.

Glaser, R. J., Kiecolt-Glaser, J., Speicher, C. E., and Holliday, J. E. Stress, loneliness and changes in herpes virus latency. *Journal of Behavioral Medicine,* 1985, *8,* 249–260.

Glaser, R., Rice, J., Speicher, C. E., Stout, J. C., and Kiecolt-Glaser, J. K. Stress depresses interferon production concomitant with a decrease in natural killer cell activity. *Behavioral Neuroscience,* 1986 *100*(5), 675–678.

Glaser, R., Thorn, B. E., Tarr, K. L., Kiecolt-Glaser, J. K., and D'Ambrosio, S. M. Effects of stress on methyltransferase synthesis: An important DNA repair enzyme. *Health Psychology,* 1985, *4*(5), 403–412.

Glasgow, R. E., and Bernstein, D. A. Behavioral treatment of smoking behavior. In C. K. Prokop and L. A. Bradley (Eds.), *Medical psychology: Contributions to behavioral medicine.* New York: Academic Press, 1981.

Glass, C. R., and Levy, L. H. Perceived psychophysiological control: The effects of power versus powerlessness. *Cognitive Therapy and Research,* 1982, *6,* 91–103.

Glass, D. C. *Behavior patterns, stress, and coronary disease.* Hillsdale, N.J.: Erlbaum, 1977.

Glass, D. C., and Singer, J. E. *Urban stress.* New York: Academic Press, 1972.

Glass, D. C., Singer, J. E., and Friedman, L. N. Psychic cost of adaptation to an environmental stressor. *Journal of Personality and Social Psychology,* 1969, *12,* 200–210.

Glass, D. C., Singer, J. E., Leonard, H. S., Krantz, D. S., Cohen, S., and Cummings, H. Perceived control of aversive stimulation and the reduction of stress responses. *Journal of Personality,* 1973, *41,* 577–595.

Goedert, J. J., Biggar, R. J., Melbye, D. L., Wilson, S., Gail, M. H., Grossman, R. J., DiGioia, R. A., Sanchez, W. C., Weiss, S. H., and Blattner, W. A. Effect of T4 count and cofactors on the incidence of AIDS in homosexual men infected with human immunodeficiency virus. *Journal of the American Medical Association,* 1987, *257,* 331–334.

Goedert, J. J., Biggar, R. J., Weiss, S. H., Eyster, M. E., Melbye, M., Wilson, S., Ginzburg, H. M., Grossman, R. J., DiGioia, R. A., Sanchez, W. C., Giron, J. A., Ebbesen, P., Gallo, R. C., and Blattner, W. A. Three year incidence of AIDS in five cohorts of HTLV-III-infected risk group members. *Science,* 1986, *231,* 992–995.

Goffman, E. *Asylums.* Garden City, N.Y.: Doubleday, 1961a.

———. *Encounters: Two studies in the sociology of interaction.* Indianapolis: Bobbs-Merrill, 1961b.

———. *Stigma.* Englewood Cliffs, N.J.: Prentice-Hall, 1963.

Goldfried, M. R., and Davison, G. C. *Clinical behavior therapy.* New York: Holt, Rinehart & Winston, 1976.

Goldiamond, I. Self-control procedures in personal behavior problems. *Psychological Reports,* 1965, *17,* 851–868.

Goldstein, A. P., and Stein, N. *Prescriptive psychotherapies.* Elmsford, N.Y.: Pergamon, 1976.

Gordis, L. Methodologic issues in the measurement of patient compliance. In D. L. Sackett and R. B. Haynes (Eds.), *Compliance with therapeutic regimens.* Baltimore: Johns Hopkins University Press, 1976.

Gordis, L., Markowitz, M., and Lillienfield, A. M. Why patients don't follow medical advice: A study of children on long-term antistreptococcal prophylaxis. *Journal of Pediatrics,* 1969, *75,* 957–968.

Gore, S. The influence of social support and related variables in ameliorating the consequences of job loss. Ph.D. diss., University of Pennsylvania, 1973.

Grace, W. J., and Graham, D. T. Relationship of specific attitudes and emotions to certain bodily diseases. *Psychosomatic Medicine,* 1952, *14,* 242–251.

Graham, D. T. Psychosomatic medicine. In N. S. Greenfield and R. A. Sternbach (Eds.), *Handbook of psychophysiology.* New York: Holt, Rinehart & Winston, 1972.

Graham, D. T., Kabler, J. D., and Graham, F. K. Physiological responses to the suggestion of attitudes specific for hives and hypertension. *Psychosomatic Medicine,* 1962, *24,* 159–169.

Graham, D. T., Lundy, R. M., Benjamin, L. S., Kabler, J. D., Lewis, W. C., Kunich, N. C., and Graham, F. K. Specific attitudes in initial interviews with patients having different "psychosomatic" diseases. *Psychosomatic Medicine,* 1962, *24,* 257–266.

Graham, D. T., Stern, J. A., and Winokur, G. Experimental investigation of the specificity hypotheses in psychosomatic disease. *Psychosomatic Medicine,* 1958, *20,* 446–457.

Green, G. M., and Carolin, D. The depressant effect of cigarette smoke on the in vitro antibacterial activity of alveolar macrophages. *New England Journal of Medicine,* 1967, *276,* 421–427.

Green, L. W. Health education models. In J. D. Matarazzo, S. M. Weiss, J. A. Herd, N. E. Miller, and S. M. Weiss (Eds.), *Behavioral health: A handbook of health enhancement and disease prevention.* New York: Wiley, 1984.

Greenberg, C. I., and Baum, A. Compensatory response to anticipated densities. *Journal of Applied Social Psychology,* 1979, *9,* 1–12.

Greene, W. A. The psychosocial setting of the development of leukemia and lymphoma. *Annals of the New York Academy of Sciences,* 1966, *125,* 794–801.

Greene, W. A., Betts, R. F., and Ochitull, H. N. Psychosocial factors and immunity: Preliminary report. Paper presented at the annual meeting of the American Psychosomatic Society, Washington, D.C., 1978.

Greene, W. H., Betts, R. F., Ochitill, H. N., Iker, H. P., and Douglas, R. G. Psychosocial factors and immunity: Preliminary report. *Psychosomatic Medicine*, 1974, *40*, 87.

Greer, S. E., and Calhoun, J. F. Learned helplessness and depression in acutely distressed community residents. *Cognitive Therapy and Research*, 1983, *7*, 205–222.

Grieco, A. Cutting the risks for STD's. *Medical Aspects of Human Sexuality*, March 1987, 70–84.

Griffiths, R. R., Bigelow, G. E., and Liebson, I. The relationship of social factors to ethanol self-administration in alcoholics. In P. E. Nathan, G. A. Marlatt, and T. Loberg (Eds.), *Alcoholism: New directions in behavioral research and treatment*. New York: Plenum, 1978.

Grinker, R. R., and Spiegel, J. P. *War neuroses*. Philadelphia: Blakiston, 1945.

Grinker, R. R., Willerman, B., Bradley, A., and Fastovsky, A. A study of psychological predisposition to the development of operational fatigue. *American Journal of Orthopsychiatry*, 1946, *16*, 191–214.

Gruchow, H. W. Catecholamine activity and infectious disease episodes. *Journal of Human Stress*, 1979, *5*(3), 11–17.

Gruen, W. Effects of brief psychotherapy during the hospitalization period on the recovery process in heart attacks. *Journal of Consulting and Clinical Psychology*, 1975, *43*, 223–232.

Grunberg, N. E. The effects of nicotine and cigarette smoking on food consumption and taste preferences. *Addictive Behavior*, 1982, *7*, 317–331.

———. Behavioral and biological factors in the relationship between tobacco use and body weight. In E. S. Katkin and S. B. Manuck (Eds.), *Advances in behavioral medicine*, vol. 2. Greenwich, Conn.: JAI Press, 1986.

———. Behavioral factors in preventive medicine and health promotion. In W. Gordon, A. Herd, and A. Baum (Eds.), *Perspectives on behavioral medicine*, vol. 3. New York: Academic Press, 1988.

Gutterman, E. M., Erhardt, A. A., Markowitz, J. S., and Link, B. G. Vulnerability to stress among women with in utero Diethylstilbesterol (DES) exposed daughters. *Journal of Human Stress*, 1985, *11*, 103–110.

Hackett, T. P., and Weisman, A. D. Reactions to the imminence of death. In G. H. Grosser, H. Wechsler, and H. Greenblatt (Eds.), *The threat of impending disaster*. Cambridge, Mass.: M.I.T. Press, 1964.

Haefner, D. P., and Kirscht, J. P. Motivational and behavioral effects of modifying health beliefs. *Public Health Reports*, 1970, *85*, 478–484.

Haft, J. I. Cardiovascular injury induced by sympathetic catecholamines. *Progress in Cardiovascular Diseases*, 1974, *17*, 73–86.

Haggard, E. A. Some conditions determining adjustment during and readjustment following experimentally induced stress. In S. S. Tomkins (Ed.), *Contemporary psychopathology*. Cambridge, Mass.: Harvard University Press, 1946.

Hall, E. T. *The hidden dimension*. New York: Doubleday, 1966.

Hall, S. M., and Hall, R. G. Clinical series in behavioral treatment of obesity. *Health Psychology*, 1982, *1*, 359–372.

Halstead, W. C. *Brain and intelligence*. Chicago: University of Chicago Press, 1947.

Hambling, J. Psychosomatic aspects of arterial hypertension. *British Journal of Medical Psychology*, 1952, *25*, 39–47.

Hamburg, D. A., Elliott, G. R., and Parron, D. L. *Health and behavior: Frontiers of research in the biobehavioral sciences*. Washington, D.C.: National Academy Press, 1982.

Hanson, D. R., and Gottesman, L. I. The genetics, if any, of infantile autism and childhood schizophrenia. *Journal of Autism and Childhood Schizophrenia*, 1976, *6*, 209–234.

Hanusa, B. A., and Schulz, R. Attributional mediation of learned helplessness.

Journal of Personality and Social Psychology, 1977, *35,* 602–611.

Harburg, E., Erfurt, J. D., Haunstein, L. S., Chape, C., Schull, W. J., and Schork, M. A. Socioecologic stress, suppressed hostility, skin color and black-white male blood pressure: Detroit. *Psychosomatic Medicine,* 1973, *35,* 276–296.

Hatch, J. P., Gatchel, R. J., and Harrington, R. Biofeedback: Clinical applications in medicine. In R. J. Gatchel, A. Baum, and J. E. Singer (Eds.), *Behavioral medicine and clinical psychology: Overlapping areas.* Hillsdale, N.J.: Erlbaum, 1982.

Hathaway, S. R., and McKinley, J. C. *MMPI manual.* New York: Psychological Corporation, 1943.

Hauser, R. Rapid smoking as a technique of behavior modification: Caution in the selection of subjects. *Journal of Consulting and Clinical Psychology,* 1974, *42,* 625–630.

Haynes, R. B. A critical review of the "determinants" of patient compliance with therapeutic regimens. In D. L. Sackett and R. B. Haynes (Eds.), *Compliance with therapeutic regimens.* Baltimore: Johns Hopkins University Press, 1976.

Haynes, R. B., Sackett, D. L., Gibson, E. S., Taylor, D. W., Hackett, B. C., Roberts, R. S., and Johnson, A. L. Improvement of medication compliance in uncontrolled hypertension. *Lancet,* 1976, *1,* 1265–1268.

Haynes, R. B., Taylor, D. W., and Sackett, D. L. *Compliance in health care.* Baltimore: Johns Hopkins University Press, 1979.

Haynes, S. G., and Feinleib, M. Women, work, and coronary disease: Prospective findings from the Framingham Heart Study. *American Journal of Public Health,* 1980, *70,* 133–141.

Haynes, S. G., Feinleib, M., and Kannel, W. B. The relationship of psychosocial factors to coronary heart disease in the Framingham study. III. Eight-year incidence of coronary heart disease. *American Journal of Epidemiology,* 1980, *3,* 37–58.

Haynes, S. G., Feinleib, M., Levine, S., Scotch, N., and Kannel, W. B. The relationship of psychosocial factors to coronary heart disease in the Framingham Study: Prevalence of coronary heart disease. *American Journal of Epidemiology,* 1978, *107,* 384–402.

Healey, K. M. Does preoperative instruction make a difference? *American Journal of Nursing,* 1968, *68,* 62–67.

Heirch, I., Kvale, G., Jacobsen, B. K., and Bjelke, E. Use of alcohol, tobacco and coffee, and risk of pancreatic cancer. *British Journal of Cancer,* 1983, *48*(5), 637–643.

Hellerstein, H. K., and Friedman, E. H. Sexual activity and the post-coronary patient. *Archives of Internal Medicine,* 1970, *125,* 987–999.

Henry, J. P. Understanding the early pathophysiology of essential hypertension. *Geriatrics,* 1976, *30,* 59–72.

Henry, J. P., and Cassel, J. C. Psychosocial factors in essential hypertension: Recent epidemiologic and animal experimental data. *American Journal of Epidemiology,* 1969, *90,* 171–200.

Henry, J. P., Ely, D. L., Watson, F. M. C., and Stephens, P. M. Ethological methods as applied to the measurement of emotion. In L. Levi (Ed.), *Emotions: Their parameters and measurement.* New York: Raven, 1975.

Henry, J. P., Meehan, J. P., and Stephens, P. M. The use of psychosocial stimuli to induce prolonged systolic hypertension in mice. *Psychosomatic Medicine,* 1967, *29,* 408–432.

Henry, J. P., and Stephens, J. C. *Stress, health, and the social environment.* New York: Springer-Verlag, 1977.

Henry, J. P., Stephens, P. M., and Santisteban, G. A. A model of psychosocial hypertension showing reversibility and progression of cardiovascular complication. *Circulation Research,* 1975, *36,* 156–164.

Henry, J. P., Stephens, P. M., and Walson, F. M. C. Force breeding, social disorder, and mammary tumor formation in CBA/USC mouse colonies. *Psychosomatic Medicine,* 1975, *37,* 277–283.

Herberman, R. B., and Holden, H. T. Natural cell-mediated immunity. *Advances in Cancer Research,* 1978, *27,* 305–377.

Herbst, A. L., Ulfelder, H., and Poskanzer, D. C. Adenocarcinoma of the vagina: Association of maternal stilbestrol therapy with tumor appearance in young women. *New England Journal of Medicine,* 1971, *284,* 878–881.

Herity, B., Murphy, J., Moriarty, M., Bourke, G. J., and Daly, L. Study of squamous-cell carcinoma of the cervix uteri. *Irish Journal of Medical Science,* 1982, *151*(4), 128.

Herman, C. P., and Polivy, J. Restrained eating. In A. J. Stunkard (Ed.), *Obesity.* Philadelphia: Saunders, 1980.

Heston, L. L. Psychiatric disorders in foster home reared children of schizophrenic mothers. *British Journal of Psychiatry,* 1966, *112,* 819–825.

Hetherington, A. W., and Ransom, S. W. Hypothalamic lesions and adiposity in the rat. *Anatomical Record,* 1940, 149–172.

Hieb, E., and Wang, R. Compliance: The patient's role in drug therapy. *Wisconsin Journal of Medicine,* 1974, *73,* 152–154.

Hilgard, E. R. *Hypnotic susceptibility.* New York: Harcourt, Brace and World, 1965.

————. The alleviation of pain by hypnosis. *Pain,* 1975, *1,* 213–231.

Hilgard, E. R., Atkinson, R. C., and Atkinson, R. *Introduction to psychology,* 6th ed. New York: Harcourt Brace Jovanovich, 1975.

Hilgard, E. R., and Hilgard, J. R. *Hypnosis in the relief of pain.* Los Altos, Calif.: William Kaufmann, 1975.

Hill, H. E., Kornetsky, C. G., Flanary, H. G., and Wilder, A. Effects of anxiety and morphine on the discrimination of intensities of pain. *Journal of Clinical Investigation,* 1952, *31,* 473–480.

Hinkle, L. E., Jr., and Wolff, H. G. Health and the social environment: Experimental investigations. In A. H. Leighton, J. A. Clausen, and R. W. Wilson (Eds.), *Explorations in social psychiatry.* New York: Basic Books, 1957.

Hiroto, D. S. Learned helplessness and locus of control. *Journal of Experimental Psychology,* 1974, *102,* 187–193.

Hiroto, D. S., and Seligman, M. E. P. Generality of learned helplessness in man. *Journal of Personality and Social Psychology,* 1975, *31,* 311–327.

Hirsch, J., and Knittle, J. L. Cellularity of obese and nonobese human adipose tissue. *Federation Proceedings,* 1970, *29,* 1516–1521.

Hirschorn, M. W. AIDS is not seen as a major threat by many heterosexuals on campuses. *Chronicle of Higher Education,* 1987, *33,* 1.

Hoge, V. Hospital facilities should fit the patient. In L. E. Weeks and J. R. Griffith (Eds.), *Progressive patient care.* Bulletin of the Administrative Research Services, #3, 1964.

Holbs, J. F., Connor, W. E., and Matarazzo, J. D. Lifestyle, behavioral health and heart disease. In R. J. Gatchel, A. Baum, and J. E. Singer (Eds.), *Behavioral medicine and clinical psychology: Overlapping areas.* Hillsdale, N.J.: Erlbaum, 1982.

Hokanson, J. E., and Burgess, M. The effects of three types of aggression on vascular processes. *Journal of Abnormal and Social Psychology,* 1962, *64,* 446–447.

Holland, J. C., and Tross, S. The psychosocial and neuropsychiatric sequelae of the acquired immunodeficiency syndrome and related disorders. *Annals of Internal Medicine,* 1985, *103,* 760–764.

Holman, C. W., and Muschenheim, C. *Bronchopulmonary diseases and related disorders.* New York: Harper & Row, 1972.

Holmes, T. H., and Rahe, R. H. The social readjustment rating scale. *Journal of Psychosomatic Research,* 1967, *11,* 213–218.

Holt, P. G., and Keast, D. Environmentally induced changes in immunological function: Acute and chronic effects of inhalation of tobacco smoke and other atmospheric contaminants in man and experimental animals. *Bacteriological Reviews,* 1977, *41*(1), 205–216.

Honzik, M. P. Development studies of parent–child resemblance in intelligence. *Child Development,* 1957, *28,* 215–228.

Horan, J. J., Laying, F. C., and Pursell, C. H. Preliminary study of effects of "in vivo" emotive imagery on dental discomfort. *Perceptual and Motor Skills,* 1976, *42,* 105–106.

House, J. S. Occupational stress and coronary heart disease: A review and theoretical integration. *Journal of Health and Social Behavior,* 1974, *15,* 12–27.

———. Occupational stress as a precursor to coronary disease. In W. D. Gentry and R. B. Williams, Jr. (Eds.), *Psychological aspects of myocardial infarction and coronary care.* St. Louis: C. V. Mosby, 1975.

Howard, J. H., Cunningham, D. A., and Rechnitzer, P. A. Effects of personal interaction on triglyceride, uric acid, and coronary risk among managers. *Journal of Human Stress,* 1986, *12,* 53–63.

Huber, H., Karlin, R., and Nathan, P. E. Blood alcohol level discrimination by non-alcoholics: The role of internal and external cues. *Journal of Studies of Alcoholism,* 1976, *37,* 27–39.

Hudgens, R. W. Personal catastrophe and depression. In B. S. Dohrenwend and B. P. Dohrenwend (Eds.), *Stressful life events: Their nature and effects.* New York: Wiley, 1974.

Hunt, W. A., Barnett, L. W., and Ranch, L. G. Relapse rates in addiction programs. *Journal of Clinical Psychology,* 1971, *27,* 455–456.

Hunt, W. A., and Bespalec, D. A. An evaluation of current methods for modifying smoking behavior. *Journal of Clinical Psychology,* 1974, *30,* 431–438.

Hunt, W. A., and Matarazzo, J. D. Habit mechanisms in smoking. In W. A. Hunt (Ed.), *Learning mechanisms in smoking.* Chicago: Aldine, 1970.

———. Changing smoking behavior: A critique. In R. J. Gatchel, A. Baum, and J. E. Singer (Eds.), *Behavioral medicine and clinical psychology: Overlapping areas.* Hillsdale, N. J.: Erlbaum, 1982.

Hynes, M., and Vanmarcke, E. Reliability

of embankment performance predictions. *Proceedings of the ASCE Engineering Mechanics Division Specialty Conference.* Waterloo, Canada: University of Waterloo Press, 1976.

Hyson, R. L., Ashcraft, L. J., Drugan, R. C., Grau, J. W., and Maier, S. F. Extent and control of shock affects naltrexone sensitivity of stress-induced analgesia and reactivity to morphine. *Pharmacology, Biochemistry, and Behavior,* 1982, 17(5), 1019–1025.

Ikard, F. F., Green, D. E., and Horn, D. A scale to differentiate between types of smoking as related to the management of affect. *International Journal of the Addictions,* 1969, *4,* 649–659.

Jackson, J. K. The problem of alcoholic tuberculosis patients. In P. F. Sparer (Ed.), *Personality stress and tuberculosis.* New York: International Universities Press, 1954.

Jackson, R. L., Maier, S. F., and Coon, D. J. Long-term analgesic effects of inescapable shock and learned helplessness. *Science,* 1979, *206* (4414), 91–93.

Jacob, R. G., and Chesney, M. A. Psychological and behavioral methods to reduce cardiovascular reactivity. In K. A. Matthews, S. M. Weiss, T. Detre, T. M. Dembroski, B. Falkner, S. B. Manuck, and R. B. Williams, Jr. (Eds.), *Handbook of stress, reactivity, and cardiovascular disease.* New York: Wiley, 1986.

Jacobs, M. A., Spilken, A. Z., Norman, M. M., and Anderson, L. S. Life stress and respiratory illness. *Psychosomatic Medicine,* 1970, *32,* 233–242.

Jacobson, E. *Progressive relaxation.* Chicago: University of Chicago Press, 1938.

James, W. *The principles of psychology.* New York: Holt, 1890.

Janis, I. L. *Psychological stress: Psychoanalytic and behavioral studies of surgical patients.* New York: Wiley, 1958.

———. Effects of fear arousal on attitude change: Recent developments in theory and experimental research. In L. Berkowitz (Ed.), *Advances in experimental social psy-*

chology, vol. 3. New York: Academic Press, 1967.

————. *Stress and frustration.* New York: Harcourt Brace Jovanovich, 1969.

————. *Psychological stress: Psychoanalytic and behavioral studies of surgical patients.* New York: Academic Press, 1974.

Janis, I. L., and Feschbach, S. Effects of fear-arousing communications. *Journal of Abnormal and Social Psychology,* 1953, *48,* 78–92.

Janis, I. L., and Leventhal, A. Psychological aspects of physical illness and hospital care. In B. Wolman (Ed.), *Handbook of clinical psychology.* New York: McGraw-Hill, 1965.

Janis, I. L., and Rodin, J. Attribution, control, and decision making. In G. Stone, F. Cohen, and N. Adler (Eds.), *Health psychology.* San Francisco: Jossey-Bass, 1979.

Janoff-Bulman, R. Characterological versus behavioral self blame: Inquiries into depression and rape. *Journal of Personality and Social Psychology,* 1979. *37*(10), 1798–1809.

Jarvik, M. E. Further observations on nicotine as the reinforcing agent in smoking. In W. L. Dunn, Jr. (Ed.), *Smoking behavior: Motives and incentives.* Washington, D.C.: Winston, 1973.

————. Biological influences on cigarette smoking. In *Smoking and health: A report of the Surgeon General* (DHEW Publication No. [PHS] 79-50066). Washington, D.C.: U.S. Government Printing Office, 1979.

Jeffery, R. W., Wing, R. R., and Stunkard, A. J. Behavioral treatment of obesity: The state of the art in 1976. *Behavior Therapy,* 1978, *9,* 189–199.

Jenkins, C. D. Recent evidence supporting psychologic and social risk factors for coronary disease. *New England Journal of Medicine,* 1976, *294,* 987–994, 1033–1038.

————. Behavioral risk factors in coronary artery disease. *Annual Review of Medicine,* 1978, *29,* 543–562.

————. Psychosocial and behavioral factors. In N. Kaplan and J. Stamler (Eds.), *Prevention of coronary heart disease.* Philadelphia: Saunders, 1983.

Jenkins, C. D., Rosenman, R. H., and Friedman, M. Development of an objective psychological test for the determination of the coronary-prone behavior pattern in employed men. *Journal of Chronic Diseases,* 1967, *20,* 371–379.

Jenkins, C. D., Rosenman, R. H., and Zyzanski, S. J. Prediction of clinical coronary heart disease by a test for the coronary-prone behavior pattern. *New England Journal of Medicine,* 1974, *290,* 1271–1275.

Jenkins, C. D., Zyzanski, S. J., and Rosenman, R. H. Progress toward validation of a computer-scored test for the Type A coronary-prone behavior pattern. *Psychosomatic Medicine,* 1971, *33,* 193–202.

————. Risk of new myocardial infarction in middle-aged men with manifest coronary heart disease. *Circulation,* 1976, *53,* 342–347.

Jessner, I., Blom, G., and Waldfogel, S. Emotional implications of tonsillectomy and adenoidectomy on children. *Psychoanalytic Study of Children,* 1952, *7,* 126–169.

Jessor, R., and Jessor, S. L. *Problem behavior and psychosocial development: A longitudinal study of youth.* New York: Academic Press, 1977.

Joasoo, A., and McKenzie, J. M. Stress and the immune response in rats. *International Archives of Allergy and Applied Immunology,* 1976, *50,* 659–663.

Johansson, G. Case report on female catecholamine excretion in response to examination stress. Reports from the Department of Psychology, University of Stockholm, 1977 (515).

Johnson, J. E. Effects of accurate expectations about sensations on the sensory and distress components of pain. *Journal of Personality and Social Psychology,* 1973, *27,* 261–275.

————. Stress reduction through sensation information. In I. G. Sarason and C. D. Spielberger (Eds.), *Stress and anxiety,* vol. 2. Washington, D.C.: Hemisphere, 1975.

Johnson, J. E., and Leventhal, H. Effects of accurate expectations and behavioral instructions on reactions during a noxious medical examination. *Journal of Personality and Social Psychology,* 1974, *29,* 710–718.

Johnson, J. E., Morrissey, J. F., and Leventhal, H. Psychological preparation for endoscopic examination. *Gastrointestinal Endoscopy,* 1973, *19,* 180–182.

Johnson, S., Knight, R., Marmer, D. J., and Steele, R. W. Immune deficiency in fetal alcohol syndrome. *Pediatric Research,* 1981, *15,* 908–911.

Johnson, W. D., Stokes, P., and Kaye, D. The effect of intravenous ethanol on the bactericidal activity of human serum. *Yale Journal of Medicine,* 1969, *42,* 71–85.

Jones, D. R., and Maloney, T. R. Massive eosinophic reaction to desipramine. *American Journal of Psychiatry,* 1980, *137*(1), 115–116.

Jones, M. C. Personality correlates and antecedents of drinking patterns in adult males. *Journal of Consulting and Clinical Psychology,* 1968, *32,* 2–12.

————. Personality antecedents and correlates of drinking patterns in women. *Journal of Consulting and Clinical Psychology,* 1971, *36,* 61–69.

Jones, S. L., Nation, J. R., and Massad, P. Immunization against learned helplessness in man. *Journal of Abnormal Psychology,* 1977, *86,* 75–83.

Joseph, J. G., Montgomery, S. B., Emmons, C., Kessler, R. C., Ostrow, D. G., Wortman, C. B., O'Brien, K., Eller, M., and Eshleman, S. Magnitude and determinants of behavioral risk: Longitudinal analysis of a cohort at risk for AIDS. *Psychology and Health,* 1987, *1,* 73–95.

Julius, S., and Esler, M. Autonomic nervous cardiovascular regulation in borderline hypertension. *American Journal of Cardiology,* 1975, *36,* 685–696.

Kahn, J. A., Kornfeld, D. S., Frank, K. A., Heller, S. S., and Hoar, P. F. Type A behavior and blood pressure during coronary bypass surgery. *Psychosomatic Medicine,* 1980, *42,* 407–414.

Kahn, R. L., and French, J. R. P., Jr. Status and conflict: Two themes in the study of stress. In J. E. McGrath (Ed.), *Social and psychological factors in stress.* New York: Holt, Rinehart & Winston, 1970.

Kallmann, F. J. The genetic theory of schizophrenia: An analysis of 691 schizophrenic twin index families. *American Journal of Psychiatry,* 1946, *103,* 309–322.

Kandil, O., and Borysenko, M. Decline of natural killer cell target binding and lytic activity in mice exposed to rotation stress. *Health Psychology,* 1987, *6*(2), 89–99.

Kannel, W. B. Cardiovascular disease: A multifactorial problem (Insights from the Framingham study). In M. L. Pollack and D. H. Schmidt (Eds.), *Heart disease and rehabilitation.* New York: Wiley, 1979.

————. New perspectives on cardiovascular risk factors. *American Heart Journal,* 1987, *114,* 213–219.

Kannel, W. B., Castelli, W. P., and Gordon, T. Cholesterol in the prediction of atherosclerotic disease: New perspectives based on the Framingham study. *Annals of Internal Medicine,* 1979, *90,* 85–91.

Kanner, A. D., Coyne, J. C., Schaeffer, C., and Lazarus, R. S. Comparison of two modes of stress measurement: Daily hassles and uplifts versus major life events. *Journal of Behavioral Medicine,* 1981, *4,* 1–39.

Kaplan, J. E., Spira, T. J., Fishbein, D. B., Pinsky, P. F., and Schonberger, L. B. Lymphadenopathy syndrome in homosexual men. Evidence for continuing risk of developing the acquired immunodeficiency syndrome. *Journal of the American Medical Association,* 1987, *257*(3), 335–337.

Kaplan, J. R., Adams, M. R., Clarkson, T. B., and Koritnik, D. R. Psychosocial influences on female "protection" among cynomolgous macaques. *Atherosclerosis,* 1984, *53,* 283–295.

Kaplan, J. R., Manuck, S. B., Clarkson, T. B., Lusso, F. M., and Taub, D. B. Social status, environment, and atherosclerosis in cynomolgous monkeys. *Arteriosclerosis,* 1982, *2,* 359–368.

Karasek, R., Baker, D., Marxer, F., Ahlbom, A., and Theorell, T. Job decision latitude, job demands, and cardiovascular disease: A prospective study of Swedish men. *American Journal of Public Health,* 1981, *71*(7), 694–705.

Karasek, R. A., Theorell, T. G., Schwartz, J., Pieper, C., and Alfredsson, L. Job, psychological factors and coronary heart disease: Swedish prospective findings and U.S. prevalence findings using a new occupational inference method. *Advances in Cardiology,* 1982, *29,* 62–67.

Kardiner, A., and Spiegel, H. *War stress and neurotic illness.* London: Paul B. Hoeber, 1941.

Kasl, S. V. Issues in patient adherence to health care regimens. *Journal of Human Stress,* 1975, *1,* 5–17.

Kasl, S. V., and Cobb, S. Health behavior, illness behavior, and sick role behavior, vol. 2. *Archives of Environmental Health,* 1966, *12,* 531–541.

Katkin, E. S., and Goldband, S. The placebo effect in biofeedback. In R. J. Gatchel and K. P. Price (Eds.), *Clinical applications of biofeedback: Appraisal and status.* Elmsford, N.Y.: Pergamon, 1979.

Katz, R. L., Kao, C. U., Spiegel, H., and Katz, G. J. Pain, acupuncture, hypnosis. In J. J. Bonica (Ed.), *Advances in neurology,* vol. 4. International symposium on pain. New York: Raven, 1974.

Kazdin, A. E. Covert modeling, model similarity, and reduction of avoidance behavior. *Behavior Therapy,* 1974, *5,* 325–340.

Kegeles, S. S. Some motives for seeking preventive dental care. *Journal of the American Dental Association,* 1963, *67,* 90–98.

Keller, S. Physical fitness hastens recovery from psychological stress. *Medical Science Sports Exercise,* 1980, *12,* 118–119.

Kelley, H. H. Attribution theory in social psychology. In D. Levine (Ed.), *Nebraska symposium on motivation,* vol. 15. Lincoln: University of Nebraska Press, 1967.

Kemp, A., and Berke, G. Effects of heparin and benzyl alcohol on lymphocyte-mediated cytotoxicity in vitro. *Short Communications,* 1973, *7,* 512–515.

Kendall, P. C., and Turk, D. C. Cognitive-behavioral strategies and health enhancement. In J. D. Matarazzo, S. M. Weiss, J. A. Herd, N. E. Miller, and S. M. Weiss (Eds.), *Behavioral health: A handbook of health enhancement and disease prevention.* New York: Wiley, 1984.

Kendall, R. A., and Targan, S. The dual effect of prostaglandin (PGE2) and ethanol on the natural killer cytolytic process: Effector activation and NK cell-target cell conjugate lytic inhibition. *Journal of Immunology,* 1980, *7,* 512–515.

Kety, S. S., Rosenthal, D., Wender, P. H., and Schulsinger, F. Mental illness in the biological and adoptive families of adopted schizophrenics. *American Journal of Psychiatry,* 1971, *128,* 302–306.

Keys, A. Atherosclerosis: A problem in newer public health. *Journal of Mt. Sinai Hospital,* 1953, *20,* 118–139.

Keys, A., Taylor, H. L., Blackburn, H., Brozek, J., Anderson, J., and Simonson, E. Mortality and coronary heart disease among men studied for 23 years. *Archives of Internal Medicine,* 1971, *128,* 201–214.

Kiecolt-Glaser, J. K., Fisher, L. D., Ogrocki, P., Stout, J. C., Speicher, C. E., and Glaser, R. Marital quality, marital disruption, and immune function. *Psychosomatic Medicine,* 1987, *49*(1), 13–34.

Kiecolt-Glaser, J. K., Garner, W. K., Speicher, C., Penn, G. M., Holliday, J., and Glaser, R. Psychosocial modifiers of immunocompetence in medical students. *Psychosomatic Medicine,* 1984, *46*(1), 7–14.

Kiecolt-Glaser, J. K., and Glaser, R. Psychosocial moderators of immune function. *Annals of Behavioral Medicine,* 1987, *9*(2), 16–20.

Kiecolt-Glaser, J. K., Glaser, R., Shuttleworth, E. C., Dyer, C. S., Ogrocki, P., and Speicher, C. E. Chronic stress and immunity in family caregivers of Alzheimer's disease victims. *Psychosomatic Medicine,* 1987, *49*(5), 523–535.

Kiecolt-Glaser, J. K., Glaser, R., Strain, E. C., Stout, J. C., Tarr, K. K., Holliday, J. E., and Speicher, C. E. Modulation of cellular immunity in medical students. *Journal of Behavioral Medicine,* 1986, *9,* 311–320.

Kiecolt-Glaser, J. K., Glaser, R., Williger, D., Stout, J. C., Messick, G., Sheppard, S., Ricker, D., Romisher, S. C., Friner, W., Bonnell, G., and Donnerberg, R. Psychosocial enhancement of immunocompetence in a geriatric population. *Health Psychology,* 1985, *4*(1), 24–41.

Kiecolt-Glaser, J. K., Stephens, R. E., Lipetz, P. D., Speicher, C. E., and Glaser, R. Distress and DNA repair in human lymphocytes. *Journal of Behavioral Medicine,* 1985, *8*(4), 311–320.

Killworth, D., and Bernard, H. A model of human group dynamics. *Social Science Research,* 1976, *5,* 173–224.

Kiretz, S., and Moos, R. H. Physiological effects of social environments. *Psychosomatic Medicine,* 1974, *36,* 96–114.

Kirsner, J. B. Peptic ulcer: A review of the current literature on various clinical aspects. *Gastroenterology,* 1968, *54,* 610–618.

Kiser, R. S., Khatami, M., Gatchel, R. J., Huang, X., Bhatia, K. and Altshuler, K. Z. Acupuncture relief of chronic pain syndrome correlates with increased plasma met-enkephalin concentrations. *Lancet,* 1983, *2,* 1394–1396.

Klein, D. C., and Seligman, M. E. P. Reversal of performance deficits and perceptual deficits in learned helplessness and depression. *Journal of Abnormal Psychology,* 1976, *85,* 11–26.

Klein, R. F., Kliner, V. A., Zipes, D. P., Troyer, W. G., and Wallace, A. G. Transfer from a coronary care unit. *Archives of Internal Medicine,* 1968, *122,* 104–108.

Klopfer, B., Ainsworth, M., Klopfer, W. G., and Holt, R. R. *Developments in the Rorschach technique,* vol. 1, *Techniques and theory.* Yonkers-on-Hudson, N.Y.: World Book, 1954.

Kobasa, S. C. Stressful life events, personality and health: An inquiry into hardness. *Journal of Personality and Social Psychology,* 1979, *39,* 1–11.

Konzett, H. *Jahre Osterreichische Phar-makologie Wien Med Wochenscher,* 1975, *125* (1–2 Suppl.), 1–6.

Konzett, H., Hortnagel, H., Hortnagel, L., and Winkler, H. On the urinary output of vasopressin, epinephrine and norepinephrine during different stress situations. *Psychopharmacologia,* 1971, *21,* 247–256.

Koos, E. *The health of Regionville.* New York: Columbia University Press, 1954.

Koriat, A., Melkman, R., Averill, J. R., and Lazarus, R. S. The self-control of emotional reactions to a stressful film. *Journal of Personality,* 1972, *40,* 601–619.

Korsch, B. M., Fine, R. N., and Negrete, V. F. Noncompliance in children with renal transplants. *Pediatrics,* 1978, *61,* 872–876.

Korsch, B. M., Freeman, B., and Negrete, V. F. Practical implications of doctor–patient interactions. Analysis for pediatric practice. *American Journal of Diseases of Children,* 1971, *121,* 110–114.

Korsch, B. M., Gozzi, E. K., and Francis, V. Gaps in doctor–patient communication, 1. Doctor–patient interaction and patient satisfaction. *Pediatrics,* 1968, *42,* 855–871.

Korsch, B. M., and Negrete, V. F. Doctor-patient communication. *Scientific American,* 1972, *227,* 66–74.

Krantz, D. S. Cognitive processes and recovery from heart attack: A review and theoretical analysis. *Journal of Human Stress,* 1980, *6*(3), 27–38.

Krantz, D. S., Arabian, J. M., Davia, J. E., and Parker, J. S. Type A behavior and coronary artery bypass surgery: Intraoperative blood pressure and perioperative complications. *Psychosomatic Medicine,* 1982, *44,* 273–284.

Krantz, D. S., Baum, A., and Singer, J. E. (Eds.). *Handbook of psychology and health,* vol. 3, *Cardiovascular disorders and behavior.* Hillsdale, N.J.: Erlbaum, 1983.

Krantz, D. S., Baum, A., and Wideman, M. v. Assessment of preferences for self-treatment and information in health care. *Journal of Personality and Social Psychology,* 1980, *39,* 977–990.

Krantz, D. S., Baum, A., Wideman, M. v., and Douma, M. Preferences for self treatment in health care. Paper presented at the meeting of the American Psychological Association, Montreal, Canada, 1980.

Krantz, D. S., and Blumenthal, J. *Behavioral assessment and management of cardiovascular disorders.* Sarasota, Fla.: Professional Resource Exchange, 1987.

Krantz, D. S., Contrada, R. J., LaRiccia, P. J., Anderson, J. R., Durel, L. A., Dembroski, T. M., and Weiss, T. Effects of beta-adrenergic stimulation and blockade on cardiovascular reactivity, affect, and Type A behavior. *Psychosomatic Medicine,* 1987, *49,* 146–158.

Krantz, D. S., and Deckel, A. W. Coping with coronary heart disease and stroke. In T. G. Burish and L. A. Bradley (Eds.), *Coping with chronic disease: Research and applications.* New York: Academic Press, 1983.

Krantz, D. S., and Durel, L. A. Psychobiological substrates of the Type A behavior pattern. *Health Psychology,* 1983, *2,* 393–411.

Krantz, D. S., Glass, D. C., Contrada, R., and Miller, N. E. Behavior and health. *National Science Foundation's second five-year outlook on science and technology.* Washington, D.C.: U.S. Government Printing Office, 1981.

Krantz, D. S., Glass, D. C., and Snyder, M. L. Helplessness, stress level, and the coronary-prone behavior pattern. *Journal of Experimental Social Psychology,* 1974, *10,* 284–300.

Krantz, D. S., Grunberg, N. E., and Baum, A. Health psychology. *Annual Review of Psychology.* 1985, *36,* 349–383.

Krantz, D. S., and Manuck, S. B. Acute psychophysiologic reactivity and risk of cardiovascular disease: A review and methodologic critique. *Psychological Bulletin,* 1984, *96,* 435–464.

Krantz, D. S., Sanmarco, M. I., Selvester, R. H., and Matthews, K. A. Psychological correlates of progression of atherosclerosis in men. *Psychosomatic Medicine,* 1979, *41,* 467–475.

Krantz, D. S., and Schulz, R. A model of life crisis, control, and health outcomes:

Cardiac rehabilitation and relocation of the elderly. In A. Baum and J. E. Singer (Eds.), *Advances in environmental psychology,* vol. 2. Hillsdale, N.J.: Erlbaum, 1980.

Krasnegor, N. A. *Cigarette smoking as a dependence process,* NIDA Research Monograph 23 (DHEW Publ. [ADM]79-800). Washington, D.C.: U.S. Government Printing Office, 1979.

Krasner, L. Assessment of token economy programs in psychiatric hospitals. In N. H. Miller and R. Porter (Eds.), *Learning theory and psychotherapy.* London: CIBA Foundation, 1968.

Krasnoff, A. Psychological variables and human cancer. A cross-validation study. *Psychosomatic Medicine,* 1959, *21*(4), 291–295.

Kreis, B., Peltier, A., Fournaud, S., et al. Reaction de precipitation entre certains serum humains et des extraits solubles de tabac. *Annales de Medicine Interne* (Paris), 1970, *121,* 437–440.

Kreutner, A. K. New approaches to treating dysmenorrhea. *Behavioral Medicine,* 1980, *7,* 21–25.

Krueger, R. B., Levy, E. M., Cathcart, E. S., Fox, B. H., and Black, P. H. Lymphocyte subsets in patients with major depression: Preliminary findings. *Advances,* 1984, *1,* 5–9.

Lacey, J. I. Somatic response patterning and stress: Some revisions of activation theory. In M. H. Appley and R. Trumbull (Eds.), *Psychological stress.* New York: McGraw-Hill, 1967.

LaCroix, A. Z., and Haynes, S. G. Gender differences in the health effects of workplace roles. In R. C. Barnett, L. Biener, and G. K. Baruch (Eds.), *Gender and stress.* New York: Free Press, 1987.

Landenslager, M. L., Ryan, S. M., Drugan, R. C., Hyson, R. L., and Maier, S. F. Coping and immunsuppression: Inescapable but not escapable shock suppresses lymphocyte proliferation. *Science,* 1983, *221,* 568–570.

Lando, H. A. Successful treatment of smokers with a broad-spectrum behavioral approach. *Journal of Consulting and Clinical Psychology,* 1977, *41,* 361–366.

Lang, A., and Marlatt, G. A. Problem drinking: A social learning perspective. In R. J. Gatchel, A. Baum, and J. E. Singer (Eds.), *Behavioral medicine and clinical psychology: Overlapping disciplines.* Hillsdale, N.J.: Erlbaum, 1982.

Lang, P. J. Autonomic control or learning to play the internal organs. *Psychology Today,* 1970, *4,* 39–44, 82–84.

———. A bio-informational theory of emotional imagery. *Psychophysiology,* 1979, *16,* 495–512.

Lang, P. J., Melamed, B. G., and Hart, J. A. Psychophysiological analysis of fear modification using automated desensitization procedure. *Journal of Abnormal Psychology,* 1970, *76,* 220–234.

Lange, C. The emotions. In K. Dunlap (Ed.), *The emotions.* Baltimore: Williams & Wilkins, 1922.

Lange, W. R., and Dax, E. M. HIV infection and international travel. *American Family Physician,* 1987, *36*(3), 197–204.

Langer, E. J. The illusion of control. *Journal of Personality and Social Psychology,* 1975, *32,* 311–328.

Langer, E. J., Janis, I. L., and Wolfer, J. A. Reduction of psychological stress in surgical patients. *Journal of Experimental Social Psychology,* 1975, *11,* 155–165.

Langer, E. J., and Rodin, J. The effects of choice and enhanced personal responsibility for the aged: A field experiment in an institutional setting. *Journal of Personality and Social Psychology,* 1976, *34,* 191–198.

Langer, E. J., and Roth, J. Heads I win, tails it's chance: The illusion of control as a function of the sequence of outcomes in a purely chance task. *Journal of Personality and Social Psychology,* 1975, *32,* 951–955.

Langer, E. J., and Saegert, S. Crowding and cognitive control. *Journal of Personality and Social Psychology,* 1977, *35,* 175–182.

Laux, D. C., and Klesius, P. H. Suppressive effects of caffeine on immune-response of mouse to sheep erythrocytes. *Proceedings of the Society for Experimental Biology and Medicine,* 1973, *144*(2), 633–638.

Lawler, J. E., Barker, G. F., Hubbard, J. W., and Allen, M. T. The effects of conflict on tonic levels of blood pressure in the genetically borderline hypertensive rat. *Psychophysiology,* 1980, *17,* 363–370.

Lawler, K. A., Allen, M. T., Critcher, E. C., and Standard, B. A. The relationship of physiological responses to the coronary-prone behavior pattern in children. Unpublished manuscript, undated.

Lazarus, A. A. *Behavior therapy and beyond.* New York: McGraw-Hill, 1971.

Lazarus, R. S. Story telling and the measurement of motivation: The direct versus substitutive controversy. *Journal of Consulting Psychology,* 1966, *30,* 483–487.

———. A cognitively oriented psychologist looks at biofeedback. *American Psychologist,* 1975, *30,* 553–561.

Lazarus, R. S., and Alfert, E. The short-circuiting of threat by experimentally altering cognitive appraisal. *Journal of Abnormal and Social Psychology,* 1964, *69,* 195–205.

Lazarus, R. S., and Cohen, F. Active coping processes, coping dispositions, and recovery from surgery. *Psychosomatic Medicine,* 1973, *35,* 375–389.

Lazarus, R. S., and Cohen, J. B. Environmental stress. In I. Attman and J. F. Wohlwill (Eds.), *Human behavior and the environment: Current theory and research,* vol. 2. New York: Plenum, 1977.

Lazarus, R. S., and Folkman, S. *Stress, appraisal and coping.* New York: Springer, 1984.

Lazarus, R. S., and Launier, R. Stress-related transactions between person and environment. In L. A. Pervin and M. Lewis (Eds.), *Internal and external determinants of behavior.* New York: Plenum, 1978.

Lazarus, R. S., Opton, E. M., Jr., Nomikos, M. S., and Rankin, N. O. The principle of short-circuiting of threat: Further evidence. *Journal of Personality,* 1965, *33,* 622–635.

Lemere, F., and Voegtlin, W. L. An evaluation of the aversion treatment of alcoholism. *Quarterly Journal of Studies on Alcoholism,* 1950, *71,* 199–204.

Leon, G. R. *Case histories of deviant behavior.* Boston: Holbrook, 1977.

Le Panto, R., Moroney, W., and Zenhausern, R. The contribution of anxiety to the laboratory investigation of pain. *Psychonomic Science,* 1965, *3,* 475.

Lerner, D. J., and Kannel, W. B. Patterns of coronary heart disease mortality in the sexes: A 26-year follow-up of the Framingham population. *American Heart Journal,* 1986, *111,* 383–390.

Le Shan, L. L. Psychological states as factors in the development of malignant disease: A critical review. *Journal of the National Cancer Institute,* 1959, *29,* 1–18.

Leventhal, H. Findings and theory in the study of fear communications. In L. Berkowitz (Ed.), *Advances in experimental social psychology,* vol. 5. New York: Academic Press, 1970.

Leventhal, H., and Avis, N. Pleasure, addiction, and habit: Factors in verbal report on factors in smoking behavior. *Journal of Abnormal Psychology,* 1976, *85,* 478–488.

Leventhal, H., and Cleary, P. D. The smoking problem: A review of research and theory in behavioral risk modification. *Psychological Bulletin,* 1980, *88,* 370–405.

Leventhal, H., and Hirshman, R. S. Social psychology and prevention. In G. E. Sanders and J. Suls (Eds.), *Social Psychology of Health and Illness.* Hillsdale, N.J.: Erlbaum, 1982.

Leventhal, H., Meyer, D., and Nerenz, D. The common sense representation of illness danger. In S. Rachman (Ed.), *Medical psychology,* vol. 2. New York: Pergamon Press, 1980.

Leventhal, H., Nerenz, D., and Leventhal, E. Feeling of threat and private views of illness: Factors in dehumanization in the medical care system. In A. Baum and J. E. Singer (Eds.), *Advances in environmental psychology,* vol. 4. Hillsdale, N.J.: Erlbaum, 1982.

Leventhal, H., Prohaska, T. R., and Hirshman, R. S. Preventive health behavior

across the life span. In J. C. Rosen and L. J. Solomon (Eds.), *Prevention in Health Psychology.* Hanover, N.H.: University Press of New England, 1985.

Levi, L. The urinary output of adrenalin and noradrenalin during pleasant and unpleasant emotional stress. *Psychosomatic Medicine,* 1965, *27,* 80–85.

———. Psychosocial stress and disease: A conceptual model. In E. K. Gunderson and R. H. Rahe (Eds.), *Life stress and illness.* Springfield, Ill.: Charles C. Thomas, 1974.

Levi, L. (Ed.) *Society, stress and disease: Male/female roles and relationships,* vol. 3. London: Oxford University Press, 1978.

Levine, J. D., Gordon, N. C., and Fields, H. L. The mechanism of placebo analgesia. *Lancet,* 1978, *2,* 654–657.

Levine, J. D., Gormley, J., and Fields, H. L. Observations on the analgesic effects of needle puncture (acupuncture). *Pain,* 1976, *2,* 149–159.

Levitz, L., and Stunkard, A. J. A therapeutic coalition for obesity: Behavior modification and patient self-help. *American Journal of Psychiatry,* 1974, *131,* 423–427.

Levy, S. M. Death and dying: Behavioral and social factors that contribute to the process. In T. G. Burish and L. A. Bradley (Eds.), *Coping with chronic disease: Research and applications.* New York: Academic Press, 1983.

———. Host differences in neoplastic risk. *Health Psychology,* 1983, *2,* 21–44.

Levy, S. M., Herberman, R. B., Maluish, A. M., Schlien, B., and Lippman, M. Prognostic risk assessment in primary breast cancer by behavioral and immunological parameters. *Health Psychology,* 1985, *4,* 99–113.

Ley, P. Psychological studies of doctor–patient communication. In S. Rachman (Ed.), *Contributions to medical psychology.* New York: Pergamon, 1977.

Ley, P., Bradshaw, P. W., Kincey, J., and Atherton, S. T. Increasing patients' satisfaction with communication. *British Journal of Social and Clinical Psychology,* 1976, *15,* 403–413.

Ley, P., and Spelman, M. S. *Communicating with the patient.* London: Staples Press, 1967.

Lezak, M. D. *Neuropsychological assessment.* New York: Oxford University Press, 1982.

Lichtenstein, E., and Penner, M. D. Long-term effects of rapid smoking treatment for dependent cigarette smokers. *Addictive Behaviors,* 1977, *2,* 109–112.

Lindeman, C., and Stetzer, S. Effects of preoperative visits by operating room nurses. *Nursing Research,* 1973, *22,* 4–16.

Lindeman, C. A., and VanAernam, B. Nursing intervention with the presurgical patient—The effects of structured and unstructured preoperative teaching. *Nursing Research,* 1971, *20,* 319–331.

Lindsley, D. B., and Sassamon, W. H. Autonomic activity and brain potentials associated with "voluntary control of the pilomotors." *Journal of Neurophysiology,* 1938, *1,* 342–349.

Lindzey, G., Loehlin, J., Manosevitz, M., and Thiessen, D. Behavioral genetics. *Annual Review of Psychology,* 1971, *22,* 39–94.

Lipowski, Z. J. Psychosomatic medicine in the seventies: An overview. *American Journal of Psychiatry,* 1977, *134,* 233–243.

Lipp, M. R., Looney, J. G., and Spitzer, R. L. Classifying psychophysiologic disorders: A new idea. *Psychosomatic Medicine,* 1977, *39,* 285–287.

Lipscomb, T. R., and Nathan, P. E. Effect of family history of alcoholism, drinking pattern, and tolerance on blood alcohol level discrimination. *Archives of General Psychiatry,* 1980, *37,* 571–576.

Lloyd, R. W., and Salzberg, S. C. Controlled social drinking: An alternative to abstinence as a treatment goal for some alcohol abuses. *Psychological Bulletin,* 1975, *82,* 815–842.

Locke, S. E., Hurst, M. W., Heisel, J. S., Kraus, L., and Williams, R. M. The influences of stress and other psychosocial factors on human immunity. Paper presented at the American Psychosomatic Society meeting, Boston, 1979.

Locke, S. E., Hurst, M. W., Williams, R. M., and Heisel, I. S. The influences of psychosocial factors on human cell-mediated immune function. Paper presented at the meeting of the American Psychosomatic Society, Washington, D.C., 1978.

Locke, S. E., Hurst, M. W., Heisel, J., et al. The influence of stress on the immune responses. Paper presented at the annual meeting of the American Psychosomatic Society, March 1979.

Loeser, J. D. Dorsal rhizotomy: Indicators and results. In J. J. Bonica (Ed.), *Advances in neurology: International symposium on pain,* vol. 4. New York: Raven, 1974.

Long, D. M. Use of peripheral and spinal cord stimulation in the relief of chronic pain. In J. J. Bonica and D. Albe-Fessard (Eds.), *Advances in pain research therapy,* vol. 1. New York: Raven, 1976.

Lovibond, S. H., and Caddy, G. R. Discriminated aversive control in the modification of alcoholics' drinking behavior. *Behavior Therapy,* 1970, *1,* 437–444.

Louria, D. B. Susceptibility to infection during experimental alcohol intoxication. *Transactions of the Association of American Physicians,* 1963, *76,* 102–110.

Luborsky, L., Crits-Christoph, P., Brady, J. P., Kron, R. E., Weiss, T., and Engelman, K. Antihypertensive effects of behavioral treatments and medications compared. *New England Journal of Medicine,* 1980, *302,* 586.

Lucas, R. The affective and medical effects of different preoperative interventions with heart surgery patients. *Dissertation Abstracts International,* 1975, *36,* 5763B.

Ludwig, E. G., and Collette, J. Dependency, social isolation, and mental health in a disabled population. *Social Psychiatry,* 1970, *5,* 92–95.

Luft, F., Block R., Weyman, A., Murray, Z., and Weinberger, M. Cardiovascular responses to extremes of salt intake in man. *Clinical Research,* 1978, *26,* 265A.

Lund, A. K., and Kegeles, S. Increasing adolescents' acceptance of long-term personal health behavior. *Health Psychology,* 1982, *1,* 27–43.

Lundberg, U., and Frankenhaeuser, M. Adjustment to noise stress. Reports from the Department of Psychology, University of Stockholm, 1976 (484).

Lundy, J., Raaf, J. H., Deakins, S., Waneboo, H. J., Jacobs, D. A., Lee, T., Jacobowitz, D., Spear, C., and Oettgen, H. F. The acute and chronic effects of alcohol on the human immune system. *Surgery, Gynecology and Obstetrics,* 1975, *141*(2), 212–218.

Luria, A. R. *The mind of a mnemonist.* Translated by L. Solotaroff. New York: Basic Books, 1958.

Lyles, J. N., Burish, T. G., Krozely, M. G., and Oldham, R. K. Efficacy of relaxation training and guided imagery in reducing the aversiveness of cancer chemotherapy. *Journal of Consulting and Clinical Psychology,* 1982, *50*(4), 509–524.

McAlister, A. L. Helping people quit smoking: Current progress. In A. Enelow (Ed.), *Applying behavioral science to cardiovascular disease.* New York: American Heart Association, 1975.

McAlister, A. L., Perry, C., and Macoby, N. Adolescent smoking: Onset and prevention. *Pediatrics,* 1979, *63,* 650–658.

McClelland, D. C., Atkinson, J. W., Clark, R. A., and Lowell, E. L. *The achievement motive.* New York: Appleton, 1953.

McClelland, D. C., David, W. N., Kahn, R., and Wanner, E. *The drinking man.* New York: Free Press, 1972.

McClure, C. M. Cardiac arrest through volition. *California Medicine,* 1959, *90,* 440–446.

McFall, R. M., and Lillesand, D. V. Behavior rehearsal with modeling and coaching in assertive training. *Journal of Abnormal Psychology,* 1971, *77,* 313–323.

McFall, R. M., and Marston, A. An experimental investigation of behavior rehearsal in assertive training. *Journal of Abnormal Psychology,* 1970, *76,* 295–303.

McFall, R. M., and Twentyman, C. T. Four experiments on the relative contribution of rehearsal, modeling, and coaching to assertive training. *Journal of Abnormal Psychology,* 1973, *81,* 199–218.

McGrath, J. E. *Social and psychological factors in stress.* New York: Holt, Rinehart & Winston, 1970.

McKenney, J. M., Slining, J. M., Henderson, H. R., Devins, D., and Barr, M. The effect of clinical pharmacy services on patients with essential hypertension. *Circulation,* 1973, *48,* 1104–1111.

McKinlay, J. B. Some approaches and problems in the study of the use of services: An overview. *Journal of Health and Social Behavior,* 1972, *13,* 115–152.

McKinnon, W., Baum, A., Reynolds, C. P., Silvia, C., and Jones, D. Chronic stress and immune status at Three Mile Island. Paper presented at the annual meeting of the American Psychological Association, Washington, D.C., 1986.

McKusick, L., Horstman, W., and Coates, T. AIDS and sexual behavior reported by gay men in San Francisco. *American Journal of Public Health,* 1985, *75,* 493–496.

McKusick, L., Wiley, J. A., Coates, T. J., Stall, R., Saika, G., Morin, S., Charles, K., Horstman, W., and Conant, M. A. Reported changes in the sexual behavior of men at risk for AIDS, San Francisco, 1982–84—the AIDS behavioral research project. *Public Health Reports,* 1985, *100,* 622–629.

McMahan, C. E., and Hastrup, J. L. The role of imagination in the disease process: Post-Cartesian history. *Journal of Behavioral Medicine,* 1980, *3,* 205–217.

McNamee, H. B., Mello, V. K., and Mendelson, T. H. Experimental analysis of drinking patterns of alcoholics: Concurrent psychiatric observations. *American Journal of Psychiatry,* 1968, *124,* 1063–1071.

Maguire, P., and Rutter, D. Training medical students to communicate. In A. E. Bennett (Ed.), *Communication between doctors and patients.* London: Oxford University Press, 1976.

Mahoney, M. J. *Cognition and behavior modification.* Cambridge, Mass.: Ballinger, 1974.

Mahoney, M. J., and Arnkoff, D. B. Self-management. In O. F. Pomerleau and J. P. Brady (Eds.), *Behavioral medicine: Theory and practice.* Baltimore: Williams & Wilkins, 1979.

Mahoney, M. J., and Mahoney, K. *Permanent weight control: A total solution to the dieter's dilemma.* New York: Norton, 1976.

Mahoney, M. J., Moura, N. G. M., and Wade, T. C. The relative efficacy of self-reward, self-punishment, and self-monitoring techniques for weight loss. *Journal of Consulting and Clinical Psychology,* 1973, *40,* 404–407.

Maier, S. F., Laudenslager, M. L., and Ryan, S. M. Stressor controllability, immune function, and endongenous opiates. In F. R. Brush and J. B. Overmier (Eds.), *Affect, conditioning and congition: Essays on the determinants of behavior.* Hillsdale, N.J.: Erlbaum, 1985.

Maier, S. F., Sherman, J. E., Lewis, J. W., Terman, G. W., and Liebeski, J. C. Opioid–nonopioid nature of stress-induced analgesia and learned helplessness. *Journal of Experimental Psychology—Animal Behavior Processes,* 1983, *9*(1), 80–90.

Malloy, P. E., Fairbank, J. A., and Keane, T. M. Validation of a multimethod assessment of post-traumatic stress disorder in Vietnam veterans. *Journal of Consulting and Clinical Psychology,* 1983, *4,* 488–494.

Malmo, R. B., and Shagass, C. Physiologic study of symptom mechanisms in psychiatry patients under stress. *Psychosomatic Medicine,* 1949, *11,* 25–29.

Mann, G. V. The influence of obesity on health. *New England Journal of Medicine,* 1974, *291,* 178–185, 226–232.

Mann, G. V. Diet—heart: End of an era. *New England Journal of Medicine,* 1977, *297,* 644–650.

Manuck, S. B., Kaplan, J. R., and Clarkson, T. B. Behaviorally-induced heart rate reactivity and atherosclerosis in cynomolgous monkeys. *Psychosomatic Medicine,* 1983, *45,* 95–108.

———. Stress-induced heart rate reactivity and atherosclerosis in female macaques (Abstract). *Psychosomatic Medicine,* 1985, *47,* 90.

Manuck, S. B., Kaplan, J. R., and Matthews, K. A. Behavioral antecedents of coronary heart disease and atherosclerosis. *Arteriosclerosis,* 1986, *6*(1), 1–14.

Markoff, R. A., Ryan, P., and Young, T. Endorphins and mood changes in long-distance running. *Medical Science Sports Exercise,* 1982, *14,* 11–15.

Marlatt, G. A. Alcohol, stress, and cognitive control. Paper presented at NATO-sponsored International Conference on Dimensions of Stress and Anxiety, Germany, 1975.

———. The controlled-drinking controversy: A commentary. *American Psychologist,* 1983, *38,* 1097–1110.

———. Relapse prevention: Theoretical rationale and overview of the model. In G.A. Marlatt and J.R. Gordon (Eds.), *Relapse Prevention.* New York: Guilford Press, 1985.

Marlatt, G. A., Demming, B., and Reid, J. B. Loss of control drinking in alcoholics: An experimental analogue. *Journal of Abnormal Psychology,* 1973, *81,* 233–241.

Marlatt, G. A., and Gordon, J. R. (Eds.). *Relapse prevention.* New York: Guilford Press, 1985.

Marrow, G. R. Prevalence and correlates of anticipatory nausea and vomiting in chemotherapy patients. *Journal of the National Cancer Institute,* 1982, *68,* 585–588.

Marsh, J. T., and Rasmussen, A. F., Jr. Effects of exposure to fear-producing stressors on mouse organ weights and leukocyte counts. *Federation Proceedings, Federation of American Societies for Experimental Biology,* 1959, *18,* 583.

Marshall, G. D., and Zimbardo, P. G. Affective consequences of inadequately explained physiological arousal. *Journal of Personality and Social Psychology,* 1979, *37,* 970–988.

Martelli, M. F., Auerbach, S. M., Alexander, J., and Mercuri, L. G. Stress management in the health care setting: Matching interventions with patient coping styles. *Journal of Consulting and Clinical Psychology,* 1987, *55,* 201–207.

Martin, J. L. Demographic factors, sexual behavior patterns, and HIV antibody status among New York City gay men. Paper presented at the annual meeting of the American Psychological Association, Washington, D.C., 1986.

Marston, W. V. Compliance with medical regimens: A review of the literature. *Nursing Research,* 1970, *19,* 312–323.

Maslach, C. Negative emotional biasing of unexplained arousal. *Journal of Personality and Social Psychology,* 1979, *37,* 953–969.

Maslow, A. H. *Motivation and personality.* New York: Harper & Row, 1954.

Mason, J. W. A historical view of the stress field. *Journal of Human Stress,* 1975, *1,* 22–36.

Mason, J. W., Brady, J. V., and Tolson, W. W. Behavioral adaptations and endocrine activity. In R. Levine (Ed.), *Endocrines and the central nervous system.* Baltimore: Williams & Wilkins, 1966.

Mason, J. W., Giller, E. L., Costen, T. R., Ostroff, R. B., and Podd, L. Urinary free-cortisol levels in posttraumatic stress disorder patients. *Journal of Nervous and Mental Disease,* 1986, *174,* 145–149.

Mason, J. W., Sachar, E. J., Fishman, J. R., Hamburg, D. A., and Handlon, J. H. Corticosteroid responses to hospital admission. *Archives of General Psychiatry,* 1965, *13,* 1–8.

Masters, J. C., Cerreto, M. C., and Mendlowitz, D. R. The role of the family in coping with chronic illness. In T. G. Burish and L. A. Bradley (Eds.), *Coping with chronic disease: Research and applications.* New York: Academic Press, 1983.

Masters, W. H., and Johnson, V. E. *Human sexual inadequacy.* Boston: Little, Brown, 1970.

Matarazzo, J. D. Behavioral health and behavioral medicine: Frontiers for a new health psychology. *American Psychologist,* 1980, *35,* 807–817.

———. Behavioral health: A 1990 challenge for the health sciences professions. In

J. D. Matarazzo, S. M. Weiss, J. A. Herd, N. E. Miller, and S. M. Weiss (Eds.), *Behavioral health: A handbook of health enhancement and disease prevention* New York: Wiley, 1984a.

———. Behavioral immunogens and pathogens in health and illness. In B. L. Hammonds and C. J. Scheirer (Eds.), *Psychology and health: The master lecture series,* vol. 3. Washington, D.C.: American Psychological Association, 1984b.

Matthews, K. A. Caregiver–child interactions and the Type A coronary-prone behavior pattern. *Child Development,* 1977, *48,* 1752–1756.

———. Antecedents of the Type A coronary-prone behavior pattern. In S. S. Brehm, S. M. Kassin, and F. X. Gibbons (Eds.), *Developmental social psychology: Theory and research.* New York: Oxford, 1980.

———. Psychological perspectives on the Type A behavior pattern. *Psychological Bulletin,* 1982, *91,* 293–323.

Matthews, K. A., and Angulo, J. Measurement of the Type A behavior pattern in children: Assessment of children's competitiveness, impatience-anger, and aggression. *Child Development,* 1980, *51,* 466–475.

Matthews, K. A., and Haynes, S. G. Type A behavior pattern and coronary disease risk: Update and critical evaluation. *American Journal of Epidemiology,* 1986, *123*(6), 923–960.

Matthews, K. A., and Jennings, J. R. Cardiovascular responses of boys exhibiting the Type A behavior pattern. *Psychosomatic Medicine,* 1984, *46*(6), 484–498.

Matthews, K. A., and Siegel, J. The Type A behavior pattern in children and adolescents. In A. Baum, and J. Singer (Eds.), *Handbook of psychology and health.* Hillsdale, N.J.: Erlbaum, 1987.

Matthews, K. A., Glass, D. C., Rosenman, R. H., and Bortner, R. W. Competitive drive, pattern A and coronary heart disease: A further analysis of some data from the Western Collaborative Group Study.

Journal of Chronic Diseases, 1977, *30,* 489–498.

Matthews, K. A., Rosenman, R. H., Dembroski, T. M., Harris, E. L., and MacDougall, J. M. Familial resemblance in components of the Type A behavior pattern: A reanalysis of the California Type A Twin Study. *Psychosomatic Medicine,* 1984, *46*(6), 498–511.

Matthews, K. A., Weiss, S. M., Detre, T., Dembroski, T. M., Falkner, B., Manuck, S. B., and Williams, R. B., Jr. *Handbook of stress, reactivity, and cardiovascular disease.* New York: Wiley, 1986.

Maxwell, K. W., Marcus, S., and Renzetti, A. D. Effect of tobacco smoke on phagocytic and cytopeptic activity of guinea pig alveolar macrophages. *American Review of Respiratory Illness,* 1967, *96,* 156.

May, R. M., and Anderson, R. M. Transmission dynamics of HIV infections. *Nature,* 1987, *326*(6109), 137–142.

Mayer, D. J., Price, D. D., Barber, J., and Rafii, A. Acupuncture analgesia: Evidence for activation of a pain inhibitor system as a mechanism of action. In J. J. Bonica and D. Albe-Fessard (Eds.), *Advances in pain research and therapy,* vol. 1. New York: Raven, 1976.

Mayer, T. G., Gatchel, R. J., Mayer, H., Kishino, N., Keely, J., and Mooney, V. A prospective two-year study of functional restoration in industrial low back injury utilizing objective assessment. *Journal of the American Medical Association,* 1987, *258,* 1763–1767.

Mayer, T. G., Gatchel, R. J., Kishino, N., Keeley, J., Capra, P., Mayer, H., Barnett, J., and Mooney, V. Objective assessment of spine function following industrial injury: A prospective study with comparison group and one-year follow-up. *Spine,* 1985, *10,* 482–493.

Mears, F. G., and Gatchel, R. J. *Fundamentals of abnormal psychology.* Chicago: Rand McNally, 1979.

Mechanic, D. Response factors in illness: The study of illness behavior. *Social Psychiatry,* 1966, *1,* 11–20.

————. *Medical sociology: A selective view.* New York: Free Press, 1968.

————. Social psychologic factors affecting the presentation of bodily complaints. *New England Journal of Medicine,* 1972, *286,* 1132–1139.

————. Effects of psychological distress on perceptions of physical health and use of medical and psychiatric facilities. *Journal of Human Stress,* 1978, *4*(4), 26–32.

Mechanic, D., and Jackson, D. Stress, illness behavior, and the use of general practitioner services: A study of British women. Manuscript, Department of Sociology, University of Wisconsin, 1968.

Meehl, P. E. *Research results for counselors.* St. Paul, Minn.: State Department of Education, 1951.

————. Schizotaxia, schizotypy, schizophrenia. *American Psychologist,* 1962, *17,* 827–838.

Mehrabian, A. A questionnaire measure of individual differences in stimulus screening and associated differences in arousability. *Environmental Psychology and Nonverbal Behavior,* 1977, *1,* 89–103.

Meichenbaum, D. H. Clinical implications of modifying what clients say to themselves. *University of Waterloo Research Reports in Psychology, No. 42,* December 19, 1972.

————. *Cognitive-behavior modification.* New York: Plenum, 1977.

Meichenbaum, D., and Turk, D. The cognitive-behavioral management of anxiety, anger, and pain. In P. O. Davidson (Ed.), *The behavioral management of anxiety, depression and pain.* New York: Brunner/Mazel, 1976.

Melamed, B., and Siegel, L. Reduction of anxiety in children facing hospitalization and surgery by use of filmed modeling. *Journal of Consulting and Clinical Psychology,* 1975, *43,* 511–521.

Mello, N. K. Behavioral studies of alcoholism. In B. Kessen, and H. Begleiter (Eds.), *The biology of alcoholism, physiology, and behavior,* vol. 2. New York: Plenum, 1972.

Melzack, R. *The puzzle of pain.* Harmondsworth, England: Penguin, 1973.

————. Prolonged relief of pain by brief, intense, transcutaneous somatic stimulation. *Pain,* 1975, *1,* 357–373.

Melzack, R., and Wall, P. D. Pain mechanisms: A new theory. *Science,* 1965, *150,* 971–979.

Menninger, K. A., and Menninger, W. C. Psychoanalytic observations in cardiac disorders. *American Heart Journal,* 1936, *11,* 10.

Meyer, A. J., Nash, J. D., McAlister, A. L., Maccoby, N., and Farquhar, J. W. Skills training in a cardiovascular education campaign. *Journal of Consulting and Clinical Psychology,* 1980, *48,* 129–142.

Meyer, D. L. The effects of patients' representations of high blood pressure on behavior in treatment. Ph.D. diss., University of Wisconsin, 1981.

Mikulincer, M. Attributional processes in the learned helplessness paradigm: Behavioral effects of global attributions. *Journal of Personality and Social Psychology,* 1986, *51,* 1248–1256.

Miller, D. M. A behavioral intervention program for chronic public drunkenness offenders. *Archives of General Psychiatry,* 1975, *32,* 915–918.

Miller, D. M., and Eisler, R. M. Alcohol and drug abuse. In W. E. Craighead, A. E. Kayden, and M. J. Mahoney (Eds.), *Behavior modification principles, issues, and application.* Boston: Houghton Mifflin, 1976.

Miller, D. M., and Hersen, M. Quantitative changes in alcohol consumption as a function of electrical aversive conditioning. *Journal of Clinical Psychology,* 1972, *28,* 590–593.

Miller, M. The effects of electromyographic feedback and progressive relaxation training on stress reactions in dental patients. *Dissertation Abstracts International,* 1977, *37,* 6340B.

Miller, N. E. Learning of visceral and glandular responses. *Science,* 1969, *163,* 434–445.

————. Behavioral medicine: Symbiosis

between laboratory and clinic. *Annual Review of Psychology,* 1983, *34,* 1–31.

Miller, W. R., and Seligman, M. E. P. Depression and learned helplessness in man. *Journal of Abnormal Psychology,* 1975, *84,* 228–238.

Millon, T. *Modern psychopathology.* Philadelphia: Saunders, 1969.

Millon, T., Green, C. J., and Meagher, R. B. *Millon Behavioral Health Inventory,* 3rd ed. Minneapolis: Interpretative Scoring System, 1982.

Mills, R. T., and Krantz, D. S. Information, choice, and reactions to stress: A field experiment in a blood bank with laboratory analogue. *Journal of Personality and Social Psychology,* 1979, *37,* 608–620.

Mirsky, I. A. Physiologic, psychologic, and social determinants in the etiology of duodenal ulcer. *American Journal of Digestive Diseases,* 1958, *3,* 285–314.

Mirsky, I. A., Fritterman, P., and Kaplan, S. Blood plasma pepsinogen. II. The activity of the plasma from "normal" subjects, patients with duodenal ulcer and patients with pernicious anemia. *Journal of Laboratory and Clinical Medicine,* 1952, *40,* 188–195.

Mitchell, J. (Ed.) *The ninth mental measurements yearbook.* Lincoln: University of Nebraska Press, 1985.

Monjan, A. A. Stress and immunologic competence: Studies in animals. In R. Ader (Ed.), *Psychoneuroimmunology.* New York: Academic Press, 1981.

Monjan, A., and Collector, M. Stress-induced modulation of the immune response. *Science,* 1977, *96*(1), 307–308.

Monjan, A. A., and Mandell, W. Fetal alcohol and immunity: Depression of mitogen-induced lymphocyte blastogenesis. *Neurobehavioral Toxicology,* 1980, *2,* 213–215.

Moore, J., Strube, M. J., and Lacks, P. Learned helplessness: A function of attribution style and comparative performance information. *Personality and Social Psychology Bulletin,* 1984, *10,* 526–535.

Moos, R. H., and Finney, J. W. The expanding scope of alcoholism treatment evaluation. *American Psychologist,* 1983, *38,* 1036–1044.

Morokoff, P. J., Holmes, E., and Weisse, C. S. A psychosocial program for HIV-seropositive persons. *Patient Education and Counseling,* 1987, *10,* 287–300.

Morrow, G. R. Prevalence and correlates of anticipatory nausea and vomiting in chemotherapy patients. *Journal of the National Cancer Institute,* 1982, *68,* 585–588.

Mott, F. W. *War neuroses and shell shock.* London: Oxford Medical Publications, 1919.

Mowrer, O. H., and Viek, P. An experimental analogue of fear from a sense of helplessness. *Journal of Abnormal and Social Psychology,* 1948, *43,* 193–200.

MRFIT Research Group. Multiple risk factor intervention trial: Risk factor changes and mortality results. *Journal of the American Medical Association,* 1982, *248,* 1465–1477.

Munsinger, H. The adopted child's IQ: A critical review. *Psychological Bulletin,* 1975, *82,* 623–659.

Murphy, T. M. Subjective and objective follow-up assessment of acupuncture therapy without suggestion in 100 chronic pain patients. In J. J. Bonica and D. Albe-Fessard (Eds.), *Advances in pain research and therapy,* vol. 1. New York: Raven, 1976.

Murray, H. A. *Explorations in personality.* New York: Oxford, 1938.

Nagatsu, T. *Biochemistry of catecholamines: The biochemical method.* Baltimore: University Park Press, 1973.

Nathan, P. E. The worksite as a setting for health promotion and positive lifestyle change, and Johnson & Johnson's live for life: A comprehensive positive lifestyle change. In J. D. Matarazzo, S. M. Weiss, J. A. Herd, N. E. Miller, and S. M. Weiss (Eds.), *Behavioral health: A handbook of health enhancement and disease prevention.* New York: Wiley, 1984.

Nathan, P. E., and Goldman, M. S. Problem drinking and alcoholism. In O. F. Pomerleau and J. P. Brady (Eds.), *Behav-*

ioral medicine: Theory and practice. Baltimore: Williams & Wilkins, 1979.

Nathan, P. E., and Lansky, D. Management of the chronic alcoholic: A behavioral viewpoint. In J. P. Brady and H. K. H. Brodie (Eds.), *Controversy in psychiatry.* Philadelphia: Saunders, 1978.

Nathan, P. E., and O'Brien, J. S. An experimental analysis of the behavior of alcoholics and nonalcoholics during prolonged experimental drinking. *Behavior Therapy,* 1971, *2,* 455–476.

National Cancer Institute. Cancer prevention (NIH Publication No. 84-2671). Bethesda, Md.: NIH, 1984.

National Computer Services. *Conference on the Millon Clinical Inventories.* Minnetonka, Minn., 1987.

Navia, B., Jordan, B., and Price, R. The AIDS dementia complex: I. Clinical features. *Annals of Neurology,* 1986, *19,* 517–524.

Nelson, B. Bosses face less risk than the bossed. *New York Times,* April 3, 1983.

Nemiah, J. C. Psychology and psychosomatic illness. Reflections in theory and research methodology. In J. Freyberger (Ed.), *Topics of psychosomatic research. Proceedings of 9th European Conference on Psychosomatic Research.* London: Karger, Basel, 1973.

Nemiah, J. C. Denial revisited: Reflections on psychosomatic theory. *Psychotherapy and Psychosomatics,* 1975, *26,* 140–147.

Nemiah, J. C., Freyberger, H., and Sifneos, P. Alexithymia: A view of the psychosomatic process. In O. Hill (Ed.), *Modern trends in psychosomatic medicine,* vol. 3. London: Butterworth, 1976.

Nerenz, D. R. *Control of emotional distress in cancer, chemotherapy.* Ph.D. diss. University of Wisconsin, 1980.

Neufeld, V. R. Patient education: A critique. In D. L. Sackett and R. B. Haynes (Eds.), *Compliance with therapeutic regimens.* Baltimore: Johns Hopkins University Press, 1976.

Newberry, B. H., Gildow, J., Wogan, J., et al. Inhibition of Huggins tumors by forced restraint. *Psychosomatic Medicine,* 1976, *38*(3), 155–162.

Newman, H. H., Freeman, F. N., and Holzinger, K. J. *Twins: A study of heredity and environment.* Chicago: University of Chicago Press, 1937.

Nieburgs, H. E., Weiss, J. Navarrete, M., Strax, P., Teirstein, A., Grillione, G., and Siedlecki, B. The role of stress in human and environmental oncogenesis. *Cancer Detection and Prevention,* 1979, *2*(2), 307–336.

Nisbett, R. E. Determinants of food intake in human obesity. *Science,* 1968, *159,* 1254–1255.

Nisbett, R. E., and Temoshok, L. Is there an external cognitive style? *Journal of Personality and Social Psychology,* 1976, *33,* 36–47.

Noback, C. R., and Demarest, R. J. *The nervous system: Introduction and review,* vol. 7. New York: McGraw-Hill, 1972.

Nolen-Hoeksema, S., Girgus, J. S., and Seligman, M. E. P. Learned helplessness in children: A longitudinal study of depression, achievement, and explanatory style. *Journal of Personality and Social Psychology,* 1986, *51,* 435–442.

Nomikos, M. S., Opton, E. M., Jr., Averill, J. R., and Lazarus, R. S. Surprise versus suspense in the production of stress reaction. *Journal of Personality and Social Psychology,* 1968, *8,* 204–208.

Nuckolls, K. B., Cassel, J., and Kaplan, B. H. Psychosocial assets, life crisis, and the prognosis of pregnancy. *American Journal of Epidemiology,* 1972, *95,* 431–441.

Nungester, W. J., and Klesper, R. G. A possible mechanism of lowered resistance to pneumococci infection. *Journal of Infectious Diseases,* 1939, *63,* 94–102.

Obrist, P. A., Gaebelein, C. J., Teller, E. S., Langer, A. W., Grignolo, A., Light, K. C., and McCubbin, J. A. The relationship among heart rate, carotid dP/dt, and blood pressure in humans as a function of the type of stress. *Psychophysiology,* 1978, *15,* 102–115.

Ogden, E., and Shock, N. W. Voluntary hypercirculation. *American Journal of the Medical Sciences,* 1939, *198,* 329–342.

O'Leary, M. R., Donovan, D., Krueger, K. J., and Cysenski, B. Depression and perception of reinforcement: Lack of differences in expectancy change among alcoholics. *Journal of Abnormal Psychology,* 1978, *87,* 110–112.

Osler, W. *Lectures on angina pectoris and allied states.* New York: Appleton, 1892.

Ostfeld, A., and Eaker, E. (Eds.). Measuring psychosocial variables in epidemiologic studies of cardiovascular disease (NIH Publication No. 85-2270). Bethesda, Md.: NIH, 1985.

Overmier, J. B., and Seligman, M. E. P. Effects of inescapable shock upon subsequent escape and avoidance responding. *Journal of Comparative and Physiological Psychology,* 1967, *63,* 28–33.

Oxford, J., Oppenheimer, E., and Edwards, G. Abstinence or control: The outcome for excessive drinkers two years after consultation. *Behavior Research and Therapy,* 1976, *14,* 409–418.

Page, H. *Injuries of the spine and spinal cord without apparent mechanical lesions.* London: J. and A. Churchill, 1885.

Page, L., Danion, A., and Moellering, R. C. Antecedents of cardiovascular disease in six Solomon Island societies. *Circulation,* 1970, *49,* 1132–1140.

Palmblad, J., Petrini, B., Wasserman, J., and Akerstedt, T. Lymphocyte and granulocyte reactions during sleep deprivation. *Psychosomatic Medicine,* 1970, *41,* 273–278.

Palmblad, J., Cantell, K., Strander, H., Froberg, J., Karlsson, C., Levi, L., Granstrom, M., and Unger, P. Stressor exposure and immunological response in man: Interferon producing capacity and phagocytes. *Journal of Psychosomatic Research,* 1976, *20,* 193–199.

Panayatopoulos, S., Gotsis, N., Papazoglou, N., et al. Antigenic study of Nicotiana tabacum and research on precipitins against tobacco antigens in the serum of smokers and nonsmokers. *Allergologia et Immunopathologia,* 1974, *2,* 111–114.

Pancheri, P., Bellaterra, M., Matteoli, S., Cristofari, M., Polizzi, C., and Puletti, M. Infarct as a stress agent: Life history and personality characteristics in improved versus not-improved patients after severe heart attack. *Journal of Human Stress,* 1978, *4*(4), 16–26.

Parjis, J., Joosens, J. V., Van der Linden, L., Verstreken, G., and Amer, A. K. Moderate sodium restriction and diuretics in the treatment of hypertension. *American Heart Journal,* 1973, *85,* 22–25.

Park, L. C., and Lipman, R. S. A comparison of patient dosage deviation reports with pill counts. *Psychopharmacologica,* 1964, *6,* 299–302.

Parker, S. D., Brewer, M. B., and Spencer, J. R. Natural disaster, perceived control, and attributions to fate. *Personality and Social Psychology Bulletin,* 1980, *6,* 454–459.

Parkes, C. M. *Bereavement: Studies of grief in adult life.* New York: International Universities Press, 1972.

Parsons, T. *The social system.* New York: Free Press, 1951.

Patkai, P. Catecholamine excretion in pleasant and unpleasant situations. *Acta Psychologica,* 1971, *35,* 352–363.

Pattison, E. M., Sobell, M. B., and Sobell, L. C. (Eds.). *Emerging concepts of alcohol dependence.* New York: Springer, 1977.

Paulus, P., McCain, G., and Cox, V. Death rates, psychiatric commitments, blood pressure, and perceived crowding as a function of institutional crowding. *Environmental Psychology and Nonverbal Behavior,* 1978, *3,* 107–116.

Pavlov, I. P. *Conditioned reflexes.* New York: Dover, 1927.

Penderay, M. L., Maltzman, I. M., and West, L. T. Controlled drinking by alcoholics? New findings and a reevaluation of a major affirmative study. *Science,* 1982, *217,* 169–174.

Pennebaker, J. Environmental determinants of symptom perception. Paper presented at the meeting of the American Psychological Association, New York, September 1979.

Pennebaker, J., and Brittingham, G. Environmental and sensory cues affecting the perception of physical symptoms. In A. Baum and J. E. Singer (Eds.), *Advances in environmental psychology: Environment and health,* vol. 4. Hillsdale, N.J.: Erlbaum, 1982

Pennebaker, J., and Newtson, D. The psychological impact of Mt. St. Helens. Manuscript, University of Virginia, 1981.

Perrin, G. M., and Pierce, I. R. Psychosomatic aspects of cancer—a review. *Psychosomatic Medicine,* 1959, *21*(5), 397–421.

Pervin, L. A. The need to predict and control under conditions of threat. *Journal of Personality,* 1963, *31,* 570–587.

———. *Current controversies and issues in personality.* New York: Wiley, 1978.

Peters, J. E., and Stern, R. M. Specificity of attitude hypothesis in psychosomatic medicine: A reexamination. *Journal of Psychosomatic Research,* 1971, *15,* 129–135.

Peterson, C., Rosenbaum, A. C., and Conn, M. K. Depressive mood reactions to breaking up: Testing the learned helplessness model of depression. *Journal of Social and Clinical Psychology,* 1985, *3,* 161–169.

Pettingale, K., Greer, S., and Tee, D. Serum IgA and emotional expression in breast cancer patients. *Journal of Psychosomatic Research,* 1977, *21,* 395–399.

Pickering, T. G. Personal views on mechanisms of hypertension. In J. Genest, E. Koiw, and O. Kuchel (Eds.), *Hypertension: Physiopathology and treatment.* New York: McGraw-Hill, 1977.

Pilisuk, M., and Parks, S. H. Structural dimensions of social support groups. *Journal of Psychology,* 1980, *106,* 157–177.

Pilkonis, P. A., Imler, S. D., and Rubinsky, P. Dimensions of life stress in psychiatric patients. *Journal of Human Stress,* 1985, *11,* 5–10.

Pilot, M. L., Lenkoski, L. D., Spiro, H. M., and Schaeffer, R. Duodenal ulcer in one of identical twins. *Psychosomatic Medicine,* 1957, *19,* 221–229.

Pittman, N. L., and Pittman, T. S. Effects of amount of helplessness training and internal–external locus of control on mood and performance. *Journal of Personality and Social Psychology,* 1979, *37,* 39–47.

Pliner, P. Effects of cue salience on the behavior of obese and normal subjects. *Journal of Abnormal Psychology,* 1973, *82,* 226–232.

————. Effects of liquid and solid preloads in the eating behavior of obese and normal persons. In S. Schachter and J. Rodin (Eds.), *Obese humans and rats.* Washington, D.C.: Erlbaum/Wiley, 1974.

Pliner, P., and Cappell, H. Modification of affective consequences of alcohol: A comparison of social and solitary drinking. *Journal of Abnormal Psychology,* 1974, *83,* 418–425.

Polivy, J., Scheuneman, A. L., and Carlson, K. Alcohol and tension reduction: Cognitive and physiological effects. *Journal of Abnormal Psychology,* 1976, *85,* 595–606.

Pomerleau, O. F. Behavioral factors in the establishment, maintenance, and cessation of smoking. In *Smoking and health: A report of the Surgeon General* (DHEW Publication No. [PHS] 79-50066). Washington, D.C.: U.S. Government Printing Office, 1979.

Porter, R. W., Brady, J. V., Conrad, D., Mason, J. W., Galambos, R., and McKrioch, D. Some experimental observations on gastrointestinal lesions in behaviorally conditioned monkeys. *Psychosomatic Medicine,* 1958, *20,* 379–394.

Pratt, S. A., Finley, T. N., Smith, M. H., and Ladman, A. J. A comparison of alveolar macrophages and pulmonary surfactant obtained from the lungs of human smokers and nonsmokers by endobronchial lavage. *Anatomical Record,* 1969, *163,* 497–507.

Price, J. H., Desmond, S., and Kukulka, G. High school students' perceptions and misperceptions of AIDS. *Journal of School Health,* 1985, *55*(3), 107–109.

Price, K. P. Biofeedback and migraine. In R. J. Gatchel and K. P. Price (Eds.), *Clinical applications of biofeedback: Appraisal and status.* Elmsford, N.Y.: Pergamon, 1979.

Price, K. P., and Gatchel, R. J. A perspective on clinical biofeedback. In R. J. Gatchel and K. P. Price (Eds.), *Clinical biofeedback: Appraisal and status.* Elmsford, N.Y.: Pergamon, 1979.

Purcell, K., Brady, K., Chai, H., Muser, J., Molk, L., Gordon, U., and Means, J. The effect on asthma in children of experimental separation from the family. *Psychosomatic Medicine,* 1969, *31,* 144–164.

Puska, P. Community based prevention of cardiovascular disease: The North Karelia Project. In J. D. Matarazzo, S. M. Weiss, J. A. Herd, N. E. Miller, and S. M. Weiss (Eds.), *Behavioral health: A handbook of health enhancement and disease prevention.* New York: Wiley, 1984.

Quarantelli, E. L., and Dynes, R. R. When disaster strikes. *Psychology Today,* 1972, *5*(9), 66–70.

Rabkin, J. G., and Struening, E. L. Life events, stress, and illness. *Science,* 1976, *191,* 1013–1020.

Ragland, D. R., and Brand, R. J. Type A behavior and mortality from coronary heart disease. *New England Journal of Medicine,* 1988, *318,* 65–69.

Rahe, R. H. Life changes and near-future illness reports. In L. Levi (Ed.), *Emotions: Their parameters and measurements.* New York: Raven, 1975.

Rahe, R. H. Recent life changes, emotions, and behaviors in coronary heart disease. In A. Baum and J. E. Singer (Eds.), *Handbook of psychology and health,* vol. 5, *Stress.* Hillsdale, N.J.: Erlbaum, 1987.

Rahe, R. H., Mahan, J. L., and Arthur, R. J. Prediction of near-future health change from subjects' preceeding life changes. *Journal of Psychosomatic Research,* 1970, *14,* 401–406.

Rahe, R. H., and Paasikivi, J. Psychosocial factors and myocardial infarction. II. An outpatient study in Sweden. *Journal of Psychosomatic Research,* 1971, *15,* 33–39.

Rahe, R. H., Ryman, D. H., and Ward,

H. W. Simplified scale for life change events. *Journal of Human Stress,* 1980, *6,* 22–27.

Raps, C., Peterson, C., Jones, M., and Seligman, M. Patient behavior in hospitals: Helplessness, reactance, or both. *Journal of Personality and Social Psychology,* 1982, *42,* 1036–1041.

Ratin, J. Current status of the internal-external hypothesis for obesity: What went wrong? *American Psychologist,* 1981, *36,* 361–372.

Regland, B., Cajander, S., Wiman, L. G., and Falkmer, S. Scanning electron microscopy of the bronchial mucosa in some lung diseases using bronchoscopy specimens. *Scandinavian Journal of Respiratory Diseases,* 1976, *57,* 171–182.

Rees, L. The importance of psychological, allergic, and infective factors in childhood asthma. *Schizophrenia Bulletin,* 1964, *8,* 1–11.

Reitan, R. M. Certain differential effects of left and right cerebral lesions in human adults. *Journal of Comparative and Physiological Psychology,* 1955, *48,* 474–477.

————. Psychological deficits resulting from cerebral lesions in man. In J. M. Warren and K. A. Kent (Eds.), *The frontal granular cortex and behavior.* New York: McGraw-Hill, 1964.

Reitan, R. M., and Davison, L. A. *Clinical neuropsychology: Current status and applications.* New York: Winston-Wiley, 1974.

Renneker, R. Cancer and psychotherapy. In J. Goldberg (Ed.), *Psychotherapeutic treatment of cancer patients.* New York: Free Press, 1981.

Review Panel. Coronary-prone behavior and coronary heart disease: A critical review. *Circulation,* 1981, *63,* 1199–1215.

Riley, C. S. Patients' understanding of doctors' instruction. *Medical Care,* 1966, *4,* 34–37.

Riley, V. Psychoneuroendocrine influences on immunocompetence and neoplasia. *Science,* 1981, *212,* 1100–1109.

Riley, V., Fitzmaurice, M. A., and Spackman, D. H. Animal models in biobehavioral research. Effects of anxiety stress on immunocompetence and neoplasia. In S. M. Weiss, J. A. Herd, and B. H. Fox (Eds.), *Perspectives in behavioral medicine.* New York: Academic Press, 1981.

Rimm, D. C., and Masters, J. C. *Behavior therapy: Techniques and empirical findings.* New York: Academic Press, 1974.

Rimsey, S. L., Ritzman, S. E., Mengel, E. E., et al. Skylab experiment results: Hematology studies. *Acta Astronautica,* 1975, *2,* 141–154.

Rinehart, J. J., Sagone, A. L., Baceryak, S. P., Ackerman, G. A., and LoBuglio, A. F. Effects of corticosteroid therapy on human monocyte function. *New England Journal of Medicine,* 1975, *292,* 236–241.

Ritter, B. The group treatment of children's snake phobias using vicarious and contact desensitization procedures. *Behavior Research and Therapy,* 1968, *6,* 1–6.

Rizley, R. Depression and distortion in the attribution of causality. *Journal of Abnormal Psychology,* 1978, *87,* 32–48.

Roberts, M. C. *Cancer today: Origins, prevention and treatment.* Washington, D.C.: Institute of Medicine/National Academy Press, 1984.

Rodin, J. Density, perceived choice and response to controllable and uncontrollable outcomes. *Journal of Experimental Social Psychology,* 1976, *12,* 564–578.

————. Obesity: Why the losing battle? Master lecture series on brain and behavior relationships. Presented at the meeting of the American Psychological Association, San Francisco, 1977.

————. The puzzle of obesity. *Human Nature,* 1978, *1*(2), 38–47.

Rodin, J., Elman, D., and Schachter, S. Emotionality and obesity. In S. Schachter and J. Rodin (Eds.), *Obese humans and rats.* Washington, D.C.: Erlbaum/Wiley, 1974.

Rodin, J., and Kristeller, J. L. A three-stage model of treatment continuity: Compliance, adherence and maintenance. Paper presented at the 52nd annual meeting of the Eastern Psychological Association, New York, April 1981.

Rodin, J., and Langer, E. J. Long-term effects of a control-relevant intervention with institutionalized aged. *Journal of Personality and Social Psychology*, 1977, *35*, 897–902.

Rodin, J., Rennert, K., and Solomon, S. K. Intrinsic motivation for control: Fact or fiction. In A. Baum and J. E. Singer (Eds.), *Advances in environmental psychology: Applications of personal control*, vol. 2. Hillsdale, N.J.: Erlbaum, 1980.

Rodin, J., and Slochower, J. Externality in the nonobese: The effects of environmental responsiveness on weight. *Journal of Personality and Social Psychology*, 1976, *33*, 338–344.

Rodin, J., Solomon, S., and Metcalf, J. Role of control in mediating perceptions of density. *Journal of Personality and Social Psychology*, 1978, *36*, 988–999.

Roessler, R., Cate, T. R., Lester, J. W., et al. Ego strength, life events, and antibody filters. Paper presented at the annual meeting of the American Psychoanalytic Society, March 1979.

Rogentine, G. N., Van Kammen, D. P., Fox, B. H., Doherty, J. P., Rosenblatt, J. E., Boyd, S. C., and Bunney, W. E. Psychological factors in the prognosis of malignant melanoma: A prospective study. *Psychosomatic Medicine*, 1979, *41*, 647–655.

Rogers, M. P., Dubey, D., and Reich, P. The influence of the psyche and the brain on immunity and disease susceptibility: A critical review. *Psychosomatic Medicine*, 1979, *41*, 147–164.

Roitt, I., Brostoff, J., and Male, D. *Immunology*. St. Louis: C. V. Mosby, 1985.

Rorschach, J. *Psychodiagnostics*. Berne, Switzerland: Huber, 1942.

Rose, R. M., Jenkins, C. D., and Hurst, M. W. Air traffic controller health change study (FAA Contract No. DOT-FA73WA-3211). Boston: Boston University School of Medicine, 1978.

Rosen, E., and Gregory, I. *Abnormal psychology*. Philadelphia: Saunders, 1965.

Rosenbaum, M., and Jaffee, Y. Learned helplessness: The role of individual differences in learned resourcefulness. *British Journal of Social Psychology*, 1983, *22*, 215–225.

Rosenman, R. H. The interview method of assessment of the coronary-prone behavior pattern. In T. M. Dembroski, S. M. Weiss, J. L. Shields, S. G. Haynes, and M. Feinleib (Eds.), *Coronary-prone behavior*. New York: Springer-Verlag, 1978a.

———. The role of the Type A behavior pattern in ischaemic heart disease: Modification of its effects by beta-blocking agents. *British Journal of Clinical Practice*, 1978b, *32* (Suppl. 1), 58–65.

Rosenman, R. H., Brand, R. J., Jenkins, C. D., Friedman, M., Straus, R., and Wurm, M. Coronary heart disease in the Western Collaborative Group Study: Final follow-up experience of 8½ years. *Journal of the American Medical Association*, 1975, *233*, 872–877.

Rosenman, R. H., Brand, R. J., Sholtz, R. I., and Friedman, M. Multivariate prediction of coronary heart disease during 8.5 year follow-up in the Western Collaborative Group Study. *American Journal of Cardiology*, 1976, *37*, 903–910.

Rosenman, R. H., and Friedman, M. The central nervous system and coronary heart disease. In P. M. Insel and R. H. Moos (Eds.), *Health and the social environment*. Lexington, Mass.: D. C. Health, 1974.

Rosenman, R. H., Friedman, M., and Byers, S. O. Glucose metabolism in subjects with behavior pattern A and hyperlipemia. *Circulation*, 1966, *33*, 704–707.

Rosenman, R. H., Friedman, M., Straus, R., Wurm, M., Kositchek, R., Hahn, W., and Werthessen, N. T. A predictive study of coronary heart disease: The Western Collaborative Group Study. *Journal of the American Medical Association*, 1964, *189*, 15–22.

Rosenstock, I. M. Why people use health services. *Milbank Memorial Fund Quarterly*, 1966, *44*, 94–127.

Rosenthal, D. *Genetic theory and abnormal behavior*. New York: McGraw-Hill, 1970.

Rosenthal, D., Wender, P., Kety, S. S., Welner, J., and Schulsinger, F. The adopted-away offspring of schizophrenics.

American Journal of Psychiatry, 1971, *128,* 307–311.

Roskies, E., Seraganian, P. Oseasohn, R., Martin, N., Smilga, C., and Hanley, J. A. The Montreal Type A intervention project: Major findings. *Health Psychology,* 1986, *5,* 45–69.

Ross, R., and Glomset, J. A. The pathogenesis of atherosclerosis. *New England Journal of Medicine,* 1976, *295,* 369–377, 420–425.

Ross, T. A. *Lectures on war neuroses.* London: Edward Arnold, 1941.

Roth, P. M., Caron, M. S., Ort, R. S., Berger, D. G. Albee, G. W., and Streeter, G. A. Patients' beliefs about peptic ulcer and its treatment. *Annals of Internal Medicine,* 1962, *56,* 72–80.

Roth, S., and Bootzin, R. R. Effects of experimentally induced expectancies of external control: An investigation of learned helplessness. *Journal of Personality and Social Psychology,* 1974, *29,* 253–264.

Roth, S., and Kubal, L. Effects of noncontingent reinforcement on tasks of differing importance: Facilitation of learned helplessness. *Journal of Personality and Social Psychology,* 1975, *32,* 680–691.

Rotton, J., Oszewski, D., Charleton, M., and Soler, E. Loud speech, conglomerate noise, and behavioral aftereffects. *Journal of Applied Psychology,* 1978, *63,* 360–365.

Ruble, D. N., and Brooks-Gunn, J. Menstrual symptoms: A social cognition analysis. *Journal of Behavioral Medicine,* 1979, *2,* 171–194.

Ruesch, S. The infantile personality—The core problem of psychosomatic medicine. *Psychosomatic Medicine,* 1948, *10,* 134–149.

Russell, M. A. H. Tobacco smoking and nicotine dependence. In R. J. Gibbins (Ed.), *Research advances in alcohol and drug problems,* vol. 3. New York: Wiley, 1976.

———. Tobacco dependence: Is nicotine rewarding or aversive? In *Cigarette smoking is a dependence process* (NIDA Research Monograph No. 23, DHEW Publication No. ADM 79-800). Washington, D.C.: U.S. Government Printing Office, 1979.

Sacerdote, P. Hypnosis in cancer patients. *American Journal of Clinical Hypnosis,* 1966, *9,* 100–108.

Sachs, D. P. L., Hall, R. G., and Hall, S. M. Effects of rapid smoking. Physiological evaluation of a smoking-cessation therapy. *Annals of Internal Medicine,* 1978, *88,* 639–641.

Sackett, D. L., and Haynes, R. B. *Compliance with therapeutic regimens.* Baltimore: Johns Hopkins University Press, 1976.

Sakakibara, T. Effects of brightness or darkness on carcinogenesis. *Nagoya Shiritsj Daigaku Igakkai Sasshi,* 1966, *19,* 525–547.

Salloway, J. C., and Dillon, P. B. A comparison of family network and friend network in health care utilization. *Journal of Comparative Family Studies,* 1973, *4,* 131–142.

Salter, A. *Conditioned reflex therapy.* New York: Capricorn Books, 1949.

Santamaria, B. A. G. Dysmenorrhea. *Clinical Obstetrics and Gynecology,* 1969, *12,* 708–723.

Santrock, J. W. *Life-span development,* 2nd ed. Dubuque, Iowa: William C. Brown, 1986.

Sarason, I. G., de Monchaux, C., and Hunt, T. Methodological issues in the assessment of life stress. In L. Levi (Ed.), *Emotions— Their parameters and measurement.* New York: Raven, 1975.

Sarason, I. G., Johnson, J. H., and Siegel, J. M. Assessing the impact of life changes: Development of the Life Experiences Survey. *Journal of Consulting and Clinical Psychology,* 1978, *46,* 932–946.

Saxena A. K., Sing, K. P., Srivastava, S. N., et al. Immunomodulation effects of caffeine (1,3,7-trimethylxanthine) in rodents. *Indian Journal of Experimental Biology,* 1984, *22,* 298–301.

Scarf, M. Images that heal: A doubtful idea whose time has come. *Psychology Today,* 1980, *14*(4), 32–46.

Schachter, S. *The psychology of affiliation.* Stanford, Calif.: Stanford University Press, 1959.

―――. Obesity and eating. *Science,* 1968, *161,* 751–756.

―――. *Emotion, obesity and crime.* New York: Academic Press, 1971.

―――. Pharmacological and psychological determinants of smoking. *Annals of Internal Medicine,* 1978, *88,* 104–114.

Schachter, S., Goldman, R., and Gordon, A. Effects of fear, food deprivation, and obesity on eating. *Journal of Personality and Social Psychology,* 1968, *10,* 91–97.

Schachter, S., and Rodin, J. *Obese humans and rats.* Hillsdale, N.J.: Erlbaum, 1974.

Schachter, S., Silverstein, B., Kozlowski, L. T., Perlick, D., Herman, C. P., and Liebling, B. Studies of the interaction of psychosocial and pharmacological determinants of smoking. *Journal of Experimental Psychology: General,* 1977, *106,* 3–40.

Schachter, S., and Singer, J. E. Cognitive, social, and physiological determinants of emotional state. *Psychological Review,* 1962, *69,* 379–399.

Schachter, S., and Singer, J. E. Comments on the Maslach and Marshall–Zimbardo experiments. *Journal of Personality and Social Psychology,* 1979, *37,* 989–995.

Scherwitz, L., Berton, K., and Leventhal, H. Type A assessment and interaction in the behavior pattern interview. *Psychosomatic Medicine,* 1977, *39,* 229–240.

Schildkraut, J. J. The catecholamine hypothesis of affective disorders: A review of supporting evidence. *American Journal of Psychiatry,* 1965, *122,* 509–522.

Schleifer, S. J., Keller, S. E., Camerino, M., Thornton, J. C., and Stein, M. Suppression of lymphocyte stimulation following bereavement. *Journal of the American Medical Association,* 1983, *250*(3), 374–377.

Schleifer, S. J., Keller, S., McKegney, F., and Stein, M. Bereavement and lymphocyte function. Paper presented at the American Psychiatric Association, Montreal, May 1980.

Schleifer, S. J., Keller, S. E., Meyerson, A. T., Raskin, M. J., Davis, K. L., and Stein, M. Lymphocyte function in major depressive disorder. *Archives of General Psychiatry,* 1984, *41,* 484–486.

Schmale, A. H. Relationship of separation and depression to disease. *Psychosomatic Medicine,* 1958, *20,* 259–277.

Schmale, A. H., Jr. Giving up as a final common pathway to changes in health. *Advances in Psychosomatic Medicine,* 1972, *8,* 20–40.

Schmitt, F., and Wooldridge, P. Psychological preparation of surgical patients. *Nursing Research,* 1973, *22,* 108–115.

Schmolling, P. Human reactions to the Nazi concentration camps: A summing up. *Journal of Human Stress,* 1984, *10,* 108–120.

Schneider, P., and Cable, G. Compliance clinic: An opportunity for an expanded role for pharmacists. *American Journal of Hospital Pharmacy,* 1978, *35,* 288–295.

Schneiderman, N. Animal behavior models of coronary heart disease. In D. S. Krantz, A. Baum, and J. E. Singer (Eds.), *Handbook of psychology and health,* vol. 3, *Cardiovascular disorders.* Hillsdale, N.J.: Erlbaum, 1983.

Schroeder, D. H., and Costa, P. T., Jr. Influences of life event stress on physical illness: Substantive effects or methodological flaws? *Journal of Personality and Social Psychology,* 1984, *46*(4), 853–863.

Schofield, W. The role of psychology in the delivery of health service. *American Psychologist,* 1969, *24,* 565–584.

Schultz, J. H., and Luthe, W. *Autogenic training: A psychophysiological approach in psychotherapy.* New York: Grune & Stratton, 1959.

Schulz, L. S. Classical conditioning of nausea and vomiting in cancer chemotherapy. *Proceedings of the American Society of Clinical Oncologists, 1980, 21,* 244.

Schulz, R. Effects of control and predictability on the physical and psychological well-being of the institutionalized aged.

Journal of Personality and Social Psychology, 1976, *33,* 563–573.

———. *The psychology of death, dying, and bereavement.* Reading, Mass.: Addison-Wesley, 1978.

Schulz, R., and Aderman, D. Effect of residential change on the temporal distance to death of terminal cancer patients. *Omega: Journal of Death & Dying,* 1973, *4*(2), 157–162.

Schulz, R., and Brenner, G. F. Relocation of the aged: A review and theoretical analysis. *Journal of Gerontology,* 1977, *32,* 323–333.

Schulz, R., and Hanusa, B. H. Long-term effects of control and predictability-enhancing interventions: Findings and ethical issues. *Journal of Personality and Social Psychology,* 1978, *36,* 1194–1201.

Schwartz, G. E., and Weiss, S. What is behavioral medicine? *Psychosomatic Medicine,* 1977, *36,* 377–381.

Seligman, M. E. P. *Helplessness: On depression, development, and death.* San Francisco: W. H. Freeman, 1975.

———. Learned helplessness and depression in animals and men. In J. T. Spence, R. C. Carson, and J. W. Thibaut (Eds.), *Behavioral approaches to therapy.* Morristown, N.J.: General Learning Press, 1976.

Seligman, M. E. P., and Visintainer, M. A. Tumor rejection and early experience of uncontrollable shock in the rat. In F. R. Brush and J. B. Overmier (Eds.), *Affect conditioning and cognition: Essays on the determinants of behavior.* Hillsdale, N.J.: Erlbaum, 1985.

Seligman, M. E. P., Maier, S. F., and Geer, J. The alleviation of learned helplessness in the dog. *Journal of Abnormal and Social Psychology,* 1968, *73,* 256–262.

Seligman, M. E. P., Abramson, L. Y., Semmel, A., and Von Baeyer, C. Depressive attributional style. *Journal of Abnormal Psychology,* 1979, *88,* 242–247.

Selwyn, P. A. AIDS—What is now known. Psychological aspects, treatment prospects. *Hospital Practice,* 1986, *21*(6), 125.

Selye, H. *The stress of life.* New York: McGraw-Hill, 1976.

Shapiro, A. K. Placebo effects in medicine, psychotherapy, and psychoanalysis. In A. E. Bergin, and S. L. Garfield (Eds.), *Handbook of psychotherapy and behavior change: An empirical analysis.* New York: Wiley, 1971.

Shapiro, A. P. An experimental study of comparative responses of blood pressure to different noxious stimuli. *Journal of Chronic Disease,* 1961, *13,* 293–311.

———. The non-pharmacologic treatment of hypertension. In D. S. Krantz, A. Baum, and J. E. Singer (Eds.), *Handbook of psychology and health,* vol. 3, *Cardiovascular disorders and behavior.* Hillsdale, N.J.: Erlbaum, 1983.

Shapiro, A. P., Schwartz, G. E., Ferguson, D. C. E., Redmond, D. P., and Weiss, S. M. Behavioral methods in the treatment of hypertension: I. Review of their clinical status. *Annals of Internal Medicine,* 1977. *86,* 626–636.

Sheahy, C., and Maurer, D. Transcutaneous nerve stimulation for control of pain. *Surgery and Neurosurgery,* 1974, *2,* 45–47.

Sheiner, L. B., Rosenberg, B., Marathe, V. V., and Peck, C. Differences in serum digoxin concentrations between outpatients and inpatients. An effect of compliance? *Clinical Pharmacology and Therapeutics,* 1974, *15,* 239–246.

Shekelle, R. B., Hulley, S. B., Neaton, J., et al. The MRFIT behavioral pattern study. II: Type A behavior pattern and risk of coronary death in MRFIT. *American Journal of Epidemiology,* 1985, *122,* 559–570.

Sherr, L. An evaluation of the UK Government Health Education Campaign. *Psychology and Health,* 1987, *1,* 61–72.

Sherrod, D. R. Crowding, perceived control, and behavioral aftereffects. *Journal of Applied Social Psychology,* 1974, *4,* 171–186.

Sherrod, D. R., and Downs, R. Environmental determinants of altruism: The effects of stimulus overload and perceived control on helping. *Journal of Experimental Social Psychology,* 1974, *10,* 468–479.

Sherrod, D. R., Hage, J. N., Halpern, P. L., and Moore, B. S. Effects of personal causation and perceived control on responses to an aversive environment: The more control, the better. *Journal of Experimental Social Psychology,* 1977, *13,* 14–27.

Shipley, R. H., Butt, J. H., Horwitz, B., and Farbry, J. E. Preparation for a stressful medical procedure: Effect of amount of stimulus preexposure and a coping style. *Journal of Consulting and Clinical Psychology,* 1978, *46,* 499–507.

Shor, R. E. Physiological effects of painful stimulation during hypnotic analgesia. In J. E. Gordon (Ed.), *Handbook of clinical and experimental hypnosis.* New York: Macmillan, 1967.

Shrut, S. Attitudes toward old age and death. In R. Fulton (Ed.), *Death and identity.* New York: Wiley, 1965.

Shumaker, S. A., and Grunberg, N. E. (Eds.). Proceedings of the National Working Conference on Smoking Relapse. *Health Psychology,* 1986, *5* (Suppl.).

Siegel, S. Morphine tolerance acquisition as an associate process. *Journal of Experimental Psychology: Animal Behavior Processes,* 1977, *3,* 1–13.

Sifneos, P. E. Clinical observations in some patients suffering from a variety of psychosomatic diseases. *Proceedings of the 7th European Conference on Psychosomatic Research.* London: Karger, Basel, 1967.

Silverman, N. A., Potvin, C., Alexander, J. C., and Chretien, P. B. In vitro lymphocyte reactivity and t-cell levels in chronic cigarette smokers. *Clinical and Experimental Immunology,* 1975, *22,* 285–292.

Silverstein, B., Kelley, E., Swan, J., and Kozlowski, L. Physiological predisposition towards becoming a cigarette smoker: Experimental evidence for sex differences. *Addictive Behavior,* 1982, *7,* 83–86.

Simkins, L., and Eberhage, M. Attitudes towards AIDS, herpes II, and toxic shock syndrome. *Psychological Reports,* 1984, *55,* 779–786.

Simonton, B. C., Mathews-Simonton, S., and Creighton, J. *Getting well again.* Los Angeles: J. P. Vacher, 1978.

Sims, J. H., and Baumann, D. D. The tornado threat: Coping styles of the North and South. In J. H. Sims and D. D. Baumann (Eds.), *Human behavior and the environment: Interactions between man and his physical world.* Chicago: Maaroufa Press, 1974.

Singer, J. E., and Glass, D. C. Some reflections upon losing our social psychological purity. In M. Deutsch and H. A. Hornstein (Eds.), *Applying sound psychology: Implications for research, practice, and training.* Hillsdale, N.J.: Erlbaum, 1975.

Singer, J. E., Lundberg, U., and Frankenhaeuser, M. Stress on the train: A study of urban commuting. In A. Baum, J. E. Singer, and S. Valins (Eds.), *Advances in environmental psychology,* vol. 1. Hillsdale, N.J.: Erlbaum, 1978.

Sinyor, D., Schwartz, J. G., Peronnet, F., Bisson, G., and Seraganian, P. Aerobic fitness level and reactivity to psychosocial stress. *Psychosomatic Medicine,* 1983, *45,* 205–217.

Sjoberg, L., and Persson, L. A study of attempts by obese patients to regulate eating. *Gotesberg Psychological Reports,* 1979, *7,* 12.

Sklar, L. S., and Anisman, H. Stress and cancer. *Psychological Bulletin,* 1979a, *89,* 396–406.

————. Stress and coping factors influence tumor growth. *Science,* 1979b, *205,* 513–515.

Skodak, M., and Skeels, H. M. A final follow-up study of one hundred adopted children. *Journal of Genetic Psychology,* 1949, *75,* 85–125.

Snow, B. Level of aspiration in coronary prone and noncoronary prone adults. *Personality and Social Psychology Bulletin,* 1978, *4,* 416–419.

Snyder, S. Opiate receptors and internal opiates. *Scientific American,* 1977, *236,* 44–56.

Sobell, M. B., and Sobell, L. C. Individualized behavior therapy for alcoholics. *Behavior Therapy,* 1973, *4,* 49–72.

Sokolow, M., Werdegar, D., Perloff, D. B.,

Cowan, R. M., and Brenenstuhl, H. Preliminary studies relating portably recorded blood pressures to daily life events in patients with essential hypertension. *Bibliotheca Psychiatrica et Neurologica*, 1970, *144*, 164.

Solomon, G. F. Stress and antibody response in rats. *International Archives of Allergy and Applied Immunology*, 1969, *35*, 97.

Solomon, G. F., Temoshok, L., O'Leary, A., and Zich, J. An intensive psychoimmunologic study of long-surviving persons with AIDS. Pilot work, background studies, hypotheses, and methods. *Annals of the New York Academy of Sciences*, 1987, *496*, 647–655.

Solomon, M. S., and DeJong, W. Recent sexually transmitted disease prevention efforts and their implications for AIDS health education. *Health Education Quarterly*, 1986, *13*, 4.

Southward, E. E. *Shell shock*. Boston: W. M. Leonard, 1919.

Spackman, D. H., and Riley, V. Stress effects of the LDH-virus in alternating the Gardner tumor in mice. *Proceedings of the American Association for Cancer Research*, 1975, *16*, 170.

Spagnuolo, P. J., and MacGregor, R. R. Acute ethanol effect on chemotaxis and other components of host defense. *Journal of Laboratory and Clinical Medicine*, 1975, *70*, 295–301.

Sparrow, D., Dowber, T. R., and Colson, T. The influence of cigarette smoking on prognosis after a first myocardial infarction. *Journal of Chronic Disorders*, 1978, *31*, 425.

Speisman, J., Lazarus, R. S., Mordkoff, A., and Davidson, L. Experimental reduction of stress based on ego defense theory. *Journal of Abnormal and Social Psychology*, 1964, *68*, 367–380.

Spitzer, R. L. The mental status schedule: Potential use as a criterion measure in psychotherapy research. *American Journal of Psychotherapy*, 1966, *20*, 156–164.

Spitzer, R. L., and Endicott, J. DIAGNO II: Further developments in a computer program for psychiatric diagnosis. *American Journal of Psychiatry*, 1969, *125*, 12–21.

Stacey, N. H. Inhibition of antibody-dependent cell-mediated cytotoxicity by ethanol. *Immunopharmacology*, 1984, *8*, 155–161.

Stachnik, T., Stoffelmayr, B., and Hoppe, R. B. Prevention, behavior change, and chronic disease. In T. Burish and L. A. Bradley (Eds.), *Coping with chronic disease*. New York: Academic Press, 1983.

Standard and Poor. Tobacco: Basic analyses. *Standard & Poor's Industry Survey*, May 22, 1975, 105–120.

Staub, E., Tursky, B., and Schwartz, G. E. Self-control and predictability: The effects on reactions to aversive stimulation. *Journal of Personality and Social Psychology*, 1971, *18*, 157–162.

Stavraky, K. M. Psychological factors in outcome of human cancer. *Journal of Psychosomatic Research*, 1968, *12*, 251.

Steffen, J. J., Nathan, P. E., and Taylor, H. A. Tension-reducing effects of alcohol: Further evidence and some methodological considerations. *Journal of Abnormal Psychology*, 1974, *83*, 542–547.

Stein, M., Keller, S. E., and Scheifer, S. J. Stress and immunomodulation: The role of depression and neuroendocrine function. *Journal of Immunology*, 1985, *135*(2) (suppl.), 827–833.

Stepney, R. Smoking behavior. A psychology of the cigarette habit. *British Journal of Diseases of the Chest*, 1980, *74*, 325–344.

Sternbach, R. A. *Principles of psychophysiology*. New York: Academic Press, 1966.

———. *Pain patients: Traits and treatment*. New York: Academic Press, 1974.

Sternbach, R. A., and Tursky, B. Ethnic differences among housewives in psychophysical and skin potential responses to electric shock. *Psychophysiology*, 1965, *1*, 241–246.

Sternbach, R. A., Wolf, S. R., Murphy, R. W., and Akeson, W. H. Traits of pain patients: The low-back "loser." *Psychosomatics*, 1973, *14*, 226–229.

Stoney, C. M., Davis, M. C., and Mathews, K. A. Sex differences in physiological responses to stress and coronary heart disease: A causal link? *Psychophysiology,* 1987, *24,* 127–131.

Stoney, C. M., Mathews, K. A., McDonald, R. H., and Johnson, C. A. Sex differences in acute stress response: Lipid, lipoprotein, cardiovascular and neuroendocrine adjustments. *Psychophysiology,* in press.

Stotland, E., and Blumenthal, A. The reduction of anxiety as a result of the expectation of making a choice. *Canadian Journal of Psychology,* 1964, *18,* 139–145.

Strain, J. J. Noncompliance: Its origins, manifestations, and management. *The Pharos of Alpha Omega Alpha,* 1978, *41,* 27–32.

Strain, J. J., and Hamerman, D. Ombudsmen (medical-psychiatric) rounds. *Annals of Internal Medicine,* 1978, *88,* 550–555.

Stuart, R. B. Behavioral control of overeating. *Behavior Research and Therapy,* 1967, *5,* 357–365.

Stunkard, A. J. Obesity and the denial of hunger. *Psychosomatic Medicine,* 1959, *21,* 281–289.

————. From explanation to action in psychosomatic medicine: The case of obesity. *Psychosomatic Medicine,* 1975, *37,* 195–236.

————. Behavioral medicine and beyond: The example of obesity. In O. F. Pomerleau and J. P. Brady (Eds.), *Behavioral medicine: Theory and practice.* Baltimore: Williams & Wilkins, 1979.

Stunkard, A. J., and McClaren-Hume, M. The results of treatment of obesity. *Archives of Internal Medicine,* 1958, *103,* 79–85.

Stunkard, A. J., and Mahoney, M. J. Behavioral treatment of eating disorders. In H. Leitenberg (Ed.), *Handbook of behavior modification and behavior therapy.* Englewood Cliffs, N.J.: Prentice-Hall, 1976.

Stunkard, A. J., Sorensen, T. I. A., Hanis, C., Teasdale, T. W., Chakraborty, R., Schull, W. J., and Schulsinger, F. An adoption study of human obesity. *New England Journal of Medicine,* 1986, *314*(4), 193–197.

Suchman, E. Special patterns of illness and medical care. *Journal of Health and Human Behavior,* 1965, *6,* 2–16.

Suinn, R. M. The cardiac stress management program for Type A patients. *Cardiac Rehabilitation,* 1975, *5,* 13–15.

Suinn, R. M., and Bloom, L. J. Anxiety management training for pattern A behavior. *Journal of Behavioral Medicine,* 1978, *1,* 25–35.

Sullivan, P. L., and Welsh, G. S. A technique for objective configural analysis of MMPI profiles. *Journal of Consulting Psychology,* 1952, *16,* 383–388.

Surgeon General. *Smoking and health* (DHEW Publication No. [PHS] 79-50066). Washington, D.C.: U.S. Government Printing Office, 1979.

Swenson, R. M., and Vogel, W. H. Plasma catecholamine and corticosterone as well as brain catecholamine changes during coping in rats exposed to stressful foot shock. *Pharmacology, Biochemistry and Behavior,* 1983, *18*(5), 689–693.

Syme, S. L. Life style intervention in choice-based trials. *American Journal of Epidemiology,* 1978, *108,* 87–91.

Symington, T., Currie, A. R., Curran, R. S., and Davidson, J. N. The reaction of the adrenal cortex in conditions of stress. In *Ciba Foundations Colloquia on Endocrinology,* vol. 8. Boston, Mass.: Little, Brown, 1955.

Taché, J., Selye, H., and Day, S. B. *Cancer, stress, and death.* New York: Plenum, 1979.

Tagliacozza, D. L., and Mauksch, H. O. The patient's view of the patient's role. In E. G. Jaco (Ed.), *Patients, physicians, and illness,* 2nd ed. New York: Free Press, 1972.

Taub, A. Acupuncture "anesthesia": A critical review. In J. J. Bonica and D. Albe-Fessard (Eds.), *Advances in pain research and therapy,* vol. 1. New York: Raven, 1976.

Taub, E. Self-regulation of human tissue

temperature. In G. E. Schwartz and J. Beatty (Eds.), *Biofeedback: Theory and research.* New York: Academic Press, 1977.

Taylor, D. W., Sackett, D. L., Haynes, R. B., Johnson, A. L., Gibson, E. S., and Roberts, R. S. Compliance with antihypertensive drug therapy. *Annals of the New York Academy of Science,* 1978, 390–403.

Taylor, G. J. Dr. Taylor replies. *American Journal of Psychiatry,* 1984, *141,* 1637–1638.

Taylor, S. E. Hospital patient behavior: Reactance, helplessness, or control? *Journal of Social Issues,* 1979, *35,* 156–184.

Telch, M. J., Killen J. D., McAlister, A. L., Perry, C. L., and Maccoby, N. Long-term follow-up of a pilot project on smoking prevention with adolescents. *Journal of Behavioral Medicine,* 1982, *5,* 1–8.

Temoshok, L., Sweet, D. M., and Zich, J. A three city comparison of the public's knowledge and attitudes about AIDS. *Psychology and Health,* 1987, *1,* 43–60.

Tennen, H., and Eller, S. J. Attributional components of learned helplessness and facilitation. *Journal of Personality and Social Psychology,* 1977, *35,* 265–271.

Tessler, R., and Mechanic, D. Psychological distress and perceived health status. *Journal of Health and Social Behavior,* 1978, *19,* 254–262.

Tessler, R., Mechanic, D., and Dimond, M. The effect of psychological disorders on physician utilization: A prospective study. *Journal of Health and Social Behavior,* 1976, *17,* 353–364.

Theorell, T. Life events before and after the onset of a premature myocardial infarction. In B. S. Dohrenwend and B. P. Dohrenwend (Eds.), *Stressful life events: Their nature and effects.* New York: Wiley, 1974.

Theorell, T., Knox, S., Svensson, J., and Waller, D. Blood pressure variations during a working day at age 28: Effects of different types of work and blood pressure level at age 18. *Journal of Human Stress,* 1985, *11,* 36–41.

Theorell, T., and Rahe, R. H. Psychosocial factors and myocardial infarction: An inpatient study in Sweden. *Journal of Psychosomatic Research,* 1971, *15,* 25–31.

Thimann, J. Conditioned reflex treatment of alcoholism. II. The risk of its application, its indications, contraindications and psychotherapeutic aspects. *New England Journal of Medicine,* 1949, *241,* 408–410.

Thomas, A., Chess, S., and Birch, H. The origin of personality. *Scientific American,* 1970, *223,* 102–109.

Thomas, C. B., and Duszynski, K. R. Closeness to parents and the family constellation in a prospective study of five disease states: Suicide, mental illness, malignant tumor, hypertension, and coronary heart disease. *Johns Hopkins Medical Journal,* 1974, *134,* 251–270.

Thomas, W. R., Holt, P. G., and Keast, D. Cellular immunity in mice chronically exposed to fresh cigarette smoke. *Archives of Environmental Health,* 1973, *27*(6), 372–375.

Thoresen, C. R., Friedman, M., Powell, L. H., Gill, J. J., and Ulmer, D. Altering the Type A behavior pattern in post-infarction patients. In D. S. Krantz and J. A. Blumenthal (Eds.), *Behavioral assessment and management of cardiovascular disorders.* Sarasota, Fla.: Professional Resource Exchange, 1987.

Thornton, J. W., and Powell, C. D. Immunization to and alleviation of learned helplessness in man. *American Journal of Psychology,* 1974, *87,* 351–367.

Thurlow, H. J. General susceptibility to illness: A selective review. *Canadian Medical Association Journal,* 1967, *97,* 1397–1404.

Tolman, E. C. *Collected papers in psychology.* Berkeley, Calif.: University of California Press, 1951.

Tomkins, S. S. Psychological model for smoking behavior. *American Journal of Public Health,* 1966, *56,* 17–20.

———. A modified model of smoking behavior. In E. Borgatta and R. Evans (Eds.), *Smoking, health and behavior.* Chicago: Aldine, 1968.

Toynbee, P. *Patients.* New York: Harcourt Brace Jovanovich, 1977.

Trimble, M. R. *Neuropsychiatry.* Chichester, England: Wiley, 1981.

Turk, D. C., Meichenbaum, D. H., and Berman, W. H. Application of biofeedback for the regulation of pain: A critical review. *Psychological Bulletin,* 1979, *86,* 1322–1338.

Tursky, B., and Sternbach, R. A. Further physiological correlates of ethnic differences in responses to shock. *Psychophysiology,* 1967, *4,* 67–74.

Tyroler, A., Haynes, S. G., Cobb, L. A., Irvin, W. W., James, S. A., Luller, H., Miller, R. E., Shumaker, S., Syme, S. L., and Wolf, S. Task Force 1. Environmental risk factors in coronary heart disease. *Circulation,* 1987, *76* (suppl. 1), I139–I143.

U.S. Department of Health and Human Services. *The Health Consequences of Smoking: Cardiovascular Disease* (DHEW Publication No. [PHS]84-50204). Rockville, Md.: Public Health Service Publications, 1983.

U.S. Department of Health, Education, and Welfare. Healthy people: Surgeon General's report on health promotion and disease prevention (DHEW Publication No. 79-55071). Washington, D.C.: U.S. Government Printing Office, 1979a.

————. *Proceedings of the conference on the decline in coronary heart disease mortality* Bethesda, Md.: (NIH Publication No. 79-1610).NIH, 1979b.

Van Komea, R. W., and Redd, W. H. Personality factors associated with anticipatory nausea/vomiting in patients receiving cancer chemotherapy. *Health Psychology,* 1985, *4,* 189–202.

Vickers, R. R., Hervig, L. K., Rahe, R. H., and Rosenman, R. H. Type A behavior pattern and coping and defense. *Psychosomatic Medicine,* 1981, *43,* 381–396.

Vidt, D. G. The struggle for drug compliance in hypertension. *Cardiovascular Clinics,* 1978, *9,* 243–252.

Visintainer, M. A., and Seligman, M. E. P. Fighting cancer: The hope factor. *American Health,* 1983, *2,* 58–61.

Vogler, R. E., Compton, J. V., and Weissbach, T. A. Integrated behavior change techniques for alcoholics. *Journal of Consulting and Clinical Psychology,* 1975, *43,* 233–243.

Volicer, B. J. Perceived stress levels of events associated with the experience of hospitalization. *Nursing Research,* 1973, *22,* 491–497.

Wack, J. T., and Rodin, J. Smoking and its effects on body weight and the systems of caloric regulation. *American Journal of Clinical Nutrition,* 1982, *35,* 366–380.

Waldman, R. H., Bond, J. O., Levitt, L. P., Hartwig, E. C., Prather, E. C., Baratta, R. L., Neill, J. S., and Small, P. A., Jr. An elevation of influenza immunization. Influence of route of administration and vaccine strain. *Bulletin of the World Health Organization,* 1969, *41,* 543–548.

Waldron, I., Zyzanski, S., Shekelle, R. B., Jenkins, C. D., and Tannebaum, S. Coronary-prone behavior pattern in employed men and women. *Journal of Human Stress,* 1977, *3,* 2–18.

Wallston, B. S., and Wallston, K. A. Social psychological models of health behavior: An examination and integration. In A. Baum, J. E. Singer, and S. Taylor (Eds.), *Handbook of psychology and health.* Hillsdale, N.J.: Erlbaum, 1984.

Walster, E. (1966). Assignment of responsibility for an accident. *Journal of Personality and Social Psychology,* 1966, *3*(1), 73–79.

Warheit, G. J. Occupation: A key factor in stress at the manned space center. In R. S. Eliot (Ed.), *Stress and the heart.* Mt. Kisco, N.Y.: Futura, 1974.

Weg, R. B. Changing physiology of aging. In D. S. Woodruff and J. E. Birren (Eds.), *Aging: Scientific perspectives and social issues,* 2nd ed. Monterey, Calif.: Brooks/Cole, 1983.

Weick, B. G., Ritter, S., and Ritter, R. C. Plasma catecholamines: Exaggerated elevation is associated with stress susceptibility. *Physiology and Behavior,* 1980, *24,* 869–874.

Weiner, H. *Psychobiology and human disease.* New York: Elsevier, 1977.

Weiner, H., Thaler, M., Reiser, M. F., and Mursky, I. A. Etiology of duodenal ulcer: 1. Relation of specific psychological characteristics to rate of gastric secretion (serum pepsinogen). *Psychosomatic Medicine,* 1957, *19,* 1–10.

Weisenberg, M. Cultural and racial reactions to pain. In M. Weisenberg (Ed.), *The control of pain.* New York: Psychological Dimensions, 1977a.

———. Pain and pain control. *Psychological Bulletin,* 1977b, *84,* 1004–1008.

Weiss, F., and Miller, F. G. The drive theory of social facilitation. *Psychological Review,* 1971, *78,* 44–57.

Weiss, J. M. Effects of coping response on stress. *Journal of Comparative and Physiological Psychology,* 1968, *65,* 251–260.

———. Effects of coping behavior in different warning signal conditions on stress pathology in rats. *Journal of Comparative and Physiological Psychology,* 1971a, *77,* 1–13.

———. Effects of coping behavior with and without feedback signal on stress pathology in rats. *Journal of Comparative and Physiological Psychology,* 1971b, *77,* 22–30.

Weiss, J. M., Stone, E. A., and Harrell, N. Coping behavior and brain norepinephrine level in rats. *Journal of Comparative and Physiological Psychology,* 1970, *72,* 153–160.

Wells, J. A. Chronic life situations and life change events. In A. M. Ostfeld and E. D. Eaker (Eds.), *Measuring psychosocial variables in epidemiologic studies of cardiovascular disease* (NIH Publication No. 85-2270). Bethesda, Md.: NIH, 1985.

Whitcher, S. J., and Fisher, J. D. Multidimensional reaction to therapeutic touch in a hospital setting. *Journal of Personality and Social Psychology,* 1979, *37,* 87–96.

White, R. W. Motivation reconsidered: The concept of competence. *Psychological Review,* 1959, *66,* 297–333.

Whitehead, W. E., Blackwell, B., Desilva, H., and Robinson, A. Anxiety and anger in hypertension. *Journal of Psychosomatic Research,* 1977, *21,* 383–389.

Whitehead, W. E., and Schuster, M. M.

Gastrointestinal disorders: Behavioral and physiological basis for treatment. New York: Academic Press, 1985.

Wiens, A. N., and Menustik, C. E. Treatment outcome and patient characteristics in an aversion therapy program for alcoholism. *American Psychologist,* 1983, *38,* 1089–1096.

Wilbur, J. A., and Barrow, J. G. Reducing elevated blood pressure. *Minnesota Medical,* 1969, *52,* 1303.

Wilhelmsen, L., Vedin, J. A., Elmfeldt, D., Tibbin, G., and Wilhelmsen, L. Smoking and myocardial infarction. *Lancet,* 1975, *1,* 415.

Wilkins, W. Desensitization: A reply to Morgan. *Psychological Bulletin,* 1973, *79,* 376–377.

Williams, D. A., Lewis-Faning, E., Rees, L., Jacobs, J., and Thomas, A. Assessment of the relative importance of the allergic, infective and psychological factors in asthma. *Acta Allergologista,* 1958, *12,* 376–385.

Williams, R. B., Haney, T., Gentry, W. D., and Kong, Y. Relation between hostility and arteriographically documented coronary atherosclerosis. Paper presented at the American Psychosomatic Society meetings, Washington, D.C., April 1978.

Wills, T. A. Supportive functions of interpersonal relationships. In S. Cohen and S. L. Syme (Eds.), *Social support and health.* Orlando, Fla.: Academic Press, 1985.

Wilson, G. T., and Lawson, D. M. Effects of alcohol on sexual arousal in women. *Journal of Abnormal Psychology,* 1976a, *85,* 489–497.

———. Expectancies, alcohol, and sexual arousal in male social drinkers. *Journal of Abnormal Psychology,* 1976b, *85,* 587–594.

Wishnie, H. A., Hackett, T. P., and Cassem, N. H. Psychological hazards of convalescence following myocardial infarction. *Journal of the American Medical Association,* 1971, *215,* 1292–1296.

Wittkower, E. D., and Dudek, S. Z. Psychosomatic medicine: The mind–body–society interaction. In B. Wolman (Ed.),

Handbook of general psychology. Englewood Cliffs, N.J.: Prentice-Hall, 1973.

Wolf, S. *The stomach.* New York: Oxford, 1965.

Wolf, S., and Goodell, H. (Eds.). *Stress and disease,* 2nd ed. Springfield, Ill.: Charles C. Thomas, 1968.

Wolf, S., and Wolff, H. G. *Human gastric function.* New York: Oxford, 1947.

Wolfer, J., and Visintainer, M. Pediatric surgical patients' stress responses and adjustment as a function of psychologic preparation and stress-point nursing care. *Nursing Research,* 1975, *24,* 244–255.

Wolff, H. G. Life stress and cardiovascular disorders. *Circulation,* 1950, *1,* 187–203.

Wollersheim, J. P. Effectiveness of group therapy based upon learning principles in the treatment of overweight women. *Journal of Abnormal Psychology,* 1970, *76,* 562–574.

Wolman, B. B., and Money, J. (Eds.). *Handbook of human sexuality.* Englewood Cliffs, N.J.: Prentice-Hall, 1980.

Wolpe, J. *Psychotherapy by reciprocal inhibition.* Stanford, Calif.: Stanford University Press, 1958.

Wortman, C. B. Some determinants of perceived control. *Journal of Personality and Social Psychology,* 1975, *31,* 282–294.

———. Coping with victimization: Conclusions and implications for future research. *Journal of Social Issues,* 1983, *39*(2), 195–221.

Wortman, C. B., and Brehm, J. W. Responses to uncontrollable outcomes. An integration of reactance theory and the learned helplessness model. In L. Berkowitz (Ed.), *Advances in experimental social psychology,* vol. 8. New York: Academic Press, 1975.

Wortman, C. B., and Dintzer, L. Is an attributional analysis of the learned helplessness phenomenon viable? A critique of the Abramson–Seligman–Teasdale reformulation. *Journal of Abnormal Psychology,* 1978, *87,* 75–90.

Wortman, C. B., Panciera, L., Shusterman,

L., and Hibscher, J. Attributions of causality and reactions to uncontrollable outcomes. *Journal of Experimental Social Psychology,* 1976, *12,* 301–316.

Wynder, E. L., Kajitani, T., Kuno, J., Lucas, J. C., Depalo, A., and Farrow, J. A comparison of survival rates between American and Japanese patients with breast cancer. *Surgery, Gynecology and Obstetrics,* 1963, *117*(2), 196.

Yeager, J., and Weiner, H. Observations in man. *Advances in Psychosomatic Medicine,* 1970, *6,* 40–55.

Yeates, D. B., Aspin, N., Levison, H., Jones, M. T., and Bryan, A. C. Mucociliary tracheal transport rates in man. *Journal of Applied Physiology,* 1975, *39*(3), 487–495.

Young, G. P., Weyden, M. B., Rose, I. S., and Dudley, F. J. Lymphopenic and lymphocyte transformation in alcoholics. *Experientia,* 1979, *35,* 286–269.

Zick, J., and Temoshok, L. Perceptions of social support in men with AIDS and ARC—Relationships with distress and happiness. *Journal of Applied Social Psychology,* 1987, *17*(3), 193–215.

Zimbardo, P. G. The human choice: Individuation, reason, and order versus deindividuation, impulse, and chaos. In W. J. Arnold and D. Levine (Eds.), *Nebraska symposium on motivation,* Lincoln: University of Nebraska Press, 1969.

Zola, I. K. Problems of communication, diagnosis and patient care. *Journal of Medical Education,* 1963, *10,* 829–838.

———. Culture and symptoms: An analysis of patients' presenting complaints. *American Sociological Review,* 1966, *31,* 615–630.

Zubin, J. Role of vulnerability in the etiology of schizophrenic episodes. In L. J. West and D. E. Flinn (Eds.), *Treatment of schizophrenia: Progress and prospects.* New York: Grune & Stratton, 1976.

Zubin, J., and Spring, B. Vulnerability: A new view of schizophrenia. *Journal of Abnormal Psychology,* 1977, *86,* 103–126.

Zuckerman, M. Dimensions of sensation seeking. *Journal of Consulting and Clinical Psychology,* 1971, *36,* 35–52.

GLOSSARY

acne various inflammatory diseases of the hair follicles or sebaceous glands.

acquired immune deficiency syndrome (AIDS) a disease caused by the human immunodeficiency virus (HIV) that weakens the immune system by attacking T-helper cells.

acupuncture (ak″yoo-pungk′chur) the Chinese practice of piercing specific peripheral nerves to deaden pain, anesthetize, and heal.

adrenal cortex (ah-dre′nal kor′teks) the outer layer of the adrenal gland, which secretes mineralocorticoids, androgens, and glucocorticoids.

adrenal medulla (ah-dre′nal mah-dul′ah) the innermost portion of the adrenal gland, which secretes adrenaline (epinephrine).

adrenaline (ah-dren′ah-len) see *epinephrine.*

adrenocorticotrophic hormone (ACTH) (ad-re″no-kor″teh-ko-trof′ik′ hormone) a hormone produced by the pituitary gland that stimulates the adrenal cortex to produce glucocorticoids.

alexithymia (ah-lex′-ah-thi″-me-ah) the inability of psychophysiological patients to find the words to describe their feelings.

allergy a hyperresponse to antigens characterized by inflammation.

angina pectoris (an-ji′nah pek′to-ris) chest pain, with feeling of suffocation and impending death, due most often to insufficient oxygen supply to heart tissue and brought on by effort or excitement.

Antabuse (an′tah-byoos″) trademark for a preparation of disulfiram: a whitish, odorless, tasteless powder that makes alcoholic drinks produce nausea and other unpleasant effects. Used in the treatment of alcoholism.

antibodies products of B-lymphocytes that are induced by contact with a specific antigen. Antibodies attack antigens in several different ways but can only work against the antigen for which they were produced.

antigen (an′tah-jen) anything that does not "belong" in the body and that causes an immune response. Discovery of antigens evokes an immune response against them.

anxiety disorders disorders in which the major symptom is anxiety that is felt in so many situations it appears to have no specific cause.

arousal a condition during which the bodily processes deviate from homeostasis. Arousal is mediated by the sympathetic nervous system.

arrhythmia (ah-rith′me-ah) variation from the normal heartbeat.

arteries the group of blood vessels that carry blood away from the heart.

assertiveness training training that helps people feel free to make legitimate demands and to say no. It is taught through role playing and other related tasks.

atherosclerosis (ath″er-o′skle-ro″sis) disease characterized by thickening and loss of elasticity of arterial walls.

autoimmune response reaction of the immune system against the body; instead of only attacking "nonself" foreign particles or molecules, the immune system can turn on itself or other bodily tissues.

autonomic nervous system (aw′to-nom″ik) the portion of the nervous system associated with regulation of the activity of cardiac muscle, smooth muscle, and glands.

aversion therapy the behavior therapy that pairs an unpleasant stimulus with undesirable situations so that the patient learns to avoid them.

background stressors low-magnitude, everyday events that are aversive or disruptive and that produce a chronic elevation in stress.

Barr bodies sex chromatins; masses of inactivated X chromosome material in the cells of normal females.

B-cells lymphocytes that secrete antibodies. Upon stimulation by antigen, B-cells become plasma cells and release antibodies that are directed toward the stimulating antigen.

behavioral genetics the study of individual differences in behavior that are attributable in part to differences in genetic makeup.

behavioral health an area of study that stresses individual responsibility for the maintenance of health and the prevention of illness.

behavioral immunogen (ih'myoo-no-jen) a health-protective behavioral practice.

behavioral pathogen (path'o-jen) a health-impairing habit.

benign hypertension stage (hi'per-ten"-shun) the second stage of hypertension, characterized by blood pressure that is elevated but fluctuates greatly. Hardening of the arteries begins during this stage.

biofeedback the process of learning to control the autonomic body functions using visual or auditory cues.

blood pressure the pressure of the blood on the walls of the arteries. The maximum pressure, or *systolic pressure,* occurs at the end of the stroke output of the left ventricle. The minimum pressure, or *diastolic pressure,* occurs between beats. High blood pressure is termed *hypertension*; low blood pressure is called *hypotension*.

bronchial asthma (brong'ke-al az'mah) a condition due to spasmodic contractions of the bronchi that make breathing difficult. Some cases are triggered by allergies.

carcinogenic (kar"sih-no-jen'ik) cancer causing.

cardiovascular system (kar'de-o-vas'kyooler) the system composed of the heart and the blood vessels.

Cartesian dualism (kar-te'-zhen) an argument by Descartes that the mind (or soul) is a separate entity that is parallel to and incapable of affecting physical matter or somatic process in any direct way.

catabolic process (kat"ah-bol'ik) the process by which living cells break down complex substances into simpler compounds.

cataclysmic event (kat-ah-kliz"mik) a momentous and violent event marked by overwhelming upheaval and demolition.

catecholamines (kat"eh-ko"leh-meen') a group of compounds that mimic the effects of impulses conveyed by adrenergic postganglionic fibers of the sympathetic nervous system. Epinephrine (adrenaline), norepinephrine (noradrenaline), and dopamine are catecholamines. Epinephrine and norepinephrine are secreted by the adrenal medulla and select neurons throughout the nervous system.

central nervous system (CNS) the part of the body's nervous system consisting of the brain and spinal cord.

cerebellum (ser"eh-bel'um) cranial structure involved in the coordination of movement.

chemotherapy drug treatments (e.g., for cancer) often producing uncomfortable and undesirable side effects.

cholesterol (ko-les'ter-ol) a pearly, fatlike steroid alcohol, found in animal fats and oils, bile, blood, brain tissue, milk, yolk of egg, liver, kidneys, and adrenal glands, that can accumulate to cause narrowing of arteries.

chromosome (kro'mah-som) a structure in the cell nucleus composed of a linear thread of DNA that transmits genetic information. The normal number of chromosomes in humans is 46.

cirrhosis of the liver (sir-ro'sis) group of chronic disease of the liver, and one of the top ten causes of death in the United States.

classical conditioning conditioning a subject to respond to a neutral stimulus by pairing it with a stimulus that elicits the response.

cognitive restructuring making explicit use of cognitive concepts to understand and modify overt behavior.

complement a series of enzymes that interact with one another to enhance immune response to antigens.

compliance (kom-pli-an(t)s) the act by a patient of following a physician's regimen (e.g., diet, medication, preventive behavior).

concordance rate (kahn-kord'an(t)s) the rate of occurrence of a trait, behavior action, and so on, in members of a group, particularly in pairs of twins in genetic studies.

conditioned reflex a reflex to a stimulus developed through classical conditioning.

condom (kahn'dum) a sheath or cover for the penis, worn during sexual activity to prevent infection or pregnancy.

contact desensitization (de-sen"sih-tih-za'shun) a form of *in vivo* systematic desensitization combining modeling and guided participation procedures.

contingency management (kon-tin'jen-se) a behavior modification technique that changes the frequency of a behavior by controlling the reinforcing consequences of that behavior.

control ability to affect outcomes, to regulate or otherwise influence events or occurrences.

convergence (kon-ver'jense) the act of moving toward union or uniformity.

coping behavior an adaptive way of dealing with stress or threats.

coronary heart disease (CHD) (kor'o-neh-re) disease of the heart and blood vessels (e.g., arteriosclerosis).

coronary-prone behavior (kor'o-neh-re) behavior characterizing the Type A personality. Characteristic behaviors include impatience, hostility, and hard drivingness. Coronary-prone behavior has been found to be associated with heart disease.

cortisol (kor'tih-sol) a corticosteroid produced by the adrenal cortex that plays a role in the production of carbohydrates from fatty acids, amino acids, and so on, and fat and water metabolism. It affects muscle tone and the excitation of nerve tissue and increases gastric acid secretion.

counterconditioning training to elicit a new response to replace an unwanted one.

covert sensitization (ko'-vert) aversive conditioning during which the client is taught to imagine aversive consequences after engaging in an unwanted habit.

daily hassles everyday events that often produce stress.

defensive avoidance psychological mechanism used to minimize significance of a threat and affect outcome in fear communication. It is used as an educational approach.

depersonalization (de-per'sun-al-eh-za'-shun) loss of the sense of personal identity.

depressive disorder a psychological disorder characterized by persistent dysphoria, dejection, and discouragement.

diastole (di-as'to-le) the period of dilation of the heart ventricles. It occurs between the first and the second heart sound.

diathesis stress model of illness (di-ath'eh-sis) a psychophysiological model assuming that individuals are predisposed toward a particular mental disorder and will manifest that disorder when affected by stress.

digestive system the organs in the body involved in converting food into usable chemicals. It is composed of the mouth, pharynx, stomach, intestines, and related glands.

diseases of adaptation disease conditions associated with stressful life situations (e.g., ulcers, cardiovascular disease).

dizygotic twins (di"zi-gaht'ik) fraternal twins, developed from separate fertilized ova.

Down's syndrome the most common form of mental retardation, common among individuals born with an extra chromosome in the twenty-first pair. It was formerly called Mongolism.

dyskinesia (dis"keh-ne'ze-ah) an impairment of the power to move voluntary muscles, resulting in fragmentary motions.

dyspareunia (dis"peh-roo'ne-ah) difficult or painful coitus.

eczema (ek'zih-mah) a superficial inflammation of the skin seen as redness, itching, and in some cases scaling or pigmentation.

Edwards Personal Preference Schedule a personality inventory, using a forced-choice response format to control for social desirability, developed as an alternative to the Minnesota Multiphasic Personality Inventory.

effectance motivation a concept developed by White to describe an innate need to manipulate the environment.

electrocardiogram (e-lek′tro-kar″de-o-gram″) an electrical analysis of the activity of the heart, used to reveal abnormalities in heart function.

enabling factors skills necessary to acquire health-protective behaviors.

endocrine system (en′do-krin) the system of glands and other structures that produces and secretes hormones into the circulatory system of the body.

endorphins (en-dor′fin) opiumlike substances produced in the brain and pituitary gland in response to stimulation.

eosinophils (e″o-sin′o-fil) leukocytes that attack parasites and other foreign bodies.

epinephrine (adrenaline) (ep′eh-nef′rin) a hormonal stimulator of the sympathetic nervous system secreted by the adrenal medulla.

essential hypertension (hi″per-ten′shun) an increase in blood pressure with no diagnosable organic cause.

eugenics (u-jen′iks) a science that deals with the improvement of hereditary qualities of a race or breed by selectively breeding for specific genes.

eutelegenesis (you-tel″eh-jen′eh-sis) artificial insemination by semen of a donor selected because of special characteristics for the production of superior offspring.

extinction gradual disappearance of a conditioned response when it is no longer reinforced.

fear communication as an educational approach, describing the dangers or threats of a health habit in a fear-evoking manner.

fight or flight response the body's most comprehensive reaction to extreme stress. By means of a mass-discharge response, large portions of the sympathetic nervous system are stimulated in response to a perceived stressor.

Flesch Formula a method of determining the difficulty of a written passage. The formula provides an estimate of how many people in the United States would

be able to read and understand a message.

fraternal twins nonidentical twins, developed from two separate fertilized ova.

gamete (gam′et) a mature, functional reproductive cell.

gastric ulcer (gas′trik) a lesion in the mucosal lining of the stomach.

gastritis (gas-tri′tis) inflammation of the stomach.

gastrointestinal (GI) tract (gas″tro-in-tes′-teh-nal) the organs of digestion, including the stomach, small intestine, and large intestine.

gemmule (jem′yool) a unit of living matter made up of one or more molecules having the power of growth and division.

general adaptation syndrome (GAS) reaction of the individual to excessive stress; consists of the alarm reaction, the stage of resistance, the stage of exhaustion. It was developed by Hans Selye.

genotype (jee′no-tipe) the genetic constitution of an organism; the sum total of all the genes present in an individual.

giving up-given up a response to loss of something or someone valued and/or loved. This complex, marked by reduced motivation, has been reported to precede the onset of illness.

glucocorticoids (gloo″ko-kor′teh-koid) substances produced by the adrenal cortex that raise the level of blood sugar in the body. The most important glucocorticoids are cortisol and corticosterone.

goiter (goi′ter) an enlargement of the thyroid gland causing a swelling in the front part of the neck.

gradient of reinforcement learning theory principle suggesting that the valence of a reinforcer is greater when in proximity to a behavior; it suggests that behaviors providing short-term gratification (even if health impairing in the long term) are easy to acquire and resistant to change.

Halstead-Reitan Battery (HRB) a neuropsychological test used to determine the effects of brain damage on behavior.

health psychology a field of psychology studying behavioral factors in the prevention and treatment of illness and the maintenance of health.

heuristics (hyoo-ris′tiks) the practice of using self-educating techniques (such as biofeedback) to improve performance.

hives a vascular reaction of the skin marked by the transient appearance of smooth, elevated patches that are reddish or pale and cause severe itching.

holistic approach (ho-lis′tik) a philosophy of health that considers a person as a functioning whole.

human immunodeficiency virus (HIV) (im″yoo-no-de-fish′en-se) virus presumed to be responsible for the disease AIDS.

hybrids (hi′brid) offspring of two parents that differ in one or more heritable characteristics or are of two different species.

hydrochloric acid (hi-drah-klor′ik) a water-based solution of hydrogen chloride; a strong, corrosive, irritating acid normally present in dilute form in gastric juice to facilitate the breakdown of food.

hyperphagia (hi″per-fa′je-ah) abnormally increased appetite for food frequently associated with injury to the hypothalamus.

hypertension (hi″per-ten′shun) a marked increase in diastolic and systolic blood pressure.

hypnosis a technique for inducing a trance state of heightened calmness, relaxation, and suggestibility in a subject. It can be used to reduce pain, anxiety, and fear in some situations.

hypothalamus (hi″po-thal′ah-mus) a cortical structure located beneath the thalamus that activates, controls, and integrates the peripheral autonomic functions and endocrine activity.

identical twins two individuals who develop from the same ovum and share an identical chromosome pattern.

idiopathic condition (ihd″e-o-path′ik) a condition with an unknown origin.

immunoglobulin (Ig) (im″yoo-no-glob′yoo-lin) antibodies. B-lymphocytes secrete immunoglobulins (one of five types).

inflammation bodily response to injury, wherein blood supply increases to the damaged area.

instrumental conditioning increasing the probability of a response by introducing reward or reinforcement. It is also called operant conditioning.

James-Lange theory of emotion a theory stating that the emotions we feel result from our bodies reacting to emotion-producing aspects of the environment.

Jenkins Activity Survey (JAS) a survey designed to measure Type A versus Type B behavior.

job strain a condition of stress resulting from high job demands and low job control in the occupational setting.

Klinefelter's syndrome (klin′fel-terz) a type of mental retardation associated with the sex chromosome anomaly of one extra X chromosome.

learned helplessness a psychological state resulting from repeated instances of noncontingency behavior and outcome. A person learns that events are not controllable and the feeling often generalizes to other situations. Depression has been associated with learned helplessness.

leukocytes (loo′ko-site) the white cells in the blood; they comprise most cells of the immune system.

life change units units used to measure stressfulness (positive or negative) of life experiences in the Life Experiences Survey.

Life Experiences Survey (LES) a survey to measure the stressfulness of various life events.

limbic system (lim′bik) a group of brain structures collectively concerned with autonomic functions and aspects of emotion and behavior.

locus of control the theoretical construct of perceived control over behavior. Individuals are classified as having an *internal* locus of control or an *external* locus of control.

lower motor neuron dysfunctions dysfunctions of the conducting cells that affect bodily motion.

lymph (limf) the fluid of the lymph system. It acts to drain dead antigens out of the body, to help trap antigens near lymph nodes, and to carry lymphocytes and macrophages.

lymph nodes (limf) areas in the body where the system of lymph vessels join. There are lymph nodes throughout the body, each containing lymphocytes and other immune cells.

lymphocytes (lim′feh-site) a type of white blood cell (leukocyte) that is a major component of the immune system.

There are two primary types of lymphocytes: T-cells and B-cells.

lymphokines (lim'feh-kine) substances released by lymphocytes, including interferon and interleuken-2, that help signal immune cells.

macrophages (mak'ro-faje) large leucocytes that develop from monocytes, perform phagocytic functions, and transport antigens to lymphocytes to allow lymphocytes to recognize antigens.

malignant hypertension stage (hi″per-ten'-shun) severe high blood pressure state marked by poor prognosis; the third stage of hypertension. It may involve arterial thickening, hemorrhaging, lesions, and diastolic pressure of 130 mm/Hg.

Matthews Youth Test for Health (MYTH) an instrument used to distinguish Type A and Type B behavior patterns in children.

medical model a set of assumptions that views abnormal behavior as similar to physical disease.

medulla oblongata (mah-dul'ah ob″long-gah'tah) a collection of cranial nerve cells that deal with vital bodily functions such as respiration, circulation, and special senses.

Meniere's disease (mane-yares') a disease of the inner ear that can produce deafness, vertigo, or strange sounds heard in the ears.

migraine headache (mi'grane) a vascular headache, temporal and unilateral in onset, commonly associated with irritability, nausea, vomiting, diarrhea, or constipation.

mineralocorticoid (min″er-al-o-kor'ti-koid) a corticoid secreted by the adrenal cortex that is effective in causing the retention of sodium and the loss of potassium.

Minnesota Multiphasic Personality Inventory (MMPI) a lengthy personality inventory by which an individual is diagnosed through his or her true-false replies to groups of statements indicating anxiety, depression, masculinity-femininity, paranoia, and so on.

mitogen (mi'to-jen) a substance that causes immune cells to multiply and divide. Proliferation in the face of a mitogen is used as a measure of immune system function.

modeling learning by observing and imitating the behavior of others.

Mongolism (mon'go-liz-m) see *Down's syndrome*.

monocyte (mah'no-site) a type of white blood cell (leukocyte) that engulfs and devours foreign particles.

monozygotic twins (mon'o-zi-got'ik) identical twins, developed from the same ovum and sharing identical inheritance.

morbidity the occurrence of disease or illness.

mucous colitis (myoo'kus ko-li'tis) a chronic noninflammatory disease characterized by excess passage of mucous from the gastrointestinal tract. A common disorder with a psychophysiologic basis, it is also called spastic or irritable colon.

multiaxial classification (assessment) (mul-ti-ak'se-al) a procedure used by DSM-III for measuring patients on five axes: (1) psychiatric syndrome present; (2) patient's history of personality and developmental disorders; (3) possible nonmental medical disorders; (4) severity of psychosocial stressors; and (5) highest level of adaptive functioning in past year.

Multiple Risk Factor Intervention Trial (MRFIT) an epidemiological study of high-risk men to see if modifying smoking, dietary fat intake, and high blood pressure would lower occurrence of coronary heart disease.

muscle tension headache headache originating from tension in the neck muscles where the head and neck join.

myocardial infarction (mi″o-kar'de-al infark'shun) death of the heart tissue, as a result of interruption of the blood supply to the area.

naloxone hydrochloride (nal-ak'sahn hi″-drah-klo'ride) a chemical used as a narcotic antagonist.

natural killer cells leukocytes that kill cells infected by viruses as well as other foreign cells or organisms. They do not require prior sensitization to an antigen in order to attack it.

natural selection the nonrandom reproduction of genotypes resulting from interactions among a variety of phenotypes and the environment.

need the lack of something that is required, desired, or useful; internal motivation for behavior.

neurodermatitis (nu'ro-der'mah-ti'tis) a general term for a dermatosis presumed to be due to emotional causes.

neuropsychology (nu"ro-si-kol'o-je) the branch of medicine that includes both neurology and psychology.

neutrophils (nu'tro-fil) short-lived (up to two days) leukocytes; phagocytic cells that attack bacteria. These cells do not require prior sensitization to bacteria, and migrate to areas where they are needed by chemotaxis.

nicotine (nik'eh-teen) a very poisonous, colorless, soluble fluid alkaloid obtained from tobacco or produced synthetically.

noncompliance (non-kom-pli'an(t)s) refusal by a patient to follow or cooperate with a physician's regimen.

noradrenaline (nor"ah-dren'ah-lin) see *norepinephrine*.

norepinephrine (noradrenaline) (nor"ep-eh-nef'rin) a hormone secreted by the adrenal medulla in response to hypotension.

nuclear conflict theory the psychoanalytic theory proposed by Franz Alexander to account for psychosomatic disorders.

obesity increased body weight beyond the limitation of skeletal and physical requirements as the result of an excessive accumulation of fat in the body.

observational learning the learning of patterns of behavior from the observation of others.

operant conditioning (op'eh-rant) see *instrumental conditioning*.

operationalization translation of hypotheses into the procedural and measurement terms that will be used to evaluate them.

opportunistic infections infections that under normal circumstances would not occur because of immune defenses. When the immune system is compromised, as in AIDS, these infections or diseases are more likely.

parasympathetic nervous system (par"ah-sim"pah-thet'ik) the craniosacral portion of the autonomic nervous system, important for homeostasis of the body.

pepsin (pep'sin) an enzyme present in gastric juice that catalyzes the breakdown of proteins into polypeptides.

pepsinogen (pep-sin'o-jen) the precursor of pepsin, activated in the presence of gastric acid.

perceived control the perception that one can affect outcomes and that responding can influence what happens.

peripheral nervous system (pe-rif'er-al) the portion of the nervous system consisting of the nerves and ganglia outside the brain and spinal cord.

phagocytosis (fag"o-si-to'sis) process of swallowing up antigens, breaking them down, and ridding the body of them. Three types of immune cells are phagocytes: monocytes, macrophages, and neutrophils.

phenotype (fe'no-tipe) the entire physical, biochemical, and physiological makeup of an individual as determined both genetically and environmentally.

pineal gland (pin'e-al) the site of melatonin biosynthesis.

pituitary gland (pi-tu'eh-ter"e) the "master gland" of the body, which secretes trophic hormones that regulate the proper functioning of the thyroid, gonads, adrenal cortex, and other endocrine organs.

placebo (plah-se'bo) an inactive substance given to satisfy the patient's symbolic need for drug therapy and used in controlled studies to determine the efficacy of medicinal substances.

plaque (plak) fatty material that may deposit in arteries and cause damage by narrowing passage space for blood flow.

postural hypotension (pos'yoo-ral hi"po-ten'shun) a progressive disorder beginning with symptoms of autonomic insufficiency, especially weakness when rising to an erect position.

predictability the ability to know in advance what to expect of a situation, a person's behavior, and so on.

predisposing factors factors, such as awareness and comprehension, that motivate an individual to take certain health actions.

prehypertension stage (pre-hi"per-ten'-

shun) the first stage of hypertension, characterized by responding to psychological stress with elevation of diastolic blood pressure.

primary prevention the altering of an individual's risk factors before he or she develops disease.

progressive muscle relaxation a method of achieving relaxation based on repeated contraction and relaxation of muscles.

projective techniques unstructured psychological tests in which the subject is presented with a stimulus or test item that has little or no well-defined cultural pattern of responding (e.g., the Rorschach, Thematic Apperception Test).

prospective study a study that predicts future events and then assesses the incidence of these events over time.

psoriasis (so-ri'ah-sis) a chronic skin disease characterized by circumscribed red patches covered with white scales.

psychogenic pain (si"ko-jen'ik) pain originating in the mind or in mental or emotional conflict.

psychophysiologic reactivity (si"ko-fiz"e -ah-loj'ik): the changes in individual's physiological responses, from resting levels during stress or challenge using measures such as heart rate and hormone levels in blood.

psychosomatic disorders (si"ko-so-mat'ik) another term for psychophysiological disorders.

psychosomatic medicine (si"ko-so-mat'ik) a medical approach to bodily symptoms of a psychic, emotional, or mental origin.

Rational-Emotional Therapy (RET) a form of psychotherapy focusing on the use of cognitive and emotional restructuring to foster adaptive behavior.

Raynaud's disease (ra-noz') a disease characterized by intermittent attacks of severe pallor of the fingers or toes brought on by cold or emotion.

Recurrent Coronary Prevention Project (RCPP) a clinical trial of postcoronary patients to determine if modification of Type A behavior would lessen the likelihood of recurrence of heart attack.

reinforcement (re-en-fors'ment) in classical conditioning, the process of following the conditioned stimulus with an unconditioned stimulus; in operant conditioning, the rewarding of desired responses.

reinforcing factors refers to reward or positive responses, such as peer approval, to carrying out a particular health behavior.

relapse returning to an undesirable behavior that an individual has attempted to extinguish.

relapse prevention methods that aim to avoid relapse or slips after a health behavior has been extinguished.

relaxation training a behavioral technique to aid in reducing stress through deep muscle relaxation.

respiratory system (re-speh'rah-tor"e) the tubes, organs, and structures by which breathing and air/blood gas exchange take place; nose, mouth, windpipe (trachea), bronchi, and lungs.

respondent conditioning see *classical conditioning*.

response acquiescence the tendency to agree with test items on a self-report inventory, regardless of content.

response set (bias) the tendency of an individual to respond in a particular way to questions or statements on a test.

reticular activating system (re-tik'yoo-lar) a system of cells within the medulla oblongata that control the overall degree of central nervous system activity, including wakefulness, attentiveness, and sleep.

retrospective study (reh-tro-spek'tiv) a research approach that attempts to retrace earlier events in the life of the subject.

Rorschach Inkblot Test (ror'shahk) a test in which the subject responds to a series of inkblots with associations that come to mind. Analysis of these productions enables the clinician to infer personality characteristics.

safer sex practicing methods during sexual activity to prevent exchange of bodily fluids (e.g., blood and semen).

schizophrenia (skiz"o-fre'-ne-ah) a thought disorder characterized by misinterpretation and retreat from reality, delusions, hallucinations, ambivalence, inappropriate affect, and withdrawn bizarre or regressive behavior.

secondary prevention practices intended to

halt a disease in early asymptomatic stages.

selective breeding attempting to breed species either to maintain and/or improve a trait or to breed out a trait.

self-monitoring observing and recording one's own behavior.

sensitization (sen″sih-tih-za′shun) the process by which the immune system contacts and learns to recognize an antigen.

sexual dysfunction the inability or impaired ability to experience or give sexual gratification.

shaping a form of instrumental conditioning in which at first all responses resembling the desired one are reinforced, then only closer approximations, until finally the desired response is obtained.

sick role a protected role provided by society via the medical model for an individual suffering from severe physical or mental disorder.

slip an isolated incident of returning to an undesirable health habit that has previously been extinguished.

social-desirability bias a tendency to answer questions about oneself in the socially approved manner.

social support tangible, psychoemotional, or esteem support provided for a person by social contact.

somatic nervous system (so-mat′ik) the elements of the nervous system concerned with the transmission of impulses to and from skeletal muscles, skin, eyes, and ears.

specific-attitudes theory the hypothesis proposed by Graham that certain attitudes are associated with certain psychophysiological disorders.

spinal cord the part of the vertebrate central nervous system that consists of a thick longitudinal bundle of nerve fibers extending from the brain posteriorly along the dorsal side.

stimulus control a clinical approach based on manipulation of environmental stimuli responsible for problems under treatment

stimulus substitution the classical conditioning phenomenon studied by Pavlov whereby an organism has a tendency to respond to a formerly neutral (conditioned) stimulus as if it were an unconditioned stimulus.

stress the sum of all nonspecific biological phenomena elicited by adverse external influences, including damage or defense.

stress aftereffects the effects of stress that occur after exposure to stress has ended.

stress inoculation a clinical approach intended to provide patients with skills that they can use to cope with stress.

stroke a condition with sudden onset caused by acute vascular lesion of the brain, such as hemorrhage or embolism. Also called cardiovascular accident.

Structured Interview (SI) a method for determining Type A and Type B behavior patterns.

successive approximations see *shaping*.

symptom perception the awareness of bodily sensations that might reflect illness or unusual bodily functioning.

systematic desensitization (sis-te-mat′ik de-sen′sih-tih-za′shun) a behavior therapy technique whereby the therapist systematically reduces the intensity of anxiety the patient feels and replaces it with a relaxation response.

systole (sis′to-le) the period of contraction of the ventricles of the heart.

T-cells lymphocytes that control other cells as well as kill antigens directly. T-helper cells help B-cells to make antibodies and help T-cytotoxic cells, which kill cells infected by viruses and release lymphokines to regulate other cells. T-suppressor cells also regulate other cells by suppressing their function.

tertiary prevention practices intended to stop progression of clinically manifest diseases.

testosterone (tes-tahs′teh-rone) the hormone, produced by the interstitial cells of the testes, that functions in the induction and maintenance of male secondary sex characteristics.

thalamus (thal′ah-mus) the main relay center for sensory impulses to the cerebral cortex.

Thematic Apperception Test (TAT) (themat′ik) a projective test consisting of a set of black-and-white pictures, each depicting a potentially emotion-laden situation. The subject is presented with the cards one at a time and instructed to make up a story about each situation.

token economy a behavior modification procedure in which institutionalized patients are given artificial rewards (such as poker chips) for socially constructive behavior. The tokens can be exchanged for desirable items or activities.

Turner's syndrome a syndrome in females characterized by short stature, undifferentiated gonads, and variable abnormalities associated with a defect or absence of the second sex chromosome.

twin studies tests to determine the concordance rate for monozygotic twins as compared to dizygotic twins in the diagnosis of schizophrenia.

Type A behavior a behavior pattern characterized by aggressiveness, ambitiousness, restlessness, and living under severe time pressures, associated with coronary heart patients.

Type B behavior the pattern of behavior characterized by the absence of Type A characteristics.

unconditioned reflex the response always elicited by the unconditioned stimulus in a classical conditioning experiment.

upper motor neuron dysfunctions dysfunctions occurring in the upper level of the central nervous system (e.g., cerebral palsy, incomplete spinal cord lesions, paresis).

vaginismus (vaj"eh-niz'mus) a painful spasm of the vagina due to local vigorous sensations.

veins vessels through which blood passes from various organs or parts back to the heart.

vigilance initial reaction to a fear communication in which all-out efforts are employed to combat the practice and threats of a health-impairing behavior.

XXX chromosomal type (kro"mah-so'mal) a female with an extra X chromosome. The extra chromosome may cause abnormalities in the genotype

XYY chromosomal type (kro"mah-so'mal) a male with an extra Y chromosome, considered a "super-male." The extra chromosome has been considered an important contributor to aggressive or criminal behavior.

INDEX

ABOUT THE AUTHORS

||||||||||||||||||||||||||||||||||||||||||||||||||||||||||||||||||||||||||||||||||||||||||||||||||||||||||||||||||||||||||||||||||||||||||||||||||||||||||||||||||||||||||

Robert J. Gatchel received his B.A. from the State University of New York at Stony Brook in 1969 and his Ph.D. in Clinical Psychology from the University of Wisconsin in 1973. Dr. Gatchel is currently Professor in the Division of Psychology, Department of Psychiatry at the University of Texas Health Sciences Center, Dallas. He has conducted extensive research on clinical applications of biofeedback, psycho-physiological concomitants of stress and emotion, and the etiology, assessment, and treatment of chronic pain behavior. Gatchel has authored and edited many scientific and professional publications, including *Fundamentals of Abnormal Psychology* (with F. Mears), and *Clinical Applications of Biofeedback* (with K. Price). He has served as associate editor of *Biofeedback and Self-Regulation,* on the Board of Directors of the Society for Psychophysiological Research, and is currently secretary-treasurer of that organization. He is a member or fellow of the American Psychological Association and the Academy of Behavioral Medicine Research.

Andrew Baum received his B.S. from the University of Pittsburgh and his Ph.D. from the State University of New York at Stony Brook. Dr. Baum is currently Professor in the Department of Medical Psychology at the Uniformed Services University of the Health Sciences where he is also Director of Graduate Studies for Medical Psychology and Director of the Stress Studies Center. He has conducted extensive research on stress and on various aspects of psychosocial factors in health and illness. His interests include psychological, endocrinological, and immunological changes during chronic stress and the ways in which these changes affect health and well being. He has authored or co-authored many scientific and professional publications, including *Architecture and Social Behavior* (with S. Valins), *Environmental Psychology* (with P. Bell and J. Fisher), and *Social Psychology* (with J. Fisher and J. E. Singer). He has also co-edited more than a dozen volumes including the *Handbook of Psychology and Health, Advances in Environmental Psychology,* and the series *Perspectives in Behavioral Medicine.* Baum is currently editor of the *Journal of Applied Social Psychology* and associate editor of *Health Psychology.* He was the recipient of the Annual Award from the American Psychological Association, Division of Health Psychology in 1985, was elected president of the Division of Health Psychology in 1987, and has served as secretary-treasurer of the Academy of Behavioral Medicine Research and the Council of Directors of Health Psychology Training since 1985. He is a fellow of Divisions 34 and 38 of the American Psychological Association, and is a member or fellow of the Academy of Behavioral Medicine Research, the Society for Behavioral Medicine, the Society for Experimental Social Psychology, and the American Psychosomatic Society.

David S. Krantz received his B.S. from the City College of New York and Ph.D. in psychology from the University of Texas at Austin. Dr. Krantz is currently Professor in the Department of Medical Psychology at the Uniformed Services

University of the Health Sciences, where he directs his department's course for medical students. He has conducted extensive research on behavioral factors in cardiovascular disorders and on various aspects of psychosocial stress and health. Krantz has authored or co-authored over eighty scientific and professional publications, including *Behavior, Health, and Environmental Stress* (with S. Cohen et al.) and co-edited *Behavioral Assessment and Management of Cardiovascular Disorders* (with J. Blumenthal), and *Handbook of Psychology and Health: Cardiovascular Disorders and Behavior* (with A. Baum and J. E. Singer). Dr. Krantz was the recipient of the American Psychological Association's Early Career Scientific Award in 1982, and the Annual Award from the APA Division of Health Psychology in 1981. He is an officer and/or fellow of several professional organizations, including the American Psychological Association, Academy of Behavioral Medicine Research, the American Psychosomatic Society, and the Society for Behavioral Medicine. He currently serves as an associate editor of *Health Psychology*.